CHILDREN'S COMPREHENSION PROBLEMS IN ORAL AND WRITTEN LANGUAGE

CHALLENGES IN LANGUAGE AND LITERACY

ELAINE R. SILLIMAN and C. ADDISON STONE, Series Editors

Children's Comprehension Problems in Oral and Written Language

A COGNITIVE PERSPECTIVE

Edited by

KATE CAIN *and* JANE OAKHILL

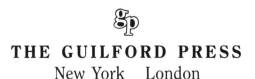

THE GUILFORD PRESS
New York   London

© 2007 The Guilford Press
A Division of Guilford Publications, Inc.
72 Spring Street, New York, NY 10012
www.guilford.com

Paperback edition 2008

Printed in the United States of America

This book is printed on acid-free paper.

Last digit is print number: 9 8 7 6 5 4 3 2

Library of Congress Cataloging-in-Publication Data

Children's comprehension problems in oral and written language : a cognitive
perspective / edited by Kate Cain, Jane Oakhill.
    p. cm.—(Challenges in language and literacy)
  Includes bibliographical references and index.
  ISBN: 978-1-59385-832-2 (paperback : alk. paper)
  ISBN: 978-1-59385-443-0 (cloth : alk. paper)
  1. Reading disability. 2. Reading comprehension. 3. Language disorders in
children—Psychological aspects. 4. Language disorders in children—
Physiological aspects. 5. Cognition disorders in children. I. Cain,
Kate. II. Oakhill, Jane.
  LB1050.5.C536 2007
  372.47—dc22

                                                          2006101602

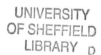

About the Editors

Kate Cain, DPhil, is a Reader in the Department of Psychology at Lancaster University. Her research and publications focus on the development of language comprehension in children, with a particular interest in the skill deficits that lead to comprehension problems. Dr. Cain's recent journal articles report investigations into the relations that exist between children's reading comprehension and their inference-making skill, knowledge of narrative structure, interpretation of figurative language, vocabulary-learning mechanisms, and memory processes. Her work has been published in the *Journal of Experimental Child Psychology, Journal of Educational Psychology, Memory and Cognition, Journal of Child Language,* and *Language and Cognitive Processes.* She is an Associate Editor of the *International Journal of Language and Communication Disorders* and the *Journal of Research in Reading.*

Jane Oakhill, DPhil, is a Professor of Experimental Psychology at the University of Sussex. Since completing her doctorate on the topic of children's problems in reading comprehension, she has worked on various research projects—including deductive reasoning in children and adults, circadian variations in human performance, and adult language comprehension—but has always maintained a research interest in children's reading comprehension, particularly individual differences. Dr. Oakhill has published widely on children's reading comprehension. Her publications include *Becoming a Skilled Reader,* with Alan Garnham, and *Children's Problems in Text Comprehension,* with Nicola Yuill. She has also coedited a number of books, notably *Reading Comprehension Difficulties: Processes and Remediation,* with Cesare Cornoldi, and *Reading Development and the Teaching of Reading: A Psychological Perspective,* with Roger Beard. In 1991 Dr. Oakhill received the British Psychological Society's Spearman Medal and was elected to a Fellowship of the Society in 2005.

Contributors

Dragana Barac-Cikoja, PhD, Gallaudet Research Institute, Gallaudet University, Washington, DC

Marcia A. Barnes, PhD, Department of Psychology, University of Guelph, Guelph, Ontario, Canada, and Department of Pediatrics, University of Toronto, Toronto, Ontario, Canada

Kristen S. Berthiaume, PhD, Department of Psychology, University of Kentucky, Lexington, Kentucky

Nicola Botting, PhD, Department of Language and Communication, University of Manchester and City University, Manchester, United Kingdom

Kate Cain, DPhil, Department of Psychology, Fylde College, Lancaster University, Lancaster, United Kingdom

Sandra B. Chapman, PhD, Center for BrainHealth, School of Behavioral and Brain Sciences, University of Texas at Dallas, Dallas, Texas

Lori G. Cook, MS, Center for BrainHealth, School of Behavioral and Brain Sciences, University of Texas at Dallas, Dallas, Texas

Maureen Dennis, PhD, Departments of Psychology and Surgery, University of Toronto, Toronto, Ontario, Canada

Jacquelyn F. Gamino, PhD, Center for BrainHealth, School of Behavioral and Brain Sciences, University of Texas at Dallas, Dallas, Texas

Crystal B. Howard, PhD, Long Beach Unified School District, Long Beach, California

Amber M. Johnston, MA, Department of Psychology, University of Guelph, Guelph, Ontario, Canada

Leonard P. Kelly, PhD, Gallaudet Research Institute, Gallaudet University, Washington, DC

Susan Leekam, PhD, Department of Psychology, University of Durham, Durham, United Kingdom

Elizabeth P. Lorch, PhD, Department of Psychology, University of Kentucky, Lexington, Kentucky

Richard Milich, PhD, Department of Psychology, University of Kentucky, Lexington, Kentucky

Jane Oakhill, DPhil, Department of Psychology, University of Sussex, Falmer, East Sussex, United Kingdom

Leilani Sáez, PhD, Department of Teacher Education, California State University Monterey Bay, Seaside, California

H. Lee Swanson, PhD, School of Education, University of California, Riverside, Riverside, California

Paul van den Broek, PhD, College of Education and Human Development, University of Minnesota, Minneapolis, Minnesota

Series Editors' Note

We are pleased to present the fifth volume in the series Challenges in Language and Literacy. In their preface to this volume, editors Kate Cain and Jane Oakhill characterize their goal as the production of a book that provides "a detailed analysis of the comprehension difficulties experienced by different groups of children that [is] accessible to a broad readership, including academics, speech–language specialists and practitioners in related disciplines, and students interested in the cognitive bases of language comprehension difficulties." The editors have fulfilled this purpose admirably; however, they have done more than this. The book indeed makes an important contribution to our understanding of the specific comprehension difficulties of various atypical child populations. However, it also contributes important data and insightful theoretical refinements to an emerging model of the various subcomponents of the comprehension process, particularly the higher-level text integration processes involved at the level of discourse and inference.

The editors are two of the foremost authorities on language comprehension as well as sensitive researchers interested in improving the skills of children with comprehension difficulties. In addition to their thoughtful orchestration of what is an integrated collection of chapters, the editors have contributed three of their own. The two initial chapters, contributed by the editors, provide an authoritative and accessible framework for conceptualizing the comprehension process and the possible impediments to comprehension. Their discussion draws comprehensively on recent research in a way that respects the complexity of the issues while simultaneously providing an accessible and engaging discussion. In the following chapters the book's various contributors, all recognized experts in the study of language processes, provide authoritative profiles of selected atypical child populations. In each of these chapters, the authors provide a state-of-the-art depiction of the target population, followed by an analysis of research—both their own and that of others—on the comprehension difficulties of that population. This synthesis is followed by a discussion of implications for future research and for clinical practice.

One hallmark of the book is its interdisciplinary scholarship in two key senses: It involves scholars from multiple disciplines, and it communicates effectively to readers from diverse disciplinary and professional backgrounds. Through its analysis of the comprehension skills and contributing subskills of discrete special child populations, the book serves to highlight key components of effective language comprehension and to identify causes of poor comprehension. As such, it speaks authoritatively to researchers interested in developing our understanding of the process of oral and written language comprehension. Second, through its detailed discussion of research on the language skills of specific atypical child populations, the book provides essential information for professionals attempting to build basic understanding of the difficulties exhibited by these populations as well as effective strategies for assessment and intervention.

Two important features of the analyses of comprehension considered in this volume include a focus on higher-level language structures (i.e., discourse) and a strong developmental focus (i.e., the notion that different processes are involved at different points in time). This latter focus moves beyond the simplistic "first-things-first" view of decoding preceding comprehension to a more nuanced view of simultaneous development of lower- and higher-order skills. In the editors' own words,

> One clear conclusion . . . is that models that presuppose that the development of basic reading skills (e.g., phonological skills and word decoding) must precede the development of comprehension skills, need to be questioned. A perspective that fits better with recent data is that comprehension skills develop simultaneously with basic language skills and have their roots in early narrative comprehension. . . . In terms of interventions, a clear implication is that we should be careful not to focus on the teaching of decoding skills to the exclusion of other skills—that is, we should not wait until children are proficient in decoding before beginning instruction in oral language skills such as vocabulary, syntax, inference making, and comprehension monitoring. (pp. 30–31)

This message resonates with recent work on early intervention; however, the various authors' proposals for targeting specific comprehension processes push recent global proposals for language enrichment toward a more articulated agenda with respect to fostering strong comprehension skills.

This volume embodies many of the themes of the larger series of which it is a part. The aim of the series is to integrate interdisciplinary perspectives on language and literacy with empirically based programs and practices for promoting effective learning outcomes in diverse students. The series is based on the premise that oral and written language skills are functionally intertwined in individual development. Understanding the complexity of this relationship requires the collaborative contributions of scholars and practitioners from multiple disciplines. The series focuses on typical and atypical language and literacy development from the preschool years to young adulthood. The goal is to provide informative, timely resources for a broad audience, including practitioners, academics, and students in the fields of language science and disorders, educational psychology, general education, special education, and learning disabilities.

We are confident that this book will do what we have in mind for the entire series, that is, stimulate the thinking and the practice of professionals devoted to the integration of work on language and literacy in myriad settings devoted to research and practice. The book is an important step forward in the integration of disciplinary perspectives on the acquisition of literacy.

C. ADDISON STONE
ELAINE R. SILLIMAN

Preface

We read to understand, or to begin to understand.
—MANGUEL (1997)

WHAT IS COMPREHENSION?

Comprehension is the ultimate aim of reading and listening: It enables us to acquire information, to experience and be aware of other (fictional) worlds, to communicate successfully, and to achieve academic success. Our goal when reading (or listening to) a text (or discourse) is usually to derive an overall interpretation of the state of affairs described, rather than simply to retrieve the meanings of individual words or sentences.[1] This goal is reflected in a factor common to all major theories of reading comprehension, which is that good comprehension involves the construction of a representation corresponding to the state of affairs described in that text, a mental model (Johnson-Laird, 1983) or a situation model (Kintsch, 1998). This representation

---

[1] Throughout this preface, we refer to text comprehension as understanding of written narratives and expository texts. Many of the same skills and processes are involved in the understanding of the same forms in spoken language, often referred to as "discourse comprehension" in the literature. We differentiate between pragmatic aspects of spoken language comprehension that are implicated in conversational interactions, where appropriate. For further discussion of pragmatics and spoken language comprehension, see the chapters by Botting (Chapter 3) and Leekam (Chapter 4) in this volume.

includes causal relations between events, the goals of protagonists, and spatial and temporal information that is relevant to the storyline (Zwaan & Radvansky, 1998). These representations are not unique to reading comprehension: They are the product of successful comprehension of spoken discourse as well.

Because literacy skills are vital to academic success, research into the language comprehension skills of children over 5 years of age has tended to focus on the skills required to become a good reading comprehender. Comprehension of written text involves processing language at many different levels. However, with the exception of translating the written symbols on the page into their spoken form, these processes are common to understanding spoken discourse as well. At the word level, the reader must decode the individual words on the page. Comprehenders of both written and spoken discourse must access the meanings of the words they read or hear. At the sentence level, the comprehender needs to work out the syntactic structure and sense of each sentence. Simply deriving the meanings of individual words and sentences is insufficient: In order to construct a mental model of the text, the comprehender needs to integrate information from different sentences to establish local coherence and to incorporate background knowledge and ideas (retrieved from long-term memory) to make sense of details that are only implicitly mentioned (Graesser, Singer, & Trabasso, 1994; Long & Chong, 2001). Consider the following (from Trabasso & Suh, 1993):

> Betty wanted to give her mother a present.
> She went to the department store.
> She found that everything was too expensive.
> Betty decided to knit a sweater.

To understand this extract in a meaningful way, the comprehender has to work out how the information expressed in the different sentences and phrases fits together, so he or she needs to establish links between the different sentences (i.e., through integration), and also to determine the meanings of pronouns such as *he* or *she* (i.e., anaphoric resolution). In the extract above, the comprehender can make links between successive sentences by establishing that *she* in sentences two and three refers to Betty, the protagonist introduced in the first sentence. Furthermore, a causal inference must be made to integrate the final sentence with the preceding text: The sweater is presumably a gift for her mother. The comprehender also needs to draw on general knowledge to supplement the information provided literally by the wording. The specific knowledge that we usually obtain presents in stores and our general knowledge about buying and selling is needed to make sense of the third sentence. In addition to these processes, skilled comprehenders will check their understanding of the text as they read, which can help them to identify, for example, whether or not they have worked out the correct referent for a pronoun or whether they need to make an inference. This latter process is referred to as comprehension monitoring.

WHAT HAPPENS
WHEN COMPREHENSION BREAKS DOWN?

When comprehension does not proceed smoothly, background knowledge may not be brought to bear on the interpretation of events, the inferences necessary to fully understand the text may not be made, pronouns may not be resolved, and causality may not be established. As a consequence, a complete and integrated representation of a text's meaning will not be constructed and the readers (or the listeners) may fail to get the point—for example, they may not appreciate the reason for Betty's trip to the department store or her decision to knit a sweater.

We all have had experiences of comprehension failure. For some of us that experience may have arisen at school—for example, failing to grasp the main point of a story in a foreign language because there were too many unknown key words or not understanding how an electrical circuit works because we lacked the fundamental knowledge about the electrochemistry of cells. Failures of comprehension do not always arise in educational settings. Have you ever wondered why a sentence in a book does not make sense and then realized that you have mistakenly turned over two pages, or have you found the plot of a thriller hard to follow because you missed the first 10 minutes of the movie?

For many individuals, language comprehension difficulties occur on a regular basis and may go unnoticed. Many children with reading comprehension difficulties develop accurate and fluent word-reading ability so that on a measure of word reading their ability appears good. For some readers and listeners, a failure to fully comprehend may not be apparent until they are required to recall or apply that information—for example, in a formal test. This is because some individuals with comprehension difficulties do not monitor their comprehension; that is, they do not check their understanding as they read or listen. Others may lack the skills and strategies needed to remedy any failures to understand.

For these individuals, comprehension failures may affect more significant aspects of their lives than reading novels in foreign languages or following the twists and turns in the plot of a thriller. Poor comprehension can limit the ability to communicate effectively and to acquire new information and advance knowledge. As a consequence, the poor comprehender may have reduced chances of academic success and have access to fewer employment opportunities. For these reasons, a better understanding of the causes of comprehension failure is needed.

OVERVIEW OF THIS VOLUME

In this volume, we have brought together a collection of research on a diverse range of populations who experience written and spoken language comprehension difficulties. There are four parts. Part I serves as an introduction in two ways. Chapter 1 details the development of written and spoken language comprehension in early childhood and identifies the skills and processes that must be acquired to be a successful comprehender. Chapter 2 examines the language profile of children with poor comprehension, details the strengths and weaknesses of the different methodologies that can be used to test theories of causality, and examines evidence that key skill impairments are causally implicated in comprehension failure.

Part II is devoted to children with developmental disorders: specific language impairment, autism spectrum disorder, attention-deficit/hyperactivity disorder, and learning disabilities. Part III contains three chapters. Chapters 7 and 8 explore the language comprehension impairments of children who have suffered neurological damage: children with spina bifida myelomeningocele and children who have suffered pediatric traumatic brain injury. Chapter 9 offers a contrast: The focal population is children with hearing impairment. We discuss the common themes and the educational and research implications of these findings in the single chapter that is Part IV. This chapter is authored by the editors, but incorporates feedback from all the contributors to this volume.

Our aim for this volume was to provide a detailed analysis of the comprehension difficulties experienced by different groups of children that was accessible to a broad readership, including academics, speech–language specialists and practitioners in related disciplines, and students interested in the cognitive bases of language comprehension difficulties. Each chapter begins with an overview of the written and spoken language comprehension difficulties experienced by each population, followed by a detailed examination of the research evidence concerning different skills and processes that might explain the language comprehension problems experienced by these populations. In addition to the theoretical interpretation of the latest research findings, each chapter concludes with a discussion of the practical implications that arise.

A common picture emerges: These diverse populations experience many of the same language comprehension problems. Furthermore, the findings that come out of these three research areas are shown to be relevant not only to the assessment and treatment of comprehension difficulties in the specific population under consideration; each set of findings also informs models of typical function by identifying the cognitive functions that are crucial to success in language comprehension. We hope that the work presented in this volume will stimulate further research that will lead to a better understanding of the causes of comprehension failure and how best to remediate it.

REFERENCES

Graesser, A. C., Singer, M., & Trabasso, T. (1994). Constructing inferences during narrative text comprehension. *Psychological Review, 101,* 371–395.

Johnson-Laird, P. N. (1983). *Mental models.* Cambridge, UK: Cambridge University Press.

Kintsch, W. (1998). *Comprehension: A paradigm for cognition.* New York: Cambridge University Press.

Long, D. L., & Chong, J. L. (2001). Comprehension skill and global coherence: A paradoxical picture of poor comprehenders' abilities. *Journal of Experimental Psychology: Learning, Memory, and Cognition, 27,* 1424–1429.

Manguel, A. (1997). *A history of reading.* London: Flamingo.

Trabasso, T., & Suh, S. (1993). Understanding text: Achieving explanatory coherence through on-line inferences and mental operations in working memory. *Discourse Processes, 16,* 3–34.

Zwaan, R. A., & Radvansky, G. A. (1998). Situation models in language comprehension and memory. *Psychological Bulletin, 123,* 162–185.

Contents

PART I

Comprehension Processes and Impairments in Typically Developing Children

The comprehension of written and spoken language is a complex task that involves many different cognitive skills and processes. Before children begin reading instruction, they already have well-developed language comprehension skills that will aid them in their acquisition of word recognition and comprehension skills. Spoken language comprehension skills serve as a foundation for developing reading comprehension, but do not in themselves guarantee success in reading. In the next two chapters we provide an introduction to typical and atypical development of language comprehension and focus on the skills that aid the comprehension of written text. We examine the development of word-, sentence-, and discourse-level skills and how these might limit the development of effective and efficient reading comprehension. We also examine the language and cognitive deficits in a population with specific reading (and listening) comprehension problems.

Chapter 1 considers the skills that are common to reading and listening comprehension and how they develop. A common basis for competence in written and spoken language comprehension is recognized in a model of reading ability that has been highly influential in recent years, the Simple View of Reading (Hoover & Gough, 1990).

1

This model proposes that reading ability is the product of word-reading ability and listening comprehension. Thus reading comprehension can be limited by either poor word reading and/or by poor oral language comprehension. Although understanding what we read is crucial to academic success, there have been relatively few studies of how early language development influences later reading comprehension. We focus on longitudinal studies, including our own recent work, which are able to inform the course of development and provide a more detailed analysis of the contributions of different language skills to reading development. Chapter 1 ends with a discussion of the abilities that underpin comprehension skill and the practical implications for the teaching of comprehension.

In Chapter 2, we consider the difficulties experienced by "typically" developing children with a specific reading comprehension deficit. We term these children "typically" developing, because they do not have the developmental disorders, neurological damage, or sensory impairments of the populations considered in Parts II and III. Our own research has focused, in detail, on children with a specific reading comprehension deficit: children who have developed age-appropriate word-reading skills but whose reading comprehension skills lag behind. These children's difficulties extend beyond the written word to impaired comprehension of spoken narratives. Their ability to produce coherent narratives is also impaired. In this chapter we consider the nature and the source of difficulties experienced by these children in several key text- and discourse-level processing skills that affect their ability to integrate information and construct a coherent meaning-based representation of text. We present a catalogue of preserved and impaired language skills in this population but we focus on research that has used designs that enable us to disentangle cause and effect, namely, research that includes a comprehension–age match comparison group, longitudinal studies of poor comprehenders, and interventions.

REFERENCE

Hoover, W. A., & Gough, P. B. (1990). The simple view of reading. *Reading and Writing, 2,* 127–160.

CHAPTER 1

Introduction to Comprehension Development

JANE OAKHILL
KATE CAIN

This chapter provides an overview of the research into the development of children's reading comprehension skills—skills that are crucial for academic success. Before children begin reading instruction, they already have well-developed language comprehension skills that will aid them in their acquisition of word recognition and reading comprehension skills, although there are well-documented developments in oral language skills during the primary school years (Garton & Pratt, 1998). Indeed, comprehension of language, whether written or spoken, is a complex task that involves many different cognitive skills and processes.

Skills in spoken language comprehension serve as a foundation for developing reading comprehension, but do not in themselves guarantee success in reading. Clearly, reading comprehension depends on listening comprehension: In order to read a language with adequate comprehension, one has to understand that language in its spoken form. Therefore, general language comprehension will constrain the development of reading comprehension. Although there is a relation between reading and listening comprehension, the strength of the relation changes with age. Correlations between reading and listening comprehension are generally low in beginning readers (e.g., Curtis, 1980; Sticht & James, 1984), but gradually increase and reach asymptote in high school when decoding differences are small (Sticht & James, 1984). For college students, correlations of between .82 and .92 have been found (Gernsbacher, Varner, & Faust, 1990; Palmer, MacLeod, Hunt, & Davidson, 1985).

These studies support the view that we might expect an individual's reading comprehension to develop to the same level as his or her listening comprehension, once limitations in word decoding are overcome. This view has been termed the "simple view" of reading by Gough and colleagues (see, e.g., Gough & Tunmer, 1986). However, typical text is not "speech written down": written and spoken language differ along a number of dimensions, so there are reasons why beginning readers might have problems that are specific to reading. One problem is that written language makes use of syntactic constructions and vocabulary that may not be familiar to children from their everyday spoken interactions (see, e.g., Cunningham, 2005; Garton & Pratt, 1998; Reid, 1970, 1983). In addition, written language is "decontextualized"–that is, it is typically not about the "here and now." Garton and Pratt (1998) also suggest that written language demands the integration of information across extended tracts of discourse in a manner that spoken language usually does not. (Of course, in a spoken interaction, the listener can stop and ask the speaker for clarification if a referent is not clear. But the text cannot be interrogated.)

Thus, written language will make demands on the reader that are not apparent in spoken language comprehension, which possibly goes some way in explaining why many children who are, apparently, perfectly competent speakers and comprehenders of spoken language have problems with reading comprehension (see, e.g., Cain & Oakhill, Chapter 2, this volume). In a review of research on word-reading fluency and comprehension, Paris, Carpenter, Paris, and Hamilton (2005) conclude that although low levels of word-reading fluency are positively correlated with low levels of reading comprehension, it is incorrect to conclude that fluent word reading will ensure good reading comprehension: The data clearly show that it does not. In addition, strategic processing (e.g., rereading, reading difficult text more slowly) is likely to be an ability that is important for text, but not for listening, comprehension (or, at least, the strategies that aid comprehension are likely to be quite different in the two modalities).

Nevertheless, reading and listening comprehension share many components, and it is very likely that some common language skills underlie both. Thus, it follows that the components of spoken language comprehension that contribute to language comprehension will be important in the development of successful reading comprehension. Comprehension of spoken language will require competence at many different levels: phonology, semantics, syntax, and pragmatics (see, e.g., Bishop, 1997). It is reasonable, then, to suppose that these components also influence the understanding of written language. We explore each of these different areas in more detail below.

The language base of (word) reading and reading disabilities has been extensively researched (see Blachman, 1997; Brady & Shankweiler, 1991; Catts & Kamhi, 1999, 2005). A strong link between language abilities and reading has been shown (e.g., Bradley & Bryant, 1983; Liberman & Shankweiler, 1985; Stanovich, 1988; Vellutino, Scanlon, Small, & Tanzman, 1991), and, in particular, there is strong evidence for a relation between phonological skills and reading development and disorders (e.g., Brady & Shankweiler, 1991; Muter, Hulme, Snowling, & Taylor, 1998; Torgesen, Wagner, & Rashotte, 1994). However, most of this work maps the relation between phonological skills and the reading of words.

In comparison, relatively few studies examine how early language influences later reading comprehension. In particular, aspects of language such as vocabulary and grammar are likely to influence reading development. Vocabulary knowledge is likely to be important both in learning to recognize individual words (Plaut, McLelland, Seidenberg, & Patterson, 1996; Nation & Snowling, 1998a) and in text comprehension (McKeown, Beck, Omanson, & Perfetti, 1983; Stahl, 1983). Grammatical skills might also aid word recognition through the use of context (Tunmer, 1989) and may contribute to the development of reading comprehension (e.g., Bowey, 1986; Perfetti, 1985). In addition, a number of higher-order discourse skills are likely to contribute to the development of reading comprehension, including inference, metacognitive skills, and understanding text structure (e.g., Oakhill & Cain, 2004).

There are many studies of the predictors of word-reading skill, including metastudies (Scarborough, 1998), but few such studies of comprehension. In the studies that are available, the precise relation between different aspects of language skill and later reading comprehension is not clear-cut. One reason for the lack of consensus is that these studies typically focus on only a few language skills, and few have assessed the same set of skills. An additional problem is that many researchers fail to find a relation between language skills and subsequent reading development simply because they do not look for such a relation (see Dickinson, McCabe, Anastasopoulos, Peisner-Feinberg, & Poe, 2003). Indeed, often language variables are relegated to the status of control variables (a clear exception is the study by Chaney, 1998, which is discussed below, in the section on vocabulary and syntax). Thus, it is quite possible that the contributions of oral language skills to later reading development have been underestimated. A further problem that might help to account for the lack of consensus in the findings is that there is also substantial variation in the reading outcome measures used to assess reading achievement (see, e.g., Cutting & Scarborough, 2006; Paris & Stahl, 2005).

In this chapter, we aim to provide a more detailed analysis of the contributions of different language skills to reading development. We consider the evidence for a link between oral language and reading comprehension at the word level (phonological skills and word decoding), at the sentence level (semantics and syntax), and at the text level (narrative skills in both comprehension and production), and we also consider the role of metalinguistic skills in reading development. Obviously, some studies have explored a single skill and others have explored many different language skills. In these latter cases, we include the study in the section to which it seems to make the most important contribution.

LONGITUDINAL STUDIES: SOME METHODOLOGICAL ISSUES

Many studies of comprehension development have relied on concurrent evaluations of language and reading abilities (Gottardo, Stanovich, & Siegel, 1996; Lombardino, Riccio, Hynd, & Pinheiro,1997; Vellutino et al., 1991). But in such studies it is difficult, if not impossible, to determine whether it is language that is influencing reading or vice versa. A few studies have looked at the relation longitudinally (Catts, Fey, Zhang, & Tomblin, 1999; Muter, Hulme, Snowling, & Stevenson, 2004; Willson & Rupley, 1997). We include both types of study in this review, but we emphasize the longitudinal studies because of their potential for illuminating causal issues (see below).

Longitudinal studies that track the course of changes in comprehension skill can provide important information about the causal relations among the component skills of comprehension, and thus about the course of development. Here, we provide a brief overview of our own longitudinal study, which we also refer to in the appropriate sections. This study provides data on the reading development of the same group of children over a 4-year period from ages 7–8 (Year 3), 8–9 (Year 4), and 10–11 (Year 6). At each of these ages, we took measures of reading comprehension and word reading accuracy, using the Neale Analysis of Reading Ability–Revised (Neale, 1989). We also took measures of general verbal ability (Times 1 and 3 only), memory, and specific reading-related skills such as phonemic awareness (phoneme deletion), vocabulary (British Picture Vocabulary Scale), syntax (Test for Reception of Grammar), and measures of three comprehension-related skills: inference making, comprehension monitoring (assessed by the ability to detect inconsistencies in text), and story structure understanding (assessed by the ability to reconstruct a story from a set of jumbled sentences). Thus, we included measures of IQ, memory, word- and sentence-level comprehension skills, and text- and discourse-level comprehension skills. We believe that this study is unique in that it includes measures of these important subskills of comprehension, rather than simply a global measure of narrative comprehension (or production).

The results of multiple regression were applied to a causal path diagram to show the pattern and strength of relations among the various skills across time. A preliminary account of the results of these analyses can be found in Oakhill and Cain (2007) and Perfetti, Landi, and Oakhill (2005). They can be summarized briefly as follows. Initial reading comprehension skill was a strong predictor of later comprehension, and verbal ability (vocabulary and Verbal IQ) also made significant unique contributions to the prediction of comprehension ability across time. Nevertheless, three distinct predictors of reading comprehension emerged, either through direct or indirect links: answering inferential questions, monitoring comprehension, and understanding story structure. These factors predicted comprehension at a later time even after the autoregressive effect of comprehension (i.e., the prediction of comprehension at later times from comprehension at earlier times) was controlled. With word-reading accuracy as the dependent variable, the pattern was quite different. The significant predictors were previous measures of reading accuracy and a phoneme deletion measure taken at Time 1. From these analyses a picture of skill development emerges in which certain components of comprehension are predictive of general comprehension skill. Early abilities in inference skill, comprehension monitoring, and story structure understanding all predict performance on a later global assessment of comprehension skill independently of the contribution of earlier comprehension skill.

The inclusion of the relevant autoregressor (i.e., the measure of the skill being predicted—in this case, comprehension—at an earlier time point) in the above analyses is particularly important for causal hypotheses. De Jong and van der Leij (2002) have argued that any additional effects of variables after the inclusion of the autoregressive effect can be taken as support for a causal relation between those variables and the outcome measure. To make this more concrete: In the analyses described above, we found that inference skill accounted for variance in reading comprehension at a later time point, over and above the autogressive effect of reading comprehension. This result rules out the possibility that the relation between earlier inference skills and reading comprehension in Year 6 was due simply to their association with earlier reading comprehension.

A general issue with longitudinal studies is that the results that emerge often depend on what variables are entered and what outcome measures are used. Catts et al. (1999), for instance, argue that IQ, and in particular Full Scale IQ, should not be controlled because it is a very general measure whose relation to reading is not clearly defined. Thus, a variable such as IQ may account for a large proportion of variance without really "explaining" anything. Indeed, in Catts et al.'s study, although measures of phonological processing and oral language accounted for unique variance in reading comprehension over and above that contributed by Full Scale IQ (47.4%), the variance accounted for was substantially reduced relative to a model in which IQ was not included, and this was particularly the case with oral language. The selection of different control variables has contributed to different patterns of results. In particular, Dickinson et al. (2003) have pointed out that many studies include language measures as "control variables," thus excluding examination of their independent contribution to comprehension skill and reading more generally. As they state, "Quite possibly, important interrelationships exist that have been unexplored, ignored, or relegated to the level of nuisance by virtue of statistical control procedures" (p. 469). Of course, there are circumstances in which one might want to control for language ability, but it is relatively rarely that such variables are considered as informative predictors in their own right.

There are also implications concerning the type of comprehension test that is used as an outcome measure. For instance, Cutting and Scarborough (2006) compared three comprehension assessments that are commonly used in the United States: the (reading) comprehension subtests from the Gates–MacGinitie Reading Test–Revised (G-M; MacGinitie, MacGinitie, Maria, & Dreyer, 2000); the Gray Oral Reading Test–Third Edition (GORT-3; Wiederholt & Bryant, 1992); and the Wechsler Individual Achievement Test (WIAT; Wechsler, 1992). They found that the unique contributions of word recognition/decoding skill varied across comprehension measures, with nearly twice as much variance accounted for in WIAT scores (11.9%) than in G-M (6.1%) and GORT-3 (7.5%) scores. Furthermore, the percentage of variance uniquely explained by oral language proficiency varied substantially across tests. This percentage was similar for the WIAT and GORT-3 (each 9%), but higher for the G-M (15%). There were also indications in the data that the different measures of reading comprehension make differential demands on vocabulary knowledge and sentence-processing abilities.

FACTORS THAT INFLUENCE COMPREHENSION DEVELOPMENT

Word- and Sentence-Level Skills

Phonological Skills/Word Decoding

As mentioned above, most of the work on phonological skills and reading development has focused—rightly—on the relation to word reading. Since the focus of this chapter is reading comprehension, we do not consider the extensive evidence for a link between phonological awareness and the development of word reading (for a recent brief review, see Dickinson et al., 2003). Studies that have looked at the relation between phonological skills and comprehension have produced mixed effects, perhaps because of differences in the nature of the comprehension assessment and, in particular, its reliance on word recognition skills (see Cutting & Scarborough, 2006, discussed above).

Manis, Seidenberg, and Doi (1999) explored the relation between phonological skills, rapid automatized naming (RAN: digits and numbers), and the development of word reading and comprehension after 1 year between first and second grade. They found that their measure of phonological skills (sound deletion) accounted for substantial variance in comprehension skill 1 year later (even when the autoregressive effect of earlier comprehension had been taken into account) and, as would be expected, also accounted for variance in later word-reading skill. By contrast, the measures of RAN had little influence on later comprehension, and none at all when the autoregressor was taken into account.

Parrila, Kirby, and McQuarrie (2004) included measures of phonological processing, articulation rate, verbal short-term memory, and naming speed (color naming), plus assessments of both word reading and passage comprehension, in their longitudinal study of children from first to third grade. They found that naming speed in kindergarten predicted passage comprehension (and word recognition) in all three later grades. Phonological awareness was also predictive, but, in line with other studies, its influence declined across grades. Word identification was also a significant predictor of later comprehension, but, even with kindergarten word identification controlled, naming speed and phonological awareness independently predicted third-grade passage comprehension. The authors note, however, that the measure of comprehension they used was itself highly correlated with word recognition and that more complex measures of comprehension might not show such strong associations with phonological skills.

Some studies, in contrast (see Muter et al., 2004, discussed in the next section), have failed to find a strong relation between early phonological skills and later reading comprehension. Others have found that the relation changes quite dramatically with age. For instance, Willson and Rupley (1997) explored the development of both reading and listening comprehension between first and sixth grade. Their study was partially longitudinal in that they assessed longitudinal development across grades at four different developmental points (from 2–3, 3–4, etc.). They found that in the early grades (2–4), but not in the later grades (5 and 6), reading comprehension was primarily driven by phonemic knowledge and background knowledge of the topic of the text. By fifth and sixth grade it was knowledge of reading strategies (metacognitive strategies and use of prediction and background knowledge) that dominated the prediction of reading comprehension; this was a far more important predictor than background knowledge. This pattern of results strongly supports the idea that early comprehension will be limited by word reading, but that later in development other factors come into play.

De Jong and van der Leij (2002) also explored the contributions made by a number of skills (phonological skills, serial rapid naming, vocabulary, and listening comprehension) to later word reading and reading comprehension in a longitudinal study from first to third grade. They found that phonological abilities (specifically, phonological awareness and serial rapid naming) were highly associated with word decoding, but did not have an additional influence on the further development of word decoding after first grade. In the case of reading comprehension, early decoding, vocabulary, and listening comprehension made significant contributions to later (third-grade) reading comprehension, but the effect of listening comprehension was more important than the effect of vocabulary. De Jong and van der Leij did not initially include phonological awareness as a direct predictor of comprehension because it was highly related to word reading. However, in their discussion, they report a further analysis in which phonological awareness was used as a predictor of third-grade reading comprehension. The results showed that phonological awareness took account of a small but marginally significant amount of the variance in third-grade reading comprehension (2.7%, p = .054) after first-grade reading comprehension, word decoding, and vocabulary were controlled for. The authors suggest that this relation might occur because the phonological awareness task used (the "odd-one-out" task) has simultaneous processing and storage demands—that is, many of the characteristics of a working memory test (see Baddeley, 1986). Thus, although the result lends some support to the idea that working memory is implicated in the development of reading comprehension, further conclusions should be based on more appropriate measures of working memory. In contrast to most studies, de Jong and van der Leij included the autoregressive effect of reading comprehension in their analyses, thus enabling them to rule out the possibility that the relations of first-grade word decoding and linguistic comprehension with reading comprehension in third grade were due to their association with reading comprehension in first grade. As with our own work, discussed later, the results from de Jong and van der Leij's study also indicate that partially different determinants underlie the development of word-decoding ability and reading comprehension.

To summarize, some studies have demonstrated that phonological skills predict variance in later comprehension ability, though in most cases it is not clear whether or not they were direct predictors or were mediated by word decoding, since concurrent word decoding was not controlled for. There is substantial evidence to suggest that the relation between word-level skills and reading comprehension declines with age, and may be critically dependent on the measure of comprehension used (see Keenan, 2006).

Semantic and Syntactic Skills

Both semantic and syntactic knowledge will serve as cues for the construction of meaning from text by enabling the reader to make certain predictions about sentence constructions. Some studies have primarily explored the relation between semantic (vocabulary) skills and reading comprehension, others have looked at syntactic skills, and still others have explored both. In this section, we first consider the studies of vocabulary, then the studies of syntax, then the studies that have included both skills and language skills more generally.

SEMANTICS

Vocabulary knowledge is one of the best predictors of reading comprehension (Carroll, 1993; Davis, 1944, 1968; Thorndike, 1973). Thorndike (1973) found correlations of between .66 and .75 between reading comprehension and vocabulary knowledge. It has long been thought that a major source of new vocabulary is reading (Huey, 1908/

1968; Thorndike, 1917), presumably through a process of inferring new meanings from context, so it is likely that there is reciprocity between vocabulary acquisition and reading development. Written text is an important source of vocabulary acquisition once children become fluent readers (Cunningham, 2005; Nagy & Scott, 2000).

The precise nature of the causal link between vocabulary skills and reading comprehension is, however, unclear because the evidence is equivocal. A longitudinal study by Roth, Speece, and Cooper (2002) points to the conclusion that vocabulary is causally implicated in the development of reading comprehension. Roth et al. followed the progress of children between kindergarten and second grade to explore the relation between various aspects of language skill (structural, metalinguistic, and narrative discourse) and later reading development (including passage comprehension). They assessed structural language with measures of receptive vocabulary, word definitions, word retrieval, and tests of receptive and expressive morphology and syntax. The metalinguistic skills tested were phonological awareness and metasemantics (i.e., comprehension and production of lexical ambiguity and idioms). Their results showed that, between kindergarten and grades 1 and 2, phonological awareness did not predict reading comprehension and neither did the tests of syntax. It was semantic abilities (oral definitions and word retrieval), and the autoregressor (in fact, a measure of print awareness taken in kindergarten, which was used as a surrogate measure because comprehension could not be measured directly, and print awareness was highly correlated with first-grade reading comprehension) that best predicted later reading comprehension.

However, a study by Eldredge, Quinn, and Butterfield (1990) showed that reading comprehension is a stronger cause of general vocabulary growth than vice versa, at least in the second grade. These authors, using a cross-lagged panel design and path analysis, showed that reading comprehension measured at the beginning of the school year accounted for 47% of the variability in vocabulary measured at the end of the school year, whereas vocabulary measured at the beginning of the school year accounted for only 34% of variability in reading comprehension scores at the end of the school year. In a comparison of five different theoretical models, the authors found that the best-fitting model was one in which early comprehension skill predicted growth in vocabulary knowledge, but not vice versa. This model produced, for example, a superior fit to one in which the relation between growth in vocabulary knowledge and in comprehension was fully reciprocal. So, although some reciprocity cannot be entirely ruled out by these data, the findings clearly suggest that early reading comprehension is a stronger cause of general vocabulary growth than vice versa. One possible interpretation of this finding is that extensive reading (a possible result of better comprehension) may be instrumental in promoting vocabulary acquisition, a position supported by later studies of the relation between exposure to print and vocabulary growth (Echols, West, Stanovich, & Zehr, 1996).

A recent study by Seigneuric and Ehrlich (2005) also assessed the relative contribution of vocabulary skills to later reading comprehension and suggests a more reciprocal relation between vocabulary and comprehension skills. In addition, the authors assessed working memory and decoding skills, and explored the relations between these skills and later reading comprehension from first grade (age 7 years) to third grade (age 9 years). Their results showed that first-grade vocabulary and second-grade working memory predicted significant variance in third-grade reading comprehension, even after the autoregressive effect had been taken into account. These results are consistent with other findings that vocabulary is a strong predictor of reading comprehension in the early years of school (Bast & Reitsma, 1998; de Jong & van der Leij, 2002; Torgesen, Wagner, Rashotte, Burgess, & Hecht, 1997).

Seigneuric and Ehrlich (2005) conducted further analyses to assess whether there is a reciprocal relation between vocabulary and reading comprehension (as suggested, too, by de Jong & van der Leij, 2002). They carried out fixed-order regression analyses with vocabulary as the criterion variable. They found that first-grade reading comprehension accounted for 10% of the variance in second-grade vocabulary and 15% of the variance in third-grade vocabulary, after age and the autoregressive effect of prior vocabulary had been taken into account. These results support the conclusion that reading comprehension influences the growth of vocabulary knowledge. Taken together, their pattern of data supports the hypothesis that the relation between reading comprehension and vocabulary development is reciprocal in the early school grades.

It is not just vocabulary size, but also automaticity of access to word meanings, that is important in skilled comprehension. A causal link between vocabulary and reading comprehension is implied by models of reading that emphasize the importance of fluency and automaticity of access to word meanings (e.g., Laberge & Samuels, 1974; Perfetti & Lesgold, 1977). However, training studies have failed to provide evidence for this direct causal relation, an indication that automatic and fluent access to the meanings of the words in a text may be necessary, but not sufficient for good comprehension. Some training studies have succeeded in improving vocabulary knowledge (e.g.,

Beck, Perfetti, & McKeown, 1982; Jenkins, Pany, & Schreck, 1978; Tuinman & Brady, 1974), but few have shown corresponding increases in comprehension skill. One exception is a study by Beck et al. (1982). Those authors argued that, for vocabulary instruction to have effects on reading comprehension, it is necessary to increase not just the number of words learned, but also the fluency with which the meanings of new words can be accessed. It is also likely that effective vocabulary instruction will encourage students to use the new vocabulary in multiple ways, over an extended period of time.

Of course, reading comprehension and vocabulary may be related indirectly by a third factor. A likely candidate for such a mediator is Verbal IQ (see Anderson & Freebody, 1981). It may be that the more intelligent individuals have a greater ability to learn from context, and that this ability also enables them to develop an extensive vocabulary (for further discussion, see also Daneman, 1988). In our own longitudinal study, we found that a measure of receptive vocabulary predicted reading comprehension across time, and that it did so independently of the predictive effect of Verbal IQ (which was also a significant predictor of later comprehension). Thus, our own results suggest that the effects of vocabulary are not entirely intertwined with those of IQ.

SYNTAX

It used to be thought that children's syntactic development was more or less complete at about 5 years, but more recent work shows that their syntax continues to develop—albeit in more subtle ways—long after this age (summaries of these later developments can be found in Oakhill & Garnham, 1988, Chap. 3, and, more recently, in Garton & Pratt, 1998, Chap. 5).

Studies in this area have sometimes measured syntactic knowledge and sometimes syntactic awareness. *Syntactic knowledge* is required to extract meaning from different syntactic constructions—for example, the sort of knowledge that is needed to appreciate the meaning of active versus passive constructions. Such knowledge may be implicit. By contrast, *syntactic (or grammatical) awareness* is regarded as explicit knowledge, involving deliberate and controlled reflection on language. Syntactic awareness is not necessarily required to extract meaning, but would, for example, be used in decisions about grammatical well-formedness.

Clearly, (implicit) knowledge about syntactic forms is necessary to comprehend particular grammatical constructions, and thus might be expected to be related to comprehension level. Syntactic awareness has been proposed to influence reading ability in two different ways. Tunmer and Bowey (1984) suggested that such skills may help children to detect and correct reading errors, and thus to enhance comprehension monitoring (the topic of comprehension monitoring is considered below). Second, Tunmer and Hoover (1992) have proposed that syntactic awareness may aid word recognition if children are able to use the constraints of sentence structure to supplement their rudimentary decoding ability.

Research that has looked at the concurrent relation between syntactic awareness and reading comprehension has produced mixed results. Willows and Ryan (1986) used an oral cloze task to assess syntactic awareness. This measure was related to reading comprehension and decoding in 6- to 8-year-olds even after vocabulary ability and nonverbal IQ had been taken into account. However, semantic knowledge may have influenced performance on this task because the correct filler had to be selected on the basis of both the word's meaning (semantics) and its grammatical function. In another study with 6-year-olds, Bowey and Patel (1988) used a sentence correction task, performance on which is not necessarily reliant on semantic knowledge. In contrast to the earlier findings, performance on this measure of syntactic awareness did not account for significant variance in either reading comprehension or word-reading accuracy after individual differences in vocabulary had been taken into account.

One explanation for a relation between syntactic abilities and reading comprehension is that the two are related by phonological-processing ability. This hypothesis has been extensively explored by Shankweiler and colleagues (see Shankweiler, 1989, for a review) in relation to syntactic knowledge. According to their account, comprehension difficulties arise when children are unable to set up or to sustain a phonological representation of incoming verbal information. As a result, they experience difficulties in retaining and processing this information in verbal working memory, and thus have problems parsing syntactically complex constructions (see, e.g., Smith, Macaruso, Shankweiler, & Crain, 1989).

The relation between phonological processing and syntactic awareness was directly addressed in a study of 8-year-olds conducted by Gottardo et al. (1996). They provide evidence that comprehension difficulties are not primarily related to syntactic skills. Although they found that metasyntactic skills were related to both word recognition and reading comprehension in third graders, in support of the phonological limitation hypothesis these abilities did not account for independent variance once phonological awareness and phonological work-

ing memory had been taken into account. Thus, it may be that the relation reported between syntactic skills and reading by some authors
(Tunmer & Hoover, 1991) is epiphenomenal, and reflects a more basic
relation between phonological processing and reading ability. Unfortunately, Gottardo et al. did not investigate whether grammatical awareness made an independent contribution to reading comprehension
over and above word-reading ability. Furthermore, the length of the
sentences used in Gottardo et al.'s grammatical awareness task may
have placed heavy demands on working memory, thereby affecting the
pattern of the results (Blackmore & Pratt, 1997). A stronger test of the
relation between grammatical awareness and reading comprehension
would control for word-reading and memory skills that do not tap into
sentence-level processing.

Longitudinal studies also find only weak relations between syntactic awareness and reading comprehension. Demont and Gombert
(1996) followed children's progress from preschool (mean age 5 years,
7 months) to second grade (mean age 8 years, 8 months). They took
measures of phonological awareness, syntactic awareness, word-reading
accuracy and speed, and sentence comprehension. In general, phonological awareness better predicted later recoding and syntactic awareness better predicted later comprehension, after taking into account
the verbal and general ability assessments. Furthermore, the contribution of the syntactic measures in accounting for variance in later comprehension was less impressive than the contribution of phonological
skills to recoding.

Tunmer (1989) assessed children's syntactic awareness at the end
of the first year of school and again a year later. Performance on
measures of syntactic awareness predicted both word decoding and
listening comprehension, and these two skills in turn predicted reading comprehension. However, Blackmore and Pratt (1997) failed to
find a direct relation between preschool grammatical awareness and
later reading comprehension. Thus, the precise relation between
reading comprehension and syntactic knowledge and awareness is not
clear.

Our own recent work indicates that there might be developmental
differences in the influence of syntactic knowledge on comprehension.
In our longitudinal study, we found that syntactic ability (TROG;
Bishop, 1983) did not predict comprehension skill (or word-reading
accuracy) in 7- to 8-year-olds after vocabulary and IQ had been taken
into account, but that it explained significant variance in reading comprehension (but not reading accuracy) in the same sample of children 1
year later (Oakhill, Cain, & Bryant, 2003a).

VOCABULARY, SYNTAX, AND ORAL LANGUAGE SKILLS

A number of studies have included measures of both vocabulary knowledge and syntactic skills, often as part of a more general oral language
composite. Muter et al. (2004) followed the progress of children for 2
years after their entry into school, and assessed a number of abilities,
including phonological, grammatical, and vocabulary knowledge. They
found that early letter knowledge and phonemic sensitivity were powerful predictors of variance in later word recognition, whereas word identification skills, grammatical knowledge, and vocabulary assessed at
age 5–6 (but not phonological skills) each predicted unique variance in
reading comprehension at the end of the second year of schooling.
Thus, word identification was important in predicting comprehension,
as one might expect for younger children, as were knowledge of word
meanings and grammatical knowledge. Another important contribution of the Muter et al. (2004) study is that it highlights the need to
look at word recognition and comprehension skill separately in development, since they are predicted by different aspects of children's
underlying language skills (see also de Jong & van der Leij, 2002, and
Oakhill et al., 2003a, who make this point in greater detail).

Muter et al. (2004) report a slightly different pattern to that found
by Oakhill, Cain, and Bryant (2003b) for the younger children they
studied. In particular, Oakhill et al. did not find that vocabulary or
word-reading skills were important predictors of early comprehension
skill. However, because Muter et al. had a comprehension assessment
only at the final test point in their study, their study is not directly comparable with the study by Oakhill et al., since they were unable to take
the autoregessive effect of comprehension skill into account. It is possible that all the factors identified in these two studies influence comprehension development, with the strength of their contribution depending upon the level of the child's comprehension skill. However, studies
that carry out comparable assessments, including tests of comprehension at more than one time point, are needed to test this possibility.

Goff, Pratt, and Ong (2005) also explored the ability to predict
later comprehension of word reading, language, and memory, between
third and fifth grades. They hypothesized that orthographic processing, receptive vocabulary (PPVT; a North American version of the British Picture Vocabulary Test), and verbal working memory would independently predict reading comprehension. They also explored the
contributions of reading speed, receptive grammatical skills (TROG),
exposure to print, visuospatial working memory, and verbal learning
and retrieval. The results showed that, after controlling for age and

general intellectual ability, the word-reading and language variables (receptive vocabulary and receptive grammatical skills) were much more strongly predictive of reading comprehension than the memory variables. In line with previous findings, it was found that tasks that require the integration of new information with information stored in long-term memory were more highly predictive of comprehension skill than tasks that have only a short-term memory requirement.

Some studies have included both word- and sentence-level skills, and language skills more broadly. For example, Lombardino et al. (1997), in a study of 9-year-olds in three ability groups (reading disability, attention deficit/hyperactivity disorder [ADHD] without reading disability, and typical readers), found that, across all groups, word attack skills were predicted primarily by phonemic awareness (49% of variance), with phonemic awareness and an expressive language composite (derived from the Clinical Evaluation of Language Fundamental–Revised [CELF-R]; Semel, Wiig, & Secord, 1997) accounting for 59% together. Phonemic awareness also predicted passage comprehension, and together with the expressive and receptive language composite scores accounted for 57% of variance, but expressive language alone accounted for 49% of the variance in reading comprehension. Thus, phonological skills were a far more important predictor of word recognition than of comprehension, which was best accounted for by expressive and receptive language comprehension.

Catts et al. (1999) explored the contributions made by both phonological and oral language skills to reading and reading disability in a longitudinal study from kindergarten to second grade. They took two approaches: first, they compared good and poor readers (in second grade) on measures of oral language and phonological processing in kindergarten. They also used multiple-regression analyses to assess the relative contributions of phonological and oral language abilities in predicting reading achievement in the sample as a whole. They assessed oral language and phonological processing (phonological awareness and rapid naming) in kindergarten. The oral language composite used by Catts et al. included measures of vocabulary and syntax, together with a narrative story task (which required the children to comprehend, organize, and retell a story read aloud to them), and was found to be a strong predictor of later reading comprehension. Catts et al. found that phonological awareness and rapid naming accounted for independent variance in reading comprehension in second grade, but, over and above these, a composite of the oral language tasks (both receptive and expressive) accounted for a further 13.8% of variance. Thus, oral language was a far stronger predictor of later reading comprehension than either of the phonological tasks. In addition, they found that the oral language composite (a mixture of vocabulary, grammar, and discourse skills) still accounted for significant unique variance in second-grade reading comprehension even after phonological skills and Full Scale IQ had been taken into account. Unfortunately, it is impossible to say from their analyses how much the different components of the composite contributed to the prediction.

Other studies have also explored the relation between oral language skills (broadly measured, but usually including assessments of vocabulary and syntax) and later reading. Tabors, Snow, and Dickinson (2001), for instance, found consistent and strong correlations between oral narrative production, production of formal definitions, and receptive vocabulary measured at age 5 and fourth- and seventh-grade reading comprehension. Receptive vocabulary, in particular, was a strong predictor of later reading comprehension.

Evidence of the long-term contributions of early language come from a study by Chaney (1998), who found that general language proficiency (measured by the Preschool Language Scale) at age 3 was as strongly correlated with reading at age 7 (a composite of word recognition and comprehension measures) as it had been with metalinguistic and print knowledge scores at age 3. Although the contribution of general language ability on later reading was substantial, both metalinguistic skills and print knowledge at age 3 made significant contributions to reading achievement (composite) over and above the contribution of general language proficiency.

A recent structural analysis by Storch and Whitehurst (2002) of their longitudinal data explored the role of oral language from preschool through fourth grade in great detail and produced a new two-factor model of reading development that accords oral language an important developmental role. In Storch and Whitehurst's study, they attempt to provide a more conceptually coherent examination of the role of both code-related and oral language precursors to the development of reading ability. Code-related skills comprised phonological awareness, print knowledge, and emergent writing, whereas the oral language skills comprised expressive and receptive vocabulary, narrative recall, and conceptual knowledge.

Their results demonstrate a strong relation between the two domains of emergent literacy during the preschool period, consistent with other studies that have shown strong correlations between oral language skills (such as vocabulary) and code-related skills (such as phonological awareness) in young children (e.g., Chaney, 1992; Lonigan, Burgess, Anthony, & Barker, 1998). However, as formal schooling commences, the relation between oral language and code-related domains diminishes, though the code-related skills exert a strong and direct influence on beginning reading development in first grade. In second grade, reading was still heavily determined by code-related skills acquired by the end of kindergarten, and reading comprehension was also highly correlated with both word and nonword reading tasks. However, by third and fourth grade, the pattern of influence changed substantially as reading accuracy and reading comprehension could be reliably separated. Thus, later in development, reading accuracy is heavily influenced by prior word recognition and decoding. Reading comprehension, on the other hand, is determined by more varied skills: prior reading ability, but also concurrent reading accuracy and concurrent language skills. This model supports the view that sentence and text comprehension are affected by general verbal ability and oral language skills. Furthermore, the model demonstrates that oral language abilities reemerge as a strong direct force later in the process of learning to read, a relation that may have gone unnoticed in earlier studies.

In summary, the relation between these various aspects of language awareness and knowledge and reading comprehension is not very clear-cut, with mixed data. It is clear that word identification and phonological skills limit reading comprehension in the early stages, but their influence tends to diminish with age and reading progress. Vocabulary is an important predictor of later comprehension skills, and there is some evidence that the relation between vocabulary and comprehension development may be reciprocal. The role of syntactic skills is less clear, but they seem to have a lesser role than does vocabulary; there are some indications that, where found, the relations between syntactic skills and comprehension may be mediated by phonological working memory.

Metalinguistic Skills

The metalinguistic skills related to reading are many and various. Broadly, *metalinguistics* refers to the ability to manipulate the sounds (including phonological skills, discussed earlier) and meanings of words, phrases, and sentences, and includes the ability to interpret nonliteral meanings such as idioms and metaphors, and also the ability to reflect on the comprehension of a text more generally, and to repair comprehension problems. Since we considered phonological skills earlier, the focus here will be on other aspects of metalinguistic ability.

A metalinguistic skill that is more closely related to reading comprehension is the ability to reflect on what has just been read: whether it made sense, whether or not you enjoyed it, what you learnt, and what the main points were. This ability is usually referred to as *comprehension monitoring.* Comprehension monitoring, the ability to reflect on the use of language, is one of the metalinguistic skills that children acquire as their linguistic skills develop. A more general survey of recent research on the development of children's metalinguistic skills can be found in Garton and Pratt (1998, Chap. 7). However, this ability, and other strategic reading skills, tend to develop in tandem with the development of reading comprehension, rather than being a skill that is in place prior to beginning reading, and may even be a result of reading acquisition. Thus, it is dealt with quite briefly here.

In general, younger children are less likely to realize that they do not understand, and do not know what to do about it if they do realize (see Baker & Brown, 1984, and Markman, 1981, for reviews). They are, for example, unable to detect that crucial information is missing from a text. For instance, Markman (1977) assessed children's ability to detect inadequacies in instructions for how to play a game or perform a magic trick. In both cases, some crucial information was omitted. The younger children (first-graders) generally failed to realize that there was any problem with the instructions until they tried to carry them out. Older children (third-graders) realized more rapidly that the instructions were incomplete. In another study, Markman (1979) used texts that were logically inconsistent. The younger children were poor at spotting even blatant contradictions, and even the oldest (sixth-grade) children made many errors, although there was improvement with age.

Baker (1984) pointed out that the passages typically used in studies of comprehension monitoring may be problematic for different reasons. For instance, a passage may be *internally inconsistent* because there is a conflict between different pieces of information in the passage itself. Other passages may present conflicts with prior knowledge, which presents an *external* standard against which they can be evaluated. Finally, uncommon or nonsense words make passages difficult for a different reason: Some of the words are not in the child's vocabulary. The ability to monitor these different types of text problem do not necessarily develop in parallel. Garner (1981), for example, found that poorer readers are less likely to notice problems arising from internal inconsistencies than those arising from difficult vocabulary.

Baker (1984) compared spontaneous and instructed use of the three criteria for detecting comprehension problems, outlined above: internal inconsistency, external inconsistency, and vocabulary. She tested 9- and 11-year-olds (and also compared good and poor readers at each age). Half of the children were instructed about the criteria they should apply, and the other half were simply told to look for problems. Consistent with previous research, the older and better readers identified more problems than the younger and poorer readers. Interestingly, when Baker looked at the number of times a criterion was used, she found that the 9-year-old children complied with the instructions just as often as the 11-year-olds. However, they were less likely to use the criteria correctly.

Baker's findings conflict with the view that younger children are less willing to criticize written material (see, e.g., Markman & Gorin, 1981). Baker suggests, rather, that even when younger children know what problems they might encounter, they may still fail to identify them because they do not always use the criteria consistently and effectively—perhaps because they cannot cope so efficiently with the competing demands on their cognitive resources. Indeed, Ruffman (1996) has suggested that some form of information-processing limitation is important in explaining children's difficulties with comprehension monitoring. In a study that is discussed in more detail below, Vosniadou, Pearson, and Rogers (1988) showed that children's difficulties often arise because they fail to remember logically inconsistent premises. Because information-processing capabilities are known to develop with age (for a summary, see Oakhill, 1988), it is likely that children's capabilities in comprehension monitoring will show a concomitant increase.

The results from numerous studies of comprehension monitoring suggest that younger children are not building such a well-integrated model of a text or set of instructions because, if they were, they would necessarily spot inconsistencies. Indeed, it is not clear to what extent comprehension and comprehension monitoring are separate subskills or related aspects of the same process. For instance, Markman (1981) suggests that information about comprehension is often a by-product of the attempt to understand. In some cases, active comprehension monitoring may not be necessary—the reader simply needs to engage in comprehension. Vosniadou et al. (1988) also proposed that the ability to detect errors in a text is related to the ability to construct a good representation of the meaning of the passage. They asked first, third, and fifth graders to detect familiar falsehoods and unfamiliar factual contradictions in narrative texts. The children were able to detect the familiar falsehoods better than the unfamiliar contradictions, but, when familiarity was controlled, no differences were found. However, when the children's recall was compared to their comprehension monitoring, it was found that detection of inconsistencies was poorest for precisely those texts that were recalled least well. The authors conclude, therefore, that children are more likely to fail to detect inconsistencies because they do not represent the inconsistent pieces of information in memory in the first place, rather than because they are unable to compare the representations of the inconsistent parts of the text. They further suggest that younger children's difficulties in such tasks may be compounded by inadequate or incompatible prior knowledge.

In summary, children's ability to reflect on their own comprehension develops over the primary-school years. Younger children's difficulties with comprehension monitoring may be partly due to their lack of awareness of appropriate standards for evaluating their comprehension, but it is not clear whether these problems are a result of, or additional to, their difficulties with meaning representation. Older children, by contrast, use multiple standards in a flexible manner, and are more likely to build a coherent text representation that, in turn, aids their comprehension monitoring. Markman (1981) suggests that, without the ability to reflect on one's own comprehension, comprehension itself will suffer. However, others have suggested that comprehension is fundamental to monitoring. Very few studies have explored the longitudinal relation between comprehension monitoring and comprehension skill. One notable exception is the work by Chaney (1998), who found that early metalinguistic skills predicted reading ability (word recognition and comprehension combined) 4 years later, over and above the effect of general language ability. In our own longitudinal study (see Oakhill & Cain, 2007), we found that comprehension monitoring at age 8 was a significant predictor of comprehension skill at age 11, even when the autoregressive effect had been taken into account, thus indicating a possible causal link (see de Jong & van der Leij, 2002, for support for this argument). Others, however, have contested that there is a causal link between metalinguistic awareness and comprehension skill. In fact, both Vygotsky (1962) and Donaldson (1978) have argued that it is the process of learning to read that is responsible for increasing the child's language awareness, rather than the other way round. To some extent, the problems that children have with metalinguistic tasks may be related to their vocabulary skills. For instance, Gibbs (1991) showed that knowledge of word meanings can facilitate children's ability to understand figurative meanings.

Discourse-Level Skills (Narrative Understanding and Production)

Successful comprehension depends not only on identifying the words in a text, accessing their meanings, and understanding at the sentence level. The reader also needs to connect up information from different parts of the text, and make inferences to fill in missing information, in order to produce a coherent overall representation. Sometimes the skills required for this integration of text are called "higher-order skills" (as opposed to the "lower-order skills" of word recognition and meaning access).

For skilled adult readers, the making of connections in text is relatively automatic, but younger children may not make such connections for various reasons. Different authors have focused on slightly different aspects of these higher-order skills, but in all cases the component skills contribute to the same outcome: an integrated representation of the text as a whole. Some, such as van den Broek and colleagues (e.g., van den Broek, 1997) have focused on the child's developing ability to understand the causal structure of a narrative. In our own work, we have focused on different skill areas, such as inference making and understanding text structure more generally. We discuss the studies arising from each of these approaches below.

Some studies have included assessments of discourse skills, either alone (Roth et al., 2002), or as part of a broader composite (Catts et al., 1999). However, few studies have explored the relation between various aspects of discourse skill, such as inference making or the ability to understand story structures, on comprehension development. In this section, we consider some of the component processes of text comprehension and how they relate to the development of reading comprehension.

Inference and Integration

Developmental studies of inference skills show that young children are able to make the same inferences as older ones, but are less likely to do so spontaneously (they may only do so when prompted or questioned; see, e.g., Casteel & Simpson, 1991; Omanson, Warren, & Trabasso, 1978; Paris & Lindauer, 1976; Paris & Upton, 1976).

Following the pioneering work of Paris and his coworkers in this area (see, e.g., Paris & Lindauer, 1976; Paris, Lindauer, & Cox, 1977), a number of other researchers showed that the ability to make various kinds of inferences increases with age (Ackerman, 1986, 1988), though Ackerman (1988) and Ackerman and McGraw (1991) report results that led them to suggest that younger children may be making *different* inferences, but not necessarily *fewer* inferences, than older children and adults. Ackerman (1986) discusses some of the potential reasons for age-related differences in inference making. He suggests that younger children's greater tendency for nonintegrative processing directly affects their ability to establish referential cohesion, but only indirectly affects causal elaboration. Thus, even if young children were encouraged to engage in more integrative processing, their difficulties with elaborative inferencing may remain. Their difficulties may be in part related to their inability to see the need for an elaborative inference. Ackerman (1988) has attempted to look in more detail at the reasons why younger children fail to make some types of inferences. He concludes that even first graders are very well able to make at least *some* kinds of inference in *some* situations. However, young children are more dependent than older children and adults on contextual support (i.e., clues) to the inference. Developmental differences in inference making have often been attributed to differences in integration of information with age. However, Ackerman's study demonstrated that even young children are able to integrate information, at least to make the "reason inferences" that he studied. Ackerman suggests that inference failures cannot be attributed wholly to inference ability or integration or processing problems, but probably also have to do with the ways in which concept knowledge and concept prominence are organized in the listener's story representation.

A study by Barnes, Dennis, and Haefele-Kalvaitis (1996) addressed this issue, and showed that the ability to make inferences develops with age, independently of the influence of knowledge. Barnes et al. trained children (ages between 6 and 15 years) on a novel knowledge base. Once the children had learned the knowledge base to criterion, they were presented with a multiepisode story and were asked questions about it that required inferences that drew on that knowledge base. The results showed that ensuring that the knowledge base was equally available to all children did not attenuate age-related differences in inference making.

Our own work in this area (Oakhill et al., 2003b; Oakhill & Cain, 2007) has shown that inference skills contribute to later comprehension (but not to word-reading) skill between fourth and sixth grade, over and above the contributions of vocabulary, Verbal IQ, and the autoregessive effect of comprehension skill, suggesting a possible causal link. The possibility of a causal relation between inference skills and reading comprehension is also supported by a study in which we used a comprehension–age match group (Cain & Oakhill, 1999). Further details of the comprehension–age match design, and the conclusions it permits, can be found in Cain and Oakhill (Chapter 2, this volume).

Understanding Story Structure

Another important element in comprehension is understanding how the ideas in a text are related. Much of this work has focused on narratives because this is a genre that young children are most familiar with. One way to assess children's understanding of narrative structure is to get them to tell stories themselves. Children's narratives become more coherent with age (see Baker & Stein, 1981, for a review of children's developing sensitivity to logical structure and knowledge of what makes a good story). Children also expect certain types of information to occur in stories. When crucial types of information are missing, they often add them in when retelling a story, so that the retold story conforms to the story as they expected it to be. Similarly, if a story is told with the events out of order, children often restore it to a more normal order when they retell it (see, e.g., Stein, 1979).

There is a belief that narrative discourse acts to help the transition between oral language use and reading comprehension (see, e.g., Westby, 1991). Indeed, children's recall of stories indicates that tacit knowledge of the structural importance of story units is related to general reading ability (Smiley, Oakley, Worthen, Campione, & Brown, 1977). Knowledge about stories may also influence reading performance: Perfetti (1994) proposes that a possible source of comprehension failure is inadequate knowledge about text structures, which may arise because of insufficient reading experience. Peterson and Dodsworth (1991) note that narrative production is used in school to develop children's reading and writing skills. The developmental pattern is thought to progress from conversational discourse, to narrative discourse, to literacy. Indeed, narrative oral discourse and written text share many features including their more complex syntactic structures and abstract vocabulary. In addition, both are monologue language forms, and both are also forms of decontextualized language (see earlier). It is likely, then, that children's knowledge of narrative structure has an impact on their reading development.

Few researchers have directly tested the connection between narrative skill and reading. An exception is a study by Snyder and Downey (1991), who found that performance on a story-retelling task accounted for a significant portion of variance in reading comprehension in 8- to 11-year-old normally developing children. Since this study also included a group of "reading-disabled" children (who had comprehension problems), it is discussed in more detail in Cain and Oakhill (Chapter 2, this volume).

Our own work on the contribution of story structure understanding to comprehension (see Oakhill et al., 2003b; Oakhill & Cain, 2007) has shown that a measure of story structure understanding (a sentence anagram task) was a strong predictor of later comprehension skill (but not of word-reading skill) between the ages of 7 and 10, over and above the contributions of vocabulary, Verbal IQ, and the autoregressive effect. Indeed, this measure was the single best predictor of growth in comprehension skill over the same time period.

Van den Broek has also explored in some detail children's developing ability to understand the causal structure of texts (for a review, see van den Broek, 1997), and has identified developmental trends in three main aspects of comprehension: sensitivity to the general causal structure of the narrative; an increased focus on internal events such as goals, and a decreased focus on external events such as actions; and the representation of between-episode connections rather than just within-episode connections. Van den Broek and colleagues have found that even young children are guided by the causal structure of narrative, but less strongly than are older children and adults. Younger children are likely to pay attention to nonstructural features, including superficial ones such as how vivid an event is, but, with age, the role of structural features increases and that of nonstructural features decreases (van den Broek, 1997). In relation to the second aspect of development, younger children tend to focus on observable, concrete actions rather than on internal causes such as the goals of characters. In relation to the third aspect, younger children tend to connect events within an episode, but often fail to connect events across episodes in the text (Trabasso & Nickels, 1992), whereas it is usually the between-episode connections that are crucial to understanding the overall theme of the text and to constructing an integrated representation of the text overall. In general, children's ability in all three of these aspects improves with age (Bourg, Bauer, & van den Broek, 1997; Trabasso, Secco, & van den Broek, 1984; van den Broek, 1989a).

The studies described above have almost invariably used school-age children between the ages of 5 or 6 and 11, largely because it is not possible to assess the reading comprehension skills of preschool children, since they cannot read. But if one wants to know how early language skills (uncontaminated by reading progress) will influence later comprehension, then it is important to study comprehension in pre-readers. Such studies are possible, because comprehension (of narrative) can be assessed by means other than reading—for example, by picture sequences (Paris & Paris, 2003), aurally, or by means of television (van den Broek, Lorch, & Thurlow, 1996). Such alternative assessments would seem to be valid since narratives follow similar structures whether written, spoken, or televised, and there is evidence that children's developing ability to make inferences is consistent across different media (e.g., Goldman & Varnhagen, 1986; van den Broek, 1989b).

Van den Broek and colleagues (see, e.g., Kendeou et al., 2006; Kendeou, van den Broek, White, & Lynch, 2007; van den Broek et al., 2005) have directly tested the idea that comprehension skills generalize across different media, have related assessments of comprehension in different media to language skills, and have explored their contribution to later reading comprehension. In their longitudinal study, two cohorts of children (ages 4 and 6 at the outset of the study) were tested on their recall and factual and inferential comprehension of both aurally presented and televised stories. These assessments were repeated every 2 years. When the children reached 8 and 10 years, their recall and comprehension of written stories was also assessed.

Within each age group the comprehension of aural and televised stories was highly correlated, and in the older children all three types of comprehension were interrelated. In all age groups, comprehension skills were not related to basic language skills such as phonological awareness, letter and word awareness, and word recognition, but they were related to vocabulary skills. Thus, it appears that narrative skills and the skills related to word recognition develop relatively independently from an early age. The authors also explored the extent to which early narrative skills predict later comprehension. They found that narrative comprehension in preschool children (age 4) accounted for significant variance in narrative comprehension of both audio and television stories at age 6. Similarly, narrative comprehension at age 6 was predictive of comprehension of audio and televised stories at age 8, and also of reading comprehension (comprehension and recall of a narrative). Furthermore, early comprehension predicted later comprehension over and above basic language skills and vocabulary. However, it should be noted that expressive language skills were not controlled for, and both early comprehension skills and later reading comprehension were measured in part by children's spoken (i.e., expressive) summaries.

These results demonstrate that narrative language skills develop even before reading, and that there are commonalities in comprehension processes and abilities across different media. This conclusion is inconsistent with the widely held view that reading comprehension develops once decoding is in place and suggests instead that reading comprehension has its roots in early language comprehension skills. Indeed, the authors showed that comprehension in different media and word identification at age 6 made independent contributions to reading comprehension at age 8. In addition, van den Broek and colleagues' results demonstrate that these generalized comprehension processes come together with basic language skills to influence reading comprehension when the child becomes a reader. Thus, their view emphasizes the way in which both early comprehension and language skills contribute to the development of reading comprehension.

It has been shown that early narrative discourse skills predict not only later reading achievement, but are also related to academic success more generally (e.g., Feagans & Applebaum, 1986). Feagans and

Applebaum found that those children who were relatively strong in narrative skills (based on an assessment of comprehension and paraphrase skills) had better reading (both in terms of word recognition and comprehension) than those who were strong in syntax and vocabulary. The groups who were strong on narrative skills at age 6–7 also had fewer academic problems 3 years later.

It is certainly likely that children's knowledge about typical story sequences will develop with age and experience, and that such development will aid their text comprehension. It is also likely that, as children acquire knowledge, and use goal plans to interpret everyday events, they will become more adept at constructing coherent, integrated representations of such events (whether they be actual or fictional). Thus, there is ample evidence that children's ability to make inferences and to understand story structure develops during the first few years of learning to read, and there is some evidence that such skills are causally implicated in the development of comprehension skill. In addition, the work of van den Broek and colleagues indicates that such abilities precede the acquisition of reading, and are general comprehension skills that can be measured in a variety of media (not just written, but spoken and televised).

In summary, narrative comprehension and production have been shown to be predictive of later comprehension skill, and some of the specific subskills of comprehension have also been shown to be predictive. In addition, the early comprehension skills that are important in the development of later comprehension are not reading-specific but, rather, range across a variety of media, including picture stories and televised narratives.

CONCLUSIONS

When they learn to read, children progress from conversational discourse to narrative discourse, a specifically literate language form. Written text and oral narratives share many properties, including syntactic structures that are more concise and complex, and rarer and more abstract vocabulary items (see Roth et al., 2002). But, in addition, oral narratives and written text are decontextualized language forms (Dickinson & Snow, 1987; Westby, 1991). However, the development of successful reading comprehension is not solely dependent on aspects of oral language skills: memory skills, in particular, working memory and retrieval from long-term memory, and other factors that are unlikely to be crucial in oral language comprehension—for example, strategy knowledge about how and what to read—have been shown to be important predictors of reading comprehension (Willson & Rupley, 1997).

This review shows that a number of skills are implicated in the successful development of comprehension. However, the relative importance of different skills in comprehension development (phonological skills, grammatical skills, vocabulary, metalinguisitic, and other higher-order skills) perhaps change gradually during the course of development.

Scarborough (1998) has noted that the predictors of reading are likely to change with development. For instance, Speece and colleagues (see Roth, Speece, Cooper, & De la Paz, 1996; Speece, Roth, Cooper, & de la Paz, 1999) showed that phonological skills and word reading are more closely associated with earlier, rather than later, reading comprehension, whereas other linguistic skills, such as understanding narrative, have their impact later on in reading development. Similarly, Willson and Rupley (1997), who looked at word reading and comprehension between first grade and sixth grade, found that early reading comprehension was driven by phonological awareness and background knowledge, whereas how to read—strategy use—became a more important determinant of reading comprehension by sixth grade. These findings add to others that show that beyond the initial stages of reading, nonphonological language skills assume increased importance in accounting for variance in reading comprehension. In line with this suggestion, Gough, Hoover, and Peterson (1996) report a meta-analysis of studies that examined the correlations between reading comprehension, listening comprehension, and decoding skills in different age groups. They found that with an increase in age, reading comprehension became less closely related to decoding skill, and the relation between reading and listening comprehension increased. These findings suggest that reading comprehension will become more heavily dependent on the language skills that are also important in listening comprehension as children get older.

IMPLICATIONS

One clear conclusion, both from van den Broek's work and that of others (e.g., Storch & Whitehurst, 2002), discussed earlier, is that models that presuppose that the development of basic reading skills (e.g., phonological skills and word decoding) must precede the development of comprehension skills, need to be questioned. A perspective that fits better with recent data is that comprehension skills develop simultaneously with basic language skills and have their roots in early narrative comprehension. This alternative approach has implications both for reading comprehension interventions and assessment.

In terms of interventions, a clear implication is that we should be careful not to focus on the teaching of decoding skills to the exclusion of other skills—that is, we should not wait until children are proficient in decoding before beginning instruction in oral language skills such as vocabulary, syntax, inference making, and comprehension monitoring. Not only are oral language skills linked to the code-related skills that help word reading to develop, but they also provide the foundation for the development of the more-advanced language skills needed for comprehension. Research on children with oral language impairments also supports this conclusion. For example, follow-up studies of children with language impairments before they start school show that the nature of their reading problems changes over time to include problems with both decoding and comprehension (e.g., Snowling, Bishop, & Stothard, 2000; Stothard, Snowling, Bishop, Chipchase, & Kaplan, 1998).

There is already substantial evidence for the effects of early phonemic awareness training on later reading, but little work has been done on early awareness of syntactic/narrative skills and later comprehension. Clearly, more work is needed to explore the types of early intervention that will improve young children's appreciation of narrative structure, but van den Broek's work suggests that early interventions could make use of televised or aurally presented stories. Indeed, Palincsar and Brown (1984) showed that the comprehension skills of prereaders could be successfully improved with aurally presented text.

Another direct implication of van den Broek and colleagues' work relates to assessment. This work has shown that assessments of comprehension in preschool children, who are not yet able to read, are highly predictive of later reading comprehension skill. Thus, narrative understanding measured aurally, or by means of televised stories, could be used to predict future reading comprehension performance and such assessments might also be used to predict which children are likely to experience later reading comprehension difficulties (in much the same way as early measures of phonological skills have been used to predict which children might be at risk of developing dyslexia).

In sum, there is now converging evidence that there is a common basis of basic language skills that underpin the development of written, as well as spoken, language comprehension. This knowledge should lead to better specified models of how the skills crucial to successful language comprehension are acquired, and should result in concomitant progress in both interventions and assessment.

REFERENCES

Ackerman, B. P. (1986). Referential and causal coherence in the story comprehension of children and adults. *Journal of Experimental Child Psychology, 41,* 336–366.

Ackerman, B. P. (1988). Reason inferences in the story comprehension of children and adults. *Child Development, 59,* 1426–1442.

Ackerman, B. P., & McGraw, M. (1991). Constraints on the causal inferences of children and adults in comprehending stories. *Journal of Experimental Child Psychology, 51,* 364–394.

Anderson, R. C., & Freebody, P. (1981). Vocabulary knowledge. In J. T. Guthrie (Ed.), *Comprehension and teaching* (pp. 77–117). Newark, DE: International Reading Association.

Baddeley, A. (1986). *Working memory.* Oxford, UK: Oxford University Press.

Baker, L. (1984). Spontaneous versus instructed use of multiple standards for evaluating comprehension: Effects of age, reading proficiency, and type of standard. *Journal of Experimental Child Psychology, 38,* 289–311.

Baker, L., & Brown, A. I. (1984). Metacognitive skills and reading. In P. D. Pearson (Ed.), *Handbook of reading research* (Vol. 1, pp. 353–394). New York: Plenum Press.

Baker, L., & Stein, N. (1981). The development of prose comprehension skills. In C. M. Santa & B. L. Hayes (Eds.), *Children's prose comprehension: Research and practice* (pp. 7–43). Newark, DE: International Reading Association.

Barnes, M. A., Dennis, M., & Haefele-Kalvaitis, J. (1996). The effects of knowledge availability and knowledge accessibility on coherence and elaborative inferencing in children from six to fifteen years of age. *Journal of Experimental Child Psychology, 61,* 216–241.

Bast, J., & Reitsma, P. (1998). Analyzing the development of individual differences in terms of Matthew effects in reading: Results from a Dutch longitudinal study. *Developmental Psychology, 34,* 1373–1399.

Beck, I. C., Perfetti, C. A., & McKeown, G. (1982). Effects of long-term vocabulary instruction on lexical access and reading comprehension. *Journal of Educational Psychology, 74,* 506–521.

Bishop, D. V. M. (1983). *Test for the Reception of Grammar.* Manchester, UK: Chapel Press.

Bishop, D. V. M. (1997). *Uncommon understanding.* Hove, UK: Psychology Press.

Blachman, B. (Ed.). (1997). *Foundations of reading acquisition and dyslexia: Implications for early intervention.* Mahwah, NJ: Erlbaum.

Blackmore, A.M., & Pratt, C. (1997). Grammatical awareness and reading in grade 1 children. *Merrill–Palmer Quarterly, 43,* 567–590.

Bourg, T., Bauer, P., & van den Broek, P. (1997). Building the bridges: The development of event comprehension and representation. In P. van den Broek, P. Bauer, & T. Bourg (Eds.), *Developmental spans in event comprehension and representation: Bridging fictional and actual events* (pp. 385–407). Hillsdale, NJ: Erlbaum.

Bowey, J. A. (1986). Syntactic awareness in relation to reading skill and ongoing reading comprehension monitoring. *Journal of Experimental Child Psychology, 41*, 282–299.

Bowey, J. A., & Patel, R. K. (1988). Metalinguistic ability and early reading achievement. *Applied Psycholinguistics, 9*(4), 367–383.

Bradley, L., & Bryant, P. E. (1983). Categorizing sounds and learning to read: A causal connection. *Nature, 301*, 419–421.

Brady, S., & Shankweiler, D. (Eds.). (1991). *Phonological processes in literacy.* Hillsdale, NJ: Erlbaum.

Cain, K., & Oakhill, J. V. (1999). Inference making and its relation to comprehension failure. *Reading and Writing. 11*, 489–503.

Carroll, J. B. (1993). *Human cognitive abilities: A survey of factor-analytic studies.* New York: Cambridge University Press.

Casteel, M. A., & Simpson, G. B. (1991). Textual coherence and the development of inferential generation skills. *Journal of Research in Reading, 14*, 116–129.

Catts, H. W., Fey, M. F., Zhang, X., & Tomblin, J. B. (1999). Language basis of reading and reading disabilities: Evidence from a longitudinal investigation. *Scientific Studies of Reading, 3*, 331–361.

Catts, H., & Kamhi, A. (1999). *Language and reading disabilities.* Needham Heights, MA: Allyn & Bacon.

Catts, H., & Kamhi, A. (2005). *Connections between reading and language.* Mahwah, NJ: Erlbaum.

Chaney, C. (1992). Language development, metalinguistic skills, and print awareness in 3–year-old children. *Applied Psycholinguistics, 13*, 485–514.

Chaney, C. (1998). Preschool language and metalinguistic skills are links to reading success. *Applied Psycholinguistics, 19*, 433–446.

Cunningham, A. E. (2005). Vocabulary growth through independent reading and reading aloud to children. In E. H. Hiebert & M. L. Kamil (Eds.), *Teaching and learning vocabulary: Bringing research to practice* (pp. 45–68). Mahwah, NJ: Erlbaum.

Curtis, M. E. (1980). Development of components of reading skills. *Journal of Educational Psychology, 72*, 656–669.

Cutting, L. E., & Scarborough, H. S. (2006). Prediction of reading comprehension: Relative contributions of word recognition, language proficiency, and other cognitive skills can depend on how comprehension is measured. *Scientific Studies of Reading, 10*(3), 277–299.

Daneman, M. (1988). Word knowledge and reading skill. In M. Daneman, G. MacKinnon & T. G. Waller (Eds.), *Reading research: Advances in theory and practice* (Vol. 6, pp. 145–175). San Diego: Academic Press.

Davis, F. B. (1944). Fundamental factors in reading comprehension. *Psychometrika, 9*, 185–197.

Davis, F. B. (1968). Research in comprehension in reading. *Reading Research Quarterly, 3*, 499–545.

de Jong, P. F., & van der Leij, A. (2002). Effects of phonological abilities and linguistic comprehension on the development of reading. *Scientific Studies of Reading, 6*(1), 51–77.

Demont, E., & Gombert, J. E. (1996). Phonological awareness as a predictor of recoding skills and syntactic awareness as a predictor of comprehension skills. *British Journal of Educational Psychology, 66,* 315–332.

Dickinson, D. K., McCabe, A., Anastasopoulos, L., Peisner-Feinberg, E., & Poe, M. D. (2003). The comprehensive language approach to early literacy: The interrelationships among vocabulary, phonological sensitivity, and print knowledge among preschool-aged children. *Journal of Educational Psychology, 95*(3), 465–481.

Dickinson, D. K., & Snow, C. E. (1987). Interrelationships among prereading and oral language skills in kindergarten from two social classes. *Early Childhood Research Quarterly, 2,* 1–25.

Donaldson, M. (1978). *Children's minds.* Glasgow, UK: Collins.

Echols, L. D., West, R. F., Stanovich, K. E., & Zehr, K. S. (1996). Using children's literacy activities to predict growth in verbal cognitive skills: A longitudinal investigation. *Journal of Educational Psychology, 88,* 296–304.

Eldredge, J. L., Quinn, B., & Butterfield, D. D. (1990). Causal relationships between phonics, reading comprehension, and vocabulary achievement in the second grade. *Journal of Educational Research, 83,* 201–214.

Feagans, L., & Appelbaum, M. I. (1986). Validation of language subtypes in learning disabled children. *Journal of Educational Psychology, 78,* 358–364.

Garner, R. (1981). Monitoring of passage inconsistency among poor comprehenders: A preliminary test of the "piecemeal processing" explanation. *Journal of Educational Research, 74,* 159–162.

Garton, A., & Pratt, C. (1998). *Learning to be literate: The development of spoken and written language* (2nd ed.). Oxford, UK: Blackwell.

Gernsbacher, M. M., Varner, K. R., & Faust, M. E. (1990). Investigating individual differences in general comprehension skill. *Journal of Experimental Psychology: Learning, Memory and Cognition, 16,* 430–445.

Gibbs, W. R. (1991). Semantic analyzability in children's understanding of idioms. *Journal of Speech and Hearing Research, 34,* 613–620.

Goff, D., Pratt, C., & Ong, B. (2005). The relations between children's reading comprehension, working memory, language skills and components of reading decoding in a normal sample. *Reading and Writing, 18,* 583–616.

Goldman, S. R., & Varnhagen, C. K. (1986). Memory for embedded and sequential story structures. *Journal of Memory and Language, 25,* 401–418.

Gottardo, A., Stanovich, K. E., & Siegel, L. S. (1996). The relationships between phonological sensitivity, syntactic processing and verbal working memory in the reading performance of third-grade children. *Journal of Experimental Child Psychology, 63,* 563–582.

Gough, P. B., Hoover, W. A., & Peterson, C. L. (1996). Some observations on a simple view of reading. In C. Cornoldi & J. Oakhill (Eds.), *Reading comprehension difficulties: Processes and interventions* (pp. 1–13). Mahwah, NJ: Erlbaum.

Gough, P. B., & Tunmer, W. (1986) Decoding, reading and reading disability. *Remedial and Special Education, 7,* 6–10.

Huey, E. (1968) *The psychology and pedagogy of reading.* Cambridge, MA: MIT Press. (Original work published 1908)

Jenkins, J. R., Pany, D., & Schreck, J. (1978). Vocabulary and reading comprehension: Instructional effects (Technical Report No. 100). Urbana-Champaign, IL: Center for the Study of Reading.

Keenan, J. (2006, July). *How comparable are reading comprehension tests?* Paper presented at the annual meeting of the Society for the Study of Reading, Vancouver.

Kendeou, P., Lynch, J. S., van den Broek, P., Espin, C., White, M., & Kremer, K. E. (2006). Developing successful readers: Building early narrative comprehension skills through television viewing and listening. *Early Childhood Education Journal, 33*(2), 91–98.

Kendeou, P., van den Broek, P., White, M. J., & Lynch, J. (2007). Comprehension in preschool and early elementary children: Skill development and strategy interventions. In D. S. McNamara (Ed.), *Reading comprehension strategies: Theories, interventions, and technologies.* Mahwah, NJ: Erlbaum.

Laberge, D., & Samuels, S. J. (1974). Toward a theory of automatic information processing in reading. *Cognitive Psychology, 6,* 293–323.

Liberman, I. Y., & Shankweiler, D. (1985). Phonology and the problems of learning to read and write. *Remedial and Special Education, 6,* 8–17.

Lombardino, L. J., Riccio, C. A., Hynd, G. W., & Pinheiro, S. B. (1997). Linguistic deficits in children with reading disabilities. *American Journal of Speech–Language Pathology, 6,* 71–78.

MacGinitie, W. H., MacGinitie, R. K., Maria, K., & Dreyer, L. G. (2000). *Gates-MacGinitie Reading Tests* (4th ed.). Itasca, IL: Riverside Publishing.

Manis, F., Seidenberg, M. S., & Doi, L. (1999). See Dick RAN: Rapid naming and the longitudinal prediction of reading subskills in first and second graders. *Journal of the Society for the Scientific Study of Reading, 3,* 129–157.

Markman, E. M. (1977). Realizing that you don't understand: A preliminary investigation. *Child Development, 48,* 986–992.

Markman, E. M. (1979). Realizing that you don't understand: Elementary school children's awareness of inconsistencies. *Child Development, 50,* 643–655.

Markman, E. M. (1981). Comprehension monitoring. In W. P. Dickson (Ed.), *Children's oral communication skills* (pp. 61–84). London: Academic Press.

Markman, E. M., & Gorin, L. (1981). Children's ability to adjust their standards for evaluating comprehension. *Journal of Educational Psychology, 73,* 320–325.

McKeown, M. G., Beck, I. L., Omanson, R. C., & Perfetti, C. A. (1983). The effects of long-term vocabulary instruction on reading comprehension: A replication. *Journal of Reading Behavior, 25,* 3–18.

Muter, V., Hulme, C., Snowling, M. J., & Stevenson, J. (2004). Phonemes, rimes, vocabulary and grammatical skills as foundations of early reading development: Evidence from a longitudinal study. *Developmental Psychology, 40,* 665–681.

Muter, V., Hulme, C., Snowling, M. J., & Taylor, S. (1998). Segmentation, not rhyming, predicts early progress in learning to read. *Journal of Experimental Child Psychology, 71,* 3–27.

Nagy, W. E., & Scott, J. A. (2000). Vocabulary processes. In M. L. Kamil, P.

Mosenthal, P. D. Pearson, & R. Barr (Eds.), *Handbook of reading research* (Vol. 3, pp. 269–284). Mahwah, NJ: Erlbaum.

Nation, K., & Snowling, M. J. (1998a). Individual differences in contextual facilitation: Evidence from children with reading comprehension difficulties. *Child Development, 69*, 996–1011.

Nation, K., & Snowling, M. J. (1998b). Semantic processing and the development of word recognition skills: Evidence from children with reading comprehension difficulties. *Journal of Memory and Language, 39*, 85–101.

Neale, M. D. (1989). *The Neale Analysis of Reading Ability – Revised British Edition*. Windsor, UK: NFER-Nelson.

Oakhill, J. (1988). The development of children's reasoning ability: Information-processing approaches. In K. Richardson & S. Sheldon (Eds.), *Cognitive development to adolescence: A reader* (pp. 169–188). Hove, UK: Erlbaum.

Oakhill, J. V., & Cain, K. (2004) The development of comprehension skills. In T. Nunes & P. E. Bryant (Eds.), *Handbook of literacy* (pp. 155–180) Dordrecht, The Netherlands: Kluwer.

Oakhill, J. V., & Cain, K. (2007). Issues of causality in children's reading comprehension. In D. S. McNamara (Ed.), *Reading comprehension strategies: Theories, interventions, and technologies* Mahwah, NJ: Erlbaum.

Oakhill, J. V., Cain, K., & Bryant, P. E. (2003a). Dissociation of single-word reading and text comprehension skills. *Language and Cognitive Processes, 18*(4), 443–468.

Oakhill, J. V., Cain, K. E., & Bryant, P. E. (2003b, May). *Prediction of comprehension skill in the primary school years.* Paper presented at the biennial meeting of the Society for Research in Child Development, Tampa.

Oakhill, J. V., & Garnham, A. (1988). *Becoming a skilled reader.* Oxford, UK: Basil Blackwell.

Omanson, R. C., Warren, W. M., & Trabasso, T. (1978). Goals, inferences, comprehension and recall of stories by children. *Discourse Processes, 1*, 337–354.

Palincsar, A. S., & Brown, A. L. (1984). Reciprocal teaching of comprehension-fostering and monitoring activities. *Cognition and Instruction, 1*, 117–175.

Palmer, J. C., MacLeod, C. M., Hunt, E., & Davidson, J. E. (1985). Information processing correlates of reading: An individual differences analysis. *Journal of Memory and Language, 24*, 59–88.

Paris, A. H., & Paris, S. G. (2003). Assessing narrative comprehension in young children, *Reading Research Quarterly, 38*, 36–76.

Paris, S. G., Carpenter, R. D., Paris, A. H., & Hamilton, E. E. (2005). Spurious and genuine correlate of children's reading comprehension. In S. G. Paris & S. A. Stahl (Eds.), *Children's reading comprehension and assessment* (pp. 131–160). Mahwah, NJ: Erlbaum.

Paris, S. G., & Lindauer, B. K. (1976). The role of inference in children's comprehension and memory for sentences. *Cognitive Psychology, 8*, 217–227.

Paris, S. G., Lindauer, B. K., & Cox, G. L. (1977). The development of inferential comprehension. *Child Development, 48*, 1728–1733.

Paris, S. G., & Stahl, S. A. (2005). *Children's reading comprehension and assessment.* Mahwah, NJ: Erlbaum.

Paris, S. G., & Upton, L. R. (1976). Children's memory for inferential relation-ships in prose. *Child Development, 47,* 660–668.

Parrila, R., Kirby, J. R., & McQuarrie, L. (2004). Articulation rate, naming speed, verbal short-term memory, and phonological awareness: Longitu-dinal predictors of early reading development. *Scientific Studies of Reading, 8,* 3–26.

Perfetti, C. A. (1985). *Reading ability.* New York: Oxford University Press.

Perfetti, C. A. (1994). Psycholinguistics and reading ability. In M. A. Gerns-bacher (Ed.), *Handbook of psycholinguistics* (pp. 849–894). San Diego: Aca-demic Press.

Perfetti, C. A., Landi, N., & Oakhill, J. V. (2005). The acquisition of reading comprehension skill. In M. J. Snowling & C. Hulme (Eds.), *The science of reading: A handbook* (pp. 227–247). Oxford, UK: Blackwell.

Perfetti, C. A., & Lesgold, A. M. (1977). Discourse comprehension and sources of individual differences. In M. A. Just & P. A. Carpenter (Eds.), *Cognitive processes in comprehension* (pp. 141–183). Hillsdale, NJ: Erlbaum.

Peterson, C., & Dodsworth, P. (1991). A longitudinal analysis of young chil-dren's cohesion and noun specification in narratives. *Journal of Child Lan-guage, 18,* 397–415.

Plaut, D. C., McClelland, J. L., Seidenberg, M. S., & Patterson, K. (1996). Understanding normal and impaired word reading: Computational prin-ciples in quasi-regular domains. *Psychological Review, 103,* 56–115.

Reid, J. F. (1970). Sentence structure in reading primers. *Research in Education, 3,* 23–37.

Reid, J. F. (1983). Into print: Reading and language growth. In M. Donaldson, R. Grieve, & C. Pratt (Eds.), *Early childhood development and education* (pp. 151–165). Oxford, UK: Basil Blackwell.

Roth, F. P., Speece, D. L., & Cooper, D. H. (2002). A longitudinal analysis of the connection between oral language and early reading. *Journal of Educa-tional Research, 95,* 259–272.

Roth, F. P., Speece, D. L., Cooper, D. H., & De la Paz, S. (1996). Unresolved mysteries: How do metalinguistic and narrative skills connect with early reading? *Journal of Special Education, 30,* 257–277.

Ruffman, T. (1996). Reassessing children's comprehension-monitoring skills. In C. Cornoldi & J. V. Oakhill (Eds.), *Reading comprehension difficulties: Pro-cesses and intervention* (pp. 33–62). Mahwah, NJ: Erlbaum.

Scarborough, H. S. (1998). Early identification of children at risk for reading disabilities: Phonological awareness and some other promising predictors. In P. Accardo, A. Capute, & B. Shapiro (Eds.), *Specific reading disability: A view of the spectrum* (pp. 75–119). Timonium, MD: York Press.

Seigneuric, A., & Ehrlich, M.-F. (2005). Contribution of working memory capacity to children's reading comprehension: A longitudinal investiga-tion. *Reading and Writing: An Interdisciplinary Journal, 18,* 617–656.

Semel, E., Wiig, E., & Secord, W. (1987). *Clinical Evaluation of Language Fundamentals–Revised.* New York: Psychological Corporation.

Shankweiler, D. (1989). How problems of comprehension are related to diffi-culties in word reading. In D. Shankweiler & I. Y. Liberman (Eds.), *Phonol-*

ogy and reading disability: Solving the reading puzzle (pp. 35–68). Ann Arbor: University of Michigan Press.

Shankweiler, D., Crain, S., Katz, L., Fowler, A. E., Liberman, A. M., et al. (1995). Cognitive profiles of reading-disabled children: Comparison of language skills in phonology, morphology and syntax. *Psychological Science, 6,* 149–156.

Smiley, S. S., Oakley, D. D., Worthen, D., Campione, J., & Brown, A. L. (1977). Recall of thematically relevant material by adolescent good and poor readers as a function of written versus oral presentation. *Journal of Educational Psychology, 69,* 381–387.

Smith, S. T., Macaruso, P., Shankweiler, D., & Crain, S. (1989). Syntactic comprehension in young poor readers. *Applied Psycholinguistics, 10,* 420–454.

Snowling, M., Bishop, D., & Stothard, S. (2000). Is preschool language impairment a risk factor for dyslexia in adolescence? *Journal of Child Psychology and Psychiatry and Allied Disciplines, 41,* 587–600.

Snyder, L. S., & Downey, D. M. (1991). The language–reading relationship in normal and reading-disabled children. *Journal of Speech and Hearing Research, 34,* 129–140.

Speece, D. L., Roth, F. A., Cooper, D. H., & de la Paz, S. (1999). The relevance of oral language skills to early literacy: A multivariate analysis. *Applied Psycholinguistics, 20,* 167–190.

Stahl, S. (1983). Differential word knowledge and reading comprehension. *Journal of Reading Behavior, 25,* 33–50.

Stanovich, K. E. (1988). Explaining the differences between the dyslexic and the garden-variety poor reader: The phonological–core variable-difference model. *Journal of Learning Disabilities, 21,* 590–604.

Stein, N. L. (1979). How children understand stories: A developmental analysis. In L. G. Katz (Ed.), *Current topics in early childhood education* (pp. 261–290). Norwood, NJ: Ablex.

Sticht, T., & James, J. (1984). Listening and reading. In P. Pearson (Ed.), *Handbook of research on reading* (pp. 293–317). New York: Longman.

Storch, S. A., & Whitehurst, G. J. (2002). Oral language and code-related precursors to reading: Evidence from a longitudinal structural model. *Developmental Psychology, 38,* 934–947.

Stothard, S. E., Snowling, M., Bishop, D., Chipchase, M., & Kaplan, C. (1998). Language-impaired preschoolers: A follow-up into adolescence. *Journal of Speech, Language, and Hearing Research, 41,* 407–418.

Tabors, P. O., Snow, C. E., & Dickinson, D. K. (2001). Homes and schools together: Supporting language and literacy development. In D. K. Dickinson & P. O. Tabors (Eds.), *Beginning literacy with language* (pp. 313–334). Baltimore: Brookes.

Thorndike, E. L. (1917). Reading as reasoning: A study of mistakes in paragraph reading. *Journal of Educational Psychology, 8,* 323–332.

Thorndike, R. L. (1973). *Reading comprehension education in fifteen countries.* New York: Wiley.

Torgesen, J. K., Wagner, R. K., & Rashotte, C. A. (1994). Longitudinal studies of phonological processing and reading. *Journal of Learning Disabilities,* 27, 276–286.

Torgesen, J. K., Wagner, R. K., Rashotte, C. A., Burgess, S., & Hecht, S. (1997). Contributions of phonological awareness and rapid automatic naming ability to the growth of word-reading skills in second- to fifth-grade children. *Scientific Studies of Reading, 1,* 161–185.

Trabasso, T., & Nickels, M. (1992). The development of goal plans of action in the narration of a picture story. *Discourse Processes, 15,* 249–275.

Trabasso, T., Secco, T., & van den Broek, P. (1984). Causal cohesion and story coherence. In H. Mandl, N. L. Stein, & T. Trabasso (Eds.), *Learning and comprehension of text* (pp. 83–111). Hillsdale, NJ: Erlbaum.

Tuinman, J. J., & Brady, M. E. (1974). How does vocabulary account for variance on reading comprehension tests?: A preliminary instructional analysis. In P. Nacke (Ed.), *Twenty-third National Reading Conference yearbook* (pp. 176–184). Clemson, SC: National Reading Conference.

Tunmer, W. E. (1989). The role of language-related factors in reading disability. In D. Shankweiler & I. Y. Liberman (Eds.), *Phonology and reading disability: solving the puzzle* (pp. 91–131). Ann Arbor: University of Michigan Press.

Tunmer, W. E., & Bowey, J. A. (1984). Metalinguistic awareness and reading acquisition. In W. E. Tunmer, C. Pratt, & M. L. Herriman (Eds.), *Metalinguistic awareness in children* (pp. 144–168). New York: Springer-Verlag.

Tunmer, W. E., & Hoover, W. A. (1992). Cognitive and linguistic factors in learning to read. In P. B. Gough, L. C. Ehri, & R. Treiman (Eds.), *Reading acquisition* (pp. 175–214). Hillsdale, NJ: Erlbaum.

Tunmer, W. E., Nesdale, A. R., & Wright, A. D. (1987). Syntactic awareness and reading acquisition. *British Journal of Developmental Psychology, 5*(1), 25–34.

van den Broek, P. W. (1989a). Causal reasoning and inference making in judging the importance of story statements. *Child Development, 60,* 286–297.

van den Broek, P. W. (1989b). The effects of causal structure on the comprehension of narratives: Implications for education. *Reading Psychology: An International Quarterly, 10,* 19–44.

van den Broek, P. (1997). Discovering the cements of the universe: The development of event comprehension from childhood to adulthood. In P. van den Broek, P. Bauer, & T. Bourg (Eds.), *Developmental spans in event comprehension: Bridging fictional and actual events* (pp. 321–342). Mahwah, NJ: Erlbaum.

van den Broek, P., Kendeou, P., Kremer, K., Lynch, J. S., Butler, J., White, M. J., et al. (2005). Assessment of comprehension abilities in young children. In S. G. Paris & S. A. Stahl (Eds.), *Children's reading comprehension and assessment* (pp. 107–130). Mahwah, NJ: Erlbaum.

van den Broek, P., Lorch, E. P., & Thurlow, R. (1996). Children's and adult's memory for television stories: The role of causal factors, story-grammar categories, and hierarchical level. *Child Development, 67,* 3010–3028.

Vellutino, F., & Scanlon, D. (1987). Phonological coding, phonological awareness, and reading ability: Evidence from a longitudinal and experimental study. *Merrill–Palmer Quarterly, 33,* 321–363.

Vellutino, F. R., Scanlon, D. M., Pratt, A., Chen, R., & Denkla, M. (1996). Cognitive profiles of difficult-to-remediate and readily remediated poor readers: Early intervention as a vehicle for distinguishing between cognitive and experiential deficits as basic causes of specific reading disability. *Journal of Educational Psychology, 4,* 601–638.

Vellutino, F. R., Scanlon, D. M., Small, S. G., & Tanzman, M. S. (1991). The linguistic basis of reading disability: Converting written to oral language. *Text, 11,* 99–133.

Vellutino, F., Scanlon, D., & Spearing, D. (1995). Semantic and phonological coding in poor and normal readers. *Journal of Experimental Child Psychology, 59,* 76–123.

Vosniadou, S., Pearson, P. D., & Rogers, T. (1988). What causes children's failures to detect inconsistencies in text?: Representation versus comparison difficulties. *Journal of Educational Psychology, 80,* 27–39.

Vygotsky, L. S. (1962). *Thought and language.* Cambridge, MA: MIT Press.

Wechsler, D. L. (1992). *Wechsler Individual Achievement Test.* San Antonio, TX: Psychological Corporation.

Westby, C. E. (1991). Learning to talk—talking to learn: Oral–literate language differences. In C. Simon (Ed.), *Communication skills and classroom success: Therapy methodologies for language learning disabled students* (pp. 181–218). San Diego: College-Hill Press.

Wiederholt, L., & Bryant, B. (1992). *Examiner's manual: Gray Oral Reading Test-3.* Austin, TX: PRO-ED.

Willows, D. M., & Ryan, E. B. (1981). Differential utilisation of syntactic and semantic information by skilled and less skilled readers in the intermediate grades. *Journal of Educational Psychology, 73,* 607–715.

Willson, V. L., & Rupley, W. H. (1997). A structural equation model for reading comprehension based on background, phonemic and strategy knowledge. *Scientific Studies of Reading, 1,* 45–63.

CHAPTER 2

Reading Comprehension Difficulties
Correlates, Causes, and Consequences

KATE CAIN
JANE OAKHILL

Children need to develop two broad skills to become successful and independent readers: they must be able to recognize and decode the individual words on the page and they must be able to comprehend the text. Although good word-reading skills are generally considered a prerequisite for adequate reading comprehension, accurate and fluent word reading does not ensure good reading comprehension. The focus of this chapter is a group of children who show a separation between these two skills: children who have developed age-appropriate word-reading skills but whose reading comprehension skills lag behind. These children are not simply poor readers: They have a *specific comprehension deficit*. We refer to this group as "poor comprehenders."

Poor comprehenders comprise up to 10% of 7- to 11-year-olds in U.K. schools (Yuill & Oakhill, 1991). Children with a similar profile have been identified and studied by other research groups in Europe and North America (e.g., Cornoldi, de Beni, & Pazzaglia, 1996; Ehrlich & Rémond, 1997; Nation & Snowling, 1998a; Paris, Carpenter, Paris, & Hamilton, 2005; Swanson & Berninger, 1995). The comprehension difficulties experienced by this group extend beyond the written word:

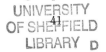
41

Their comprehension of spoken texts is also poor (Cain, Oakhill, & Bryant, 2000a; Megherbi & Ehrlich, 2005; Oakhill, 1982; Stothard & Hulme, 1992) and their ability to produce coherent narratives is impaired (Cain, 2003; Cain & Oakhill, 1996).

A wide body of research suggests that poor comprehenders have specific difficulties with many of the skills that aid the construction of a representation of the meaning of written and spoken texts. First, we consider the characteristics of poor comprehenders in relation to the different skills and processes that are involved in text comprehension. In this section we also review the skill deficits that are associated with poor comprehension. Second, we consider possible sources of poor comprehension, focusing on research designs that enable us to address issues of causality. Third, we consider the consequences of a comprehension deficit: the wider impacts that a reading and listening comprehension deficit might have on language and literacy development in general, and the implications for the prevention and remediation of comprehension difficulties. A better understanding of the reasons for these children's comprehension difficulties is not only of potential benefit to poor comprehenders themselves, in terms of remediation, this work also has the potential to inform theoretical models of language and literacy development.

CHARACTERISTICS OF POOR COMPREHENDERS

Good comprehension of a written text requires that the reader is able to recognize and decode the words on the page. Much of the research investigating children's comprehension skills has not controlled for individual differences in word-reading skill or has used measures of reading comprehension skill that are dependent on the individual's ability to read words (e.g., Forrest-Pressley & Waller, 1984; Jetton, Rupley, & Willson, 1995; Kirby & Moore, 1987; Nation & Snowling, 1999; Paris & Jacobs, 1984; Smith, Macaruso, Shankweiler, & Crain, 1989). Therefore, the extent to which such studies address children's comprehension difficulties, rather than just general reading difficulties, is unclear.

In this chapter we are concerned with children who have a *specific comprehension deficit*: children who can read accurately and fluently, but who fail to grasp the meaning of what they read. When comparing the performance of these children to children in a control group, it is important to match the two groups for their word-reading ability. The characteristics of the good and the poor comprehenders that we typically use in our own research are illustrated in the middle two columns

TABLE 2.1. Characteristics of Good and Poor Comprehenders and a Comprehension–Age Match Group

	Poor comprehenders (N = 14)	Good comprehenders (N = 14)	Comprehension–age match group (N = 14)
Chronological age	7 years, 7 months	7 years, 7 months	6 years, 7 months
Sight vocabulary[a]	37.2	37.4	34.2
Word reading accuracy in context	7 years, 9 months	7 years, 11 months	6 years, 8 months
Reading comprehension	6 years, 7 months	8 years, 1 months	6 years, 8 months

[a]Maximum score for sight vocabulary test is 45.

of Table 2.1. These groups are matched for chronological age, their ability to understand the meanings of written words, and their ability to read the words in the stories used to assess their understanding.

Comprehension is not a unitary construct: it involves the interaction between a wide range of cognitive skills and processes. Consequently, there are many different aspects of the reading process where difficulties may arise, which may, in turn, lead to comprehension failure. In this section, we provide a review of correlational studies to illustrate the range of word-, sentence-, and discourse-level skills that have been investigated in relation to children's reading comprehension difficulties.

Word-Level Skills and Processes

As discussed in the previous chapter, word reading and reading comprehension are highly correlated skills and beginner readers' understanding of written text may be limited by the efficiency with which they can read the words on the page. However, there is mounting evidence that the development of word reading and reading comprehension do not necessarily proceed hand-in-hand (Paris et al., 2005) and are in fact underpinned by different skills (de Jong & van der Leij, 2002; Oakhill, Cain, & Bryant, 2003). Clearly, when decoding and reading comprehension difficulties are concomitant, problems with understanding may arise: Slow or inaccurate word reading may leave the reader with insufficient processing capacity to compute the relations between successive words, phrases, and sentences to construct a coherent and meaningful representation of the text (Perfetti, 1994; see also Kelly & Barac-Cikoja, Chapter 9, this volume).

Phonological Skills

Phonological skills are strongly associated with word-reading development (e.g., Bradley & Bryant, 1983; Wagner & Torgesen, 1987).
Phonological processing deficits can impair the ability to retain verbal
information in working memory, which might explain the link between
poor word-reading skills and poor comprehension in some readers
(Shankweiler, 1989). There is little evidence of phonological processing
deficits in poor comprehenders. Poor comprehenders matched to their
peers for vocabulary knowledge and word-reading ability perform at a
comparable level on measures of phonological awareness, such as phoneme deletion and Spoonerism tasks (Cain, Oakhill, & Bryant, 2000b;
Stothard & Hulme, 1995). Similarly, good and poor comprehenders do
not differ in their ability to use phonological codes to support short-
term memory (Cain et al., 2000b). In contrast to children with developmental dyslexia (e.g., Hulme & Snowling, 1992), poor comprehenders
perform well on tasks that assess the ability to process the sound structure of words.

Word Reading

Work by Nation and Snowling reveals weaker word-recognition skills in
children with poor reading comprehension relative to their skilled
peers. In these studies, poor comprehenders were less able to use sentence context to read irregular words, such as *beige* and *aunt* (Nation &
Snowling, 1998a), and were less accurate at reading low-frequency exception words, such as *month* and *mold* (Nation & Snowling, 1998b).
However, although the poor comprehenders in these studies had age-
appropriate word-reading skills, they were poorer than the good
comprehenders in their ability to read words in the reading test used to
select the two groups. Thus, the differences on the experimental measures may, at least to some extent, have reflected different levels of
word-reading ability in the two groups.
    Identification of poor comprehenders who have age-appropriate
word recognition skills does not rule out the possibility that their word-
processing skills are slower and less efficient than those of good
comprehenders. Nation and Snowling found a nonsignificant tendency
for poor comprehenders to have slower word recognition skills. In
studies in which good and poor comprehenders are matched for word-
reading ability, group differences on measures of word-reading speed,
automaticity of decoding, and accuracy of nonword reading have not
been found (Stothard & Hulme, 1995; Yuill & Oakhill, 1991). Future

work should address whether there are differences between good and poor comprehenders in speed of access to phonological, orthographic, and/or semantic information.

This pattern of intact word reading and poor reading comprehension can be present in children with autism spectrum disorder (see Leekam, Chapter 4, this volume) and also children with specific language impairment, although this latter population often has both poor word-reading skill and poor reading comprehension (see Botting, Chapter 3, this volume).

Semantic Skills

Semantic skills include knowledge of word meanings as well as the efficiency of access to and retrieval of those word meanings. Comprehension of written and spoken language is dependent on knowledge of individual word meanings (McGregor, 2004) and in correlational studies good and poor comprehenders differ on measures of semantic fluency (Nation & Snowling, 1998b). It is tempting to reason that inadequate vocabulary leads to difficulties in text comprehension. However, this is not necessarily the case. Good and poor comprehenders who are matched for knowledge of written and spoken word meanings can differ on standardized measures of reading comprehension, and can also differ on experimental tests of specific comprehension skills such as inference making (Cain, Oakhill, & Lemmon, 2004).

Vocabulary knowledge may influence reading comprehension indirectly, through its relation with another variable important for comprehension: memory. Some research suggests that knowledge of word meanings may influence verbal memory, which plays an important role in supporting text representation and comprehension (Nation, Adams, Bowyer-Crane, & Snowling, 1999); other work indicates that working memory difficulties in poor comprehenders may be unrelated to any vocabulary weaknesses (Cain, 2006b).

Sentence-Level Skills and Processes

Once words have been recognized and their meanings retrieved, the meaning of the sentence must be established. Knowledge about syntactic structure can facilitate the comprehension of individual sentences. *Syntactic awareness*, the ability to reflect upon and manipulate the syntactic structure of sentences, may also be related to reading comprehension level (Bowey, 1994).

Syntactic Knowledge

Written text and spoken discourse comprise a set of connected sentences, so it perhaps not surprising that some children with text comprehension difficulties have poor syntactic knowledge (Nation, Clarke, Marshall, & Durand, 2004; Stothard & Hulme, 1992). Other research finds little support for the idea that children with text comprehension difficulties have a deficit at the sentence comprehension level (Cain & Oakhill, 2006a; Cain, Patson, & Andrews, 2005; Yuill & Oakhill, 1991). The lack of consistency between studies is unexpected because each of these studies used the same widely used standardized assessment of grammar (Test for the Reception of Grammar [TROG]; Bishop, 1983).

One not very interesting reason for this discrepancy is that differences in the group selection criteria lead to the different outcomes. Another possibility is that not all children with poor comprehension have the same profile of skill strengths and weaknesses. We consider this second possibility below.

Syntactic Awareness

Syntactic awareness is assessed by tasks that involve the manipulation of spoken sentences—for example, word order correction and error detection tasks. Much of the research investigating the relation between comprehension and syntactic awareness has used assessments that confound reading comprehension and word-reading ability. Studies that control for individual differences in word-reading skills report a specific relation between syntactic awareness and a child's reading comprehension level. For example, Gaux and Gombert (1999) found that 12-year-old poor comprehenders were impaired on several tasks, even when word-reading ability was entered as a covariate in the analyses. Bentin, Deutsch, and Liberman (1990) and Nation and Snowling (2000) have both found that poor comprehenders with intact pseudoword reading skills make a greater number of errors on measures of syntactic awareness than do good comprehenders. These studies suggest that children with poor discourse and text comprehension are impaired in their ability to correct sentences with incorrect word order or grammatical errors.

Discourse-Level Skills and Processes

There has been considerable research interest in poor comprehenders' performance on discourse-level skills that foster comprehension and facilitate the construction of meaning-based representations because these representations are central to comprehension. In this section, we consider the following skills: inference making and integration, use of cohesive devices and context, comprehension-monitoring ability, and knowledge about story structure.

Inference Making and Integration

The author of a text does not spell out every little detail: to do so would result in a rather long and boring text. As a result, the reader must generate links between different parts of a text and use his or her general knowledge to fill in missing detail, in order to construct an adequate, appropriate, and coherent representation of the text. Inference and integration skills are essential for good comprehension and the inference-making skills of poor comprehenders have received much interest (see also Barnes, Johnston, & Dennis, Chapter 7, and Botting, Chapter 3, this volume, for research on inference making in other populations with comprehension difficulties).

Early work by Oakhill revealed that less-skilled comprehenders are poor at making inferences when reading or listening to text. Relative to good comprehenders, poor comprehenders generate fewer constructive inferences, which involve integrating information from two different sentences in a text—for example, "The boy was chasing the girl. The girl ran into the playground." Infer: "The boy ran into the playground" (Oakhill, 1982). Poor comprehenders are also less likely to incorporate general knowledge with information in the text to generate simple inferences (Oakhill, 1984). Memory for the text itself does not appear to be a reason for poor comprehenders' difficulties in these studies: poor comprehenders are able to recall literal detail from the texts (Oakhill, 1982) and their inference-making difficulties are apparent even when the text is available to search through (Oakhill, 1984).

Further support for poor comprehenders' inference-making difficulties comes from a recent examination of good and poor comprehenders' performance on different types of questions on standardized assessments of reading comprehension, conducted by Bowyer-Crane and Snowling (2005). In this study, poor comprehenders were poor at answering questions tapping their ability to make cohesive inferences (similar to Oakhill's constructive inferences) relative to their performance on questions tapping literal information; good comprehenders did not differ on these two question types. Furthermore, the poor comprehenders were particularly impaired, relative to the good comprehenders, on inference questions that required elaboration of the text and those that tapped general knowledge.

We have investigated the possibility that general knowledge deficits might be a source of poor comprehenders' inference-making difficulties by using a procedure and materials constructed by Barnes and colleagues (e.g., Barnes & Dennis, 1998) that enabled strict control of individual differences in general knowledge. Children were taught a set of facts about an imaginary planet called Gan. For example, "The flowers on Gan are hot like fire," "The ponds on Gan are filled with orange juice." They then listened to a multiepisode story followed by questions that assessed their ability to generate inferences. In order to draw each inference, children had to incorporate information from the knowledge base with a story premise. Memory for the knowledge base was assessed at the end of the story and only responses to the inference questions for which the knowledge base item was recalled were included in the final analysis. Even when knowledge was controlled for in this very strict way, less-skilled comprehenders generated fewer inferences than did the skilled comprehenders (Cain, Oakhill, Barnes, & Bryant, 2001).

Cohesive Devices

Anaphors are devices that maintain cohesion between sentences and phrases in a text. An example of an anaphor is the pronoun *she* in the following: "Joe told a joke to Justine. She thought it was very funny," which refers to "Justine" (the antecedent) in the preceding part of the text. Another type of cohesive device is an *interclausal connective*, such as *so* or *because*, used to indicate the relation between different propositions or sentences. Compare "Nicola was late, so she took the bus" with "Nicola was late, because she took the bus." These linguistic cues help the reader to integrate information between sentences in a text and, in that way, are similar in kind to constructive (or cohesive) inferences.

Children with poor reading comprehension make more errors on questions that can only be answered if a pronoun has been correctly resolved relative to same-age peers—for example, "Chris lent his coat to Kate because *she* was cold. Who was cold, Chris or Kate?" (Yuill & Oakhill, 1991). They are also less likely to supply the appropriate anaphor in a cloze task—for example, "Steve gave his umbrella to Andrea in the park because _____ wanted to keep dry" (Oakhill & Yuill, 1986).

These difficulties extend to the processing of spoken discourse. Megherbi and Ehrlich (2005) used an online listening paradigm to investigate how good and poor comprehenders process pronouns in real time. The children were all age 7 years and they listened to short texts, such as: "Louise had dinner with Malcolm in a restaurant. She chatted cheerfully with. . . . " At the end of the second incomplete sentence, a probe word, *him* or *her*, was displayed on a computer screen in front of the child. The time taken to read the probe indicated that the skilled comprehenders were integrating the sentences as they were heard, using information about the gender of the pronoun, whereas the poor comprehenders were not sensitive to the information carried by pronouns.

Other work has examined how children process anaphors in extended prose. Poor comprehenders' difficulties are particularly pronounced when there is intervening text between the anaphor and its antecedent (Ehrlich & Rémond, 1997; Yuill & Oakhill, 1988). Poor use of cohesive devices is also apparent in longer, more naturalistic texts—for example, poor comprehenders are less likely to supply the correct connective (e.g., *because, after, but*) to fill in a blank space in a sentence than are good comprehenders (Cain, Patson, & Andrews, 2005). In addition, when retelling aurally presented stories, poor comprehenders are less likely to include additional connectives than are good comprehenders (Yuill & Oakhill, 1991).

Use of Context

When we read or listen to text we need to make use of contextual information to establish meaning, as well as to make local integrative links. The use of context to understand language is often considered under the umbrella term of *pragmatics* (see Leekam, Chapter 4, this volume, for a discussion of how impaired use of context may affect the comprehension of individuals with autism spectrum disorder). Poor comprehenders experience particular difficulty with the use of sentence and story context to facilitate understanding of words and phrases in text.

The first piece of evidence that poor comprehenders make less use of context when constructing meaning came from a study by Oakhill (1983). This study was designed to investigate a particular type of inference, an *instantiation*, where the reader infers a specific meaning of a common noun from the sentence context—for example, inferring that *fish* is most likely a "shark" in the following sentence: "The fish frightened the swimmer." Poor comprehenders made fewer instantiations than did good comprehenders, suggesting that they are less likely to use the semantic content of the sentence to inform meaning.

Poor comprehenders are also less able to use the context of the story to infer the meanings of single novel words. In a series of experiments, we presented good and poor comprehenders with short texts containing an unknown vocabulary item. Their task was to explain the meaning of the unknown word. For example, one of the stories began: "Bill was always very careful when riding his bike but the other day he fell off. When he looked round he saw that the problem was a *gromp*." The text provides various clues that a "gromp" is a hole or bump in the road, rather than a problem with the mechanics of the bicycle. The reader is required to integrate these contextual clues with the fact that the Bill fell off his bike to derive a meaning for the novel word. We found that poor comprehenders provided fewer correct definitions for the novel words than did good comprehenders, because they failed to take all of the necessary context into account. Similar to the work on anaphoric processing, poor comprehenders' difficulties are particularly pronounced when the novel word and the useful contextual clues are separated by filler text (see Cain, Oakhill, & Elbro, 2003, and Cain, Oakhill, & Lemmon, 2004, for further details).

Sometimes a reader may come across a phrase in a text that cannot be interpreted by reference to a single sentence. Instead, the context may provide support for the meaning of a phrase. A specific example of this use of context is young children's understanding of unfamiliar idioms. *Idioms* are expressions such as "to spill the beans" that take a figurative, rather than a literal, meaning. Young children's and poor comprehenders' understanding of an unfamiliar idiom is influenced by the context in which it appears—that is, whether the context supports a literal or a figurative interpretation of the phrase (e.g., Levorato & Cacciari, 1992; Levorato, Nesi, & Cacciari, 2004). Poor comprehenders' understanding of the figurative sense of idioms is particularly impaired for opaque idioms, such as "to be wet behind the ears" (i.e., to lack experience), where the words in the phrase provide little support for the figurative meaning (Cain, Oakhill, & Lemmon, 2005). Poor comprehenders' interpretations of these phrases are less likely to be based on the context of the story as a whole, and are sometimes nothing more than a literal interpretation of the phrase itself.

Comprehension Monitoring

The ability to monitor our understanding of text and discourse is crucial to good comprehension. If we detect that we have not fully understood a point, or find that the current idea unit does not fit with our understanding of other aspects of the text or discourse, we can take remedial steps. It may be easier to resolve a misunderstanding of spoken discourse than to resolve a misunderstanding of written text because the listener is often at liberty to interrogate the speaker. Unfortunately, with written text, the author is absent, but the reader may still be able to reread the text and/or generate an inference to resolve the problem.

The previous chapter dealt with the development of young children's ability to monitor their comprehension. One of the tasks used, the inconsistency detection task, has been employed extensively to explore the nature and extent of the comprehension-monitoring difficulties experienced by poor comprehenders. These tasks assess a child's ability to detect inconsistencies such as nonsense words, contradictory sentences, or statements that conflict with external information (general knowledge). For example, one of the stories used in our own research includes the lines "There was no moonlight, so Jill could hardly see her way" and "The moon was so bright that it lit the way" These error-detection tasks require readers to evaluate their understanding of the text because they can only detect an inconsistency if they are actively engaged in constructive processing, which requires building a model of the text's meaning and relating each new piece of information to that model as it is read. Comprehension monitoring appears to be an area of weakness for children with a specific comprehension deficit.

Ehrlich and colleagues have studied comprehension monitoring by comparing good and poor comprehenders' abilities to detect inconsistent anaphors in expository texts. In one study (Ehrlich, 1996) 12- to 15-year-olds read texts in which a noun phrase anaphor had a meaning that was contradictory to its antecedent. In the consistent version a noun phrase was repeated—for example, "The protection of existing reserves. . . . This protection. . . . " In the contradictory version, the second (anaphoric) instance of "protection" was replaced by a noun phrase with a meaning that was contrary to its intended antecedent—for this example, "wastage." Good comprehenders were more likely to detect (underline) the inconsistent anaphors than were poor comprehenders.

In further experimental work with 10-year-olds, Ehrlich, Rémond, and Tardieu (1999) found that good comprehenders spent more time reading sections of text containing inconsistent anaphors than did poor comprehenders. The good comprehenders were also more likely to look back to previous text when they encountered an inconsistent anaphor. These findings indicate that the good comprehenders spotted the inconsistency and engaged in additional processing to try to make sense of the text. Younger poor comprehenders are also less likely to spot inconsistencies in texts, particularly when the bits of inconsistent information are separated by filler text (Oakhill, Hartt, & Samols, 2005).

Knowledge of Story Structure

Narrative is the principle genre in children's early literacy experience. As a result, there has been considerable interest in how children's knowledge of narrative structure aids their developing comprehension skills. For example, Trabasso and Nickels (1992) proposed that children's understanding and production of stories can be guided by their knowledge about story organization and goal-directed actions, and Perfetti (1994) suggested that comprehension failure might arise through inadequate knowledge about how texts are structured.

The ability to appreciate the main point of a story depends on an ability to extract its gist. To assess this skill in good and poor comprehenders, we presented them with stories either aurally or as a series of pictures. After each story, children were asked to select the main point of the story from a choice of four written statements: the correct main point, the main setting, the main event, and an incorrect main point. Poor comprehenders were poor at selecting the main point of the story in both presentation conditions (Yuill & Oakhill, 1991).

Poor comprehenders also demonstrate weaknesses with elements that make a story well structured and integrated. We used an oral story production task to compare the structural coherence of good and poor comprehenders. When the story prompt was a simple topic idea—for example, "Pirates"—the poor comprehenders told stories that were more poorly organized than those produced by the good comprehenders and that were less likely to include a causally related sequence of events. Poor comprehenders were able to produce better integrated stories when required to narrate a sequence of pictures (Cain & Oakhill, 1996). A subsequent study found that poor comprehenders obtained some benefit from titles that provided goals for the story—for example, "How the pirates lost their treasure"—relative to simple titles such as "Pirates" (Cain, 2003). Cragg and Nation (2006) found that poor comprehenders produced poorer stories in a written production task, as well.

Poor comprehenders also have poor declarative knowledge about the sorts of information provided by particular story features, such as story titles, story beginnings, and story endings. These textual features can be useful aids for the reader, helping him or her to invoke relevant background information and schemas. Cain (1996) interviewed good and poor comprehenders about these features of stories. The majority of good comprehenders were able to provide appropriate examples of the sort of information contained in a story title, such as "tells you what it's about and who's in it." In contrast, less than one-quarter of the poor comprehenders were able to do so; they were more likely to respond that a title "tells you whether you like the story or not," and some poor comprehenders reported that titles do not tell the reader anything at all!

The Role of Working Memory

Working memory capacity is correlated with children's and adults' reading and listening comprehension (Cain, 2006a; Daneman & Merikle, 1996), and is impaired in children with comprehension difficulties (see Swanson, Howard, & Sáez, Chapter 6, this volume). Poor comprehenders' short-term memory store appears to be intact. They are not impaired in their ability to store a series of words or digits when compared to good comprehenders with comparable word-reading skills (Cain, 2006b; Cain et al., 2000a; Cain, Oakhill, & Lemmon, 2004; Oakhill, Yuill, & Parkin, 1986; Stothard & Hulme, 1992). In contrast, poor comprehenders are impaired on assessments of memory that require the simultaneous storage and processing of digits (e.g., Yuill, Oakhill, & Parkin, 1989) and words/sentences (de Beni & Palladino, 2000; Nation et al., 1999).

Many of the skills involved in successful comprehension, such as integration and inference, anaphoric processing, use of context, comprehension monitoring, and structuring of stories, are dependent on the storage and coordination of information in memory. Furthermore, the work discussed earlier on anaphoric resolution, inference making, and comprehension monitoring found that poor comprehenders' difficulties were more pronounced when there was intervening text between the propositions of interest.

There are good theoretical reasons to suppose that memory difficulties might underpin some of the skill deficits experienced by poor comprehenders. Swanson et al. (Chapter 6, this volume) explore the relation between this aspect of memory and comprehension failure in detail, so here we will be brief. Suffice it to say, that although there is evidence that memory impairments can arise through word-reading inefficiency, phonological processing difficulties or, perhaps, poor semantic skills, the working memory impairments of the poor comprehenders that we consider are clearly not due to such impairments. Furthermore, working memory appears to have a direct relationship with reading comprehension over and above short-term memory, word-reading ability, and vocabulary knowledge (Cain, Oakhill, & Bryant, 2004).

Are All Poor Comprehenders the Same?

We stated earlier that comprehension is not a unitary construct. That is not a particularly controversial or unique statement to make. Good comprehension relies on a wide range of language-related skills, and our review has demonstrated that many of these may be associated with poor comprehenders' reading and listening comprehension difficulties. This leads us to wonder: Are all poor comprehenders the same? That is to say, does every child with a specific reading comprehension deficit show an impairment on every one of the skills reviewed?

The brief answer is "No." There are inconsistencies across studies, most notably across those investigating word- and sentence-level skills. Some studies report differences between groups of good and poor comprehenders; others do not. These inconsistencies suggest that not all poor comprehenders experience deficits on these skills. The results of studies on discourse-level processing skills are more consistent. In general, when word-reading ability and written vocabulary knowledge are controlled, poor comprehenders demonstrate deficits on many skills that are related to the construction of meaning. On the face of it, many skills appear to be related to poor comprehenders' difficulties. Group comparisons do not, however, demonstrate that every poor comprehender presents a deficit on a given skill.

One way to explore this issue further is to examine the profiles of children identified with weak comprehension skill. If we look at the individual performance of poor comprehenders, we should find that skills fundamental to reading comprehension are impaired in the majority of children. Skill deficits that are incidental correlates should be preserved in some individuals with poor comprehension but weak in others. Cornoldi et al. (1996) examined patterns of skill strength and weakness in 11-year-old Italian schoolchildren who had weak reading comprehension skills in the presence of good decoding skills and normal intelligence. Not all poor comprehenders experienced impairments in all of the skills. For example, some children had poor working memory but good metacognitive skills, and others showed the opposite pattern.

Other work that has included examination of individual profiles also finds differences within the population of poor comprehenders. Nation et al. (2004) found that, in general, poor comprehenders were poorer at recalling sentences and providing the correct form of the irregular past tense (in a cloze task) compared to good comprehenders. However, only three (out of 23) poor comprehenders demonstrated significant impairments on both tasks, and a greater number were impaired on the recall measure than on the past tense elicitation task (11 vs. 5).

Our own examination of a group of poor comprehenders has included an examination of the word-, sentence-, and text-level skills in a group of children with a reading comprehension deficit. In this study, word-reading ability was allowed to vary and the children were not matched to good comprehenders on this variable (Cain & Oakhill, 2006a). Group comparisons between 7- to 8-year-old good and poor comprehenders (23 in each group) revealed deficits on receptive vocabulary, working memory, and several comprehension-fostering and text-processing skills: inference making, comprehension monitoring, and knowledge about story structure. The groups did not differ on syntactic knowledge. We computed z scores for these measures from a larger ($N = 102$) sample of children and used these to examine skill strengths and weaknesses in the 23 children with a significant comprehension impairment. The population of poor comprehenders was clearly heterogeneous. For example, 14 obtained scores that were below the mean of the larger sample on our measure of syntactic knowledge and nine scored above the mean; 10 scored below the mean on receptive vocabulary; 19 scored below the mean on a composite measure of the comprehension assessments and four scored above. There was no single task on which all poor comprehenders obtained below-average scores.

The (possibly) unsatisfactory conclusion from these studies is that no clear fundamental weakness has been identified. For example, some poor comprehenders may have a fundamental weakness at the sentence level that affects their text comprehension while sentence comprehension may be intact for other poor comprehenders. In addition, these studies indicate that group comparisons may obscure crucial weaknesses in the individual. We return to this point in our final section when we consider the implications for education and intervention.

We should also consider the possibility that different factors may limit reading comprehension at different stages of reading development. Evidence for this thesis comes from a study by Snyder and Downey (1991), in which they looked at the relation between phonological, lexical, sentence completion, and narrative discourse processing skills in 8- to 14-year-olds classified as good or poor readers on the basis of a silent reading comprehension test. Comparisons between the groups demonstrated that the typically developing readers outperformed the poor readers on all measures. When Snyder and Downey looked at the relative contribution of each skill to the prediction of reading comprehension, they found some interesting age differences. For the younger poor readers, speed and accuracy on the lexical measure of rapid color naming were both important predictors of reading comprehension level, along with performance on the sentence completion task. For the older poor readers, narrative discourse skills, particularly the ability to answer inference-tapping questions, were crucial. The study suggests that different factors may limit reading comprehension ability at different stages of reading development.

There is other work to support this view. For example, there is evidence that reading comprehension becomes more highly correlated with vocabulary knowledge over time (e.g., Torgesen, Wagner, Rashotte, Burgess, & Hecht, 1997), suggesting that vocabulary may be a more important determinant of reading comprehension in older than in younger children. Longitudinal work by de Jong and van der Leij (2002) suggests that phonological skills and vocabulary contribute to reading comprehension at different times in reading development. And work with much younger children finds that different skills predict reading success at different ages. For example, speech production at age 3 is an important determinant of later reading ability, whereas vocabulary and syntax when assessed at age 4 are the skills that differentiate children who go on to become good and poor readers (see Scarborough, 2005). Thus, it may be that younger readers' comprehension is limited by word- and sentence-level skills, whereas the older children's comprehension is limited by skills that foster meaning.

WHAT CAUSES POOR COMPREHENSION?

The previous section illustrated the large number of skills that are associated (or correlated) with poor comprehension. Ehri (1979) identified four different ways in which one skill may be related to another, in this case comprehension: It may be a prerequisite of reading comprehension, a facilitator, a consequence, or simply an incidental correlate. Comparisons between good and poor comprehenders do not distinguish between these alternatives. Thus, we should be wary of making causal inferences from correlational studies, even where there may be theoretical reasons to infer the direction of cause and effect. For example, poor vocabulary knowledge may be the reason for some children's failure to understand larger units of connected text and discourse; alternately, poor vocabulary skills may come about because a weakness in the ability to understand connected prose impairs the ability to consolidate and learn new word meanings in context. In this section, we consider research that has used designs that enable us to determine which, if any, of the skills that are associated with poor reading comprehension are causally related to reading comprehension development and reading comprehension difficulties. The identification of causal factors is crucial if we wish to develop interventions to help children with comprehension difficulties.

There are three (complementary) ways in which causality can be explored: by comparison of poor comprehenders with a younger comprehension–age match group, by longitudinal studies, and by studies that include an element of training or an intervention. Unfortunately, there is no one "best" method to establish which variables are causal. Each method has its limitations, so it is prudent to use all methods and to look for converging evidence as to which particular variables are causality implicated in comprehension skill.

Methods for Exploring Causality

The Comprehension–Age Match Design

The comprehension–age match design (CAM) is analogous in its logic to the reading–age match design (see Bryant & Goswami, 1986, for an overview) and has been extended to the study of comprehension (Cain et al., 2000a). This design requires three groups of participants: good and poor comprehenders, matched for chronological age and single-word reading ability, and an additional group of younger, normally developing comprehenders, selected so that their comprehension skill is at the *same absolute level* as that of the older poor comprehenders, but is normal for their age. An example of the characteristics of three such groups is provided in Table 2.1, above.

The comparison between the poor comprehenders and the CAM group is of critical interest. If the younger CAM group perform better on a measure that differentiates between good and poor comprehenders—for example, in terms of the ability to draw inferences from text—we can rule out the possibility that superior inference skills arise from superior comprehension, because the CAM group and the poor comprehenders are matched on absolute level of comprehension skill. This is, of course, a strong test, because the CAM group is, necessarily, comprised of younger children who have poorer word-reading skills than the poor comprehender group.

This design has its limitations: *it can only be used to rule out a causal link in one direction* (from comprehension ability to the skill in question) and *it cannot be used to prove a link in the opposite direction*. However, it is a relatively quick method for identifying (or ruling out) likely causal candidates, providing information that can inform the design of other, more expensive, and time-consuming methods, such as longitudinal and training studies, that can provide more robust tests of causality.

Longitudinal Studies

Longitudinal studies that track the course of changes in comprehension skill can provide additional information about the causal relations among the components of comprehension, and thus about the course of development. The aim of longitudinal studies is to measure sets of skills and abilities at different time points and then to assess two things: (1) whether or not some variables are better predictors of later comprehension skill (and growth in comprehension skill over time) than are others, and (2) whether or not a particular (early) variable is a better predictor of comprehension skill over time than (early) comprehension skill is a predictor of that variable. Longitudinal studies of reading comprehension development are discussed in detail by Oakhill and Cain (Chapter 1, this volume). In this chapter, we consider both prospective and retrospective longitudinal studies. *Prospective studies* are those that have either tracked the progress of poor comprehenders over time to determine the wider consequences of poor comprehension (Cain & Oakhill, 2006b), or sought to determine which early skills predict later comprehension problems, whereas *retrospective longitudinal studies* explore which skills in the early years are deficient in children subsequently identified with a comprehension deficit (Catts, Adlof, & Ellis Weismer, 2006).

In a longitudinal study, it is necessary to determine whether or not the skill of interest—for example, vocabulary—predicts later comprehension performance over and above level of comprehension at the start of the study. It is not always possible to measure the skill of interest at the earliest time point in order to take this into account in the statistical analysis. For example, most 5-year-olds would score poorly on a measure of reading comprehension because their word-reading skills would limit their performance. However, it is possible to take measures of the underlying construct—for example, narrative comprehension or listening comprehension. For an example of this approach, see van den Broek et al. (2005). Another limitation of longitudinal designs is that a skill identified as a predictor of later competence might achieve its effects indirectly, through a mediating skill. For example, early phonological awareness might appear to predict later reading comprehension, but the relationship might only be indirect because phonological awareness is a strong predictor of a more likely causal influence: word-reading ability. It is therefore important to consider many different theoretically possible relations when selecting the variables to be assessed in a longitudinal design. However, clearly there is a limit on the number of different assessments that can be conducted with each participant.

Training and Intervention Studies

These studies test the efficacy of a particular type of intervention or skill training. First, a skill is identified on both theoretical and empirical grounds as a causal candidate of good comprehension. A group of poor comprehenders is then trained on that skill, and their performance, not only on the skill that has been trained but also on a standardized measure of comprehension ability, is compared with that of another group. The comparison group can comprise good comprehenders who participated in the same training and/or poor comprehenders who received a different training regime of comparable type or duration. If the poor comprehenders' comprehension level is found to improve more than that of either comparison group, it is assumed that the trained skill is causally implicated in the improvement in their comprehension. For example, if an intervention designed to improve poor comprehenders' inference-making ability led to greater gains in their reading comprehension relative to the improvement seen in a group of poor comprehenders, we might conclude that a deficit in inference-making ability was the cause of the poor comprehenders' difficulties.

Training studies are considered by some to be the true test of causality. Unfortunately, as with the other two designs, there are limitations that should be borne in mind when interpreting the results. The training effect might not have arisen because of a direct improvement in the skill being trained. For example, many inferences rely on the integration of information presented in the text with the reader's general knowledge. If children are taught how to identify where and when inferences are required, does improvement arise because of their better integration skills or because of an increased ability to identify clues in a text? Another possibility is that the training leads to improved activation of relevant general knowledge when reading. When we consider the complexity of some of the skills that are associated with good comprehension, it is obvious that a clear test of one skill may not always be possible. It is important to consider how training might influence performance indirectly, through a common mediating variable.

Evidence for Causal Relations

In this section we evaluate the evidence for causal relations between reading comprehension and the different potential causes of poor comprehension, outlined previously. We discuss word- and sentence-level skills first, followed by a more detailed discussion of discourse-level comprehension-fostering skills, which have been the focus of a greater number of research studies.

Word- and Sentence-Level Skills

There is no strong evidence that the efficiency of word reading is impaired in all children with comprehension difficulties. For that reason, word-level skills have not been a focus of training studies involving children with specific comprehension difficulties and there have been no studies investigating the efficiency of word-reading skills with a comprehension–age match design. Although training studies have focused on discourse-level comprehension-fostering skills, such as inference generation, the training given to "control" groups has, on occasion, targeted word-level skills (e.g., Yuill & Oakhill, 1991). The performance of these "control" groups supports the idea that word-reading fluency is not the underlying cause of the comprehension problems experienced by poor comprehenders.

Yuill and Oakhill (1988) compared the efficacy of inference training with two different types of control intervention, one of which involved training children to read key words in the text quickly and accurately. The training in rapid decoding clearly worked: This group of children were subsequently faster on a test of reading speed than the children who received the inference training. However, the rapid decoding training did not lead to a significant improvement in reading comprehension level.

Despite the high correlations that have been found between performance on vocabulary tests and reading comprehension (Carroll, 1993), there has been limited assessment of a causal relation between vocabulary impairments and specific comprehension deficits. One reason for the lack of studies is that it is possible (and indeed a necessary selection criterion by some research groups) to find children who have a difficulty understanding connected prose, even when their knowledge of word meanings is matched to that of peers (Cain et al., 2005; Ehrlich et al., 1999; Stothard & Hulme, 1992). Thus, there has not been a strong theoretical reason to investigate vocabulary knowledge as a causal factor of the difficulties experienced by this particular population of poor comprehenders.

Work on sentence-level skills has looked at both knowledge of syntax and syntactic awareness. In a retrospective longitudinal study, Catts et al. (2006) found that children with good word-reading skills but poor comprehension in eighth grade had weaker vocabulary knowledge and also weaker grammatical knowledge than same-age good comprehenders in second and fourth grade. These children also had weaker comprehension skills at the earlier time point, so the study does not address the direction of causality between the two skills. Layton, Robinson, and Lawson (1998) have successfully trained syntactic awareness in 8- to 10-year-olds. However, the effects did not lead to improvements in word-reading accuracy or reading comprehension and the poor comprehenders obtained comparable benefits to good comprehenders.

Feagans and Applebaum (1986) conducted a prospective longitudinal study that included assessments of word-, sentence-, and discourse-level skills. The aim of the study was to explore the impact of different types of language deficit on subsequent educational performance. Children with different profiles of strength and weakness in semantic, syntactic, and narrative skills were identified. The children with the best educational outcome had the highest relative scores in semantics and syntax at outset; children who had deficits in narrative comprehension skill (based on the ability to act out and summarize stories) did most poorly on later assessments of reading comprehension.

The studies reviewed thus far provide little support for the hypothesis that poor word- and sentence-level skills lead to specific, rather than more general, comprehension deficits. In the next section, we consider the causal relations between reading comprehension and discourse-level skills in more detail.

Discourse-Level Skills

The three discourse-level skills considered here are inference and integration, comprehension monitoring, and narrative structuring skills, which have all been the subject of causal investigations.

As outlined above, poor comprehenders' difficulties with inference making are well documented. Inference making is considered crucial to good comprehension, and weak inference and integration skills are associated with individual differences in adult's comprehension (Long, Oppy, & Seely, 1994, 1997). However, we need to establish whether weak inference-making skills are a cause or a consequence of poor comprehension.

A study using the CAM design rules out the latter possibility. We compared the performance of poor comprehenders with that of a younger CAM group on two types of inference: those that required the integration of information from different sentences in a text and those that required the integration of background knowledge with information in the text to fill in details that are only mentioned implicitly (Cain & Oakhill, 1999). The children read short stories and answered questions after each one to tap these two types of inference and also memory for explicit details in the text. The poor comprehenders were poorer than the CAM group at both types of inference question, although the difference was only statistically significant for the questions tapping inferences that involved integrating information from different parts of the text. These data suggest that (1) skill at drawing inferences is not simply a by-product of reading comprehension skill because the poor comprehenders and the CAM group were matched for reading comprehension level, (2) and identify inference making as a candidate cause of good comprehension.

The findings from two training studies provide further support for this proposed direction of causality. In one, 7- to 8-year-old good and poor comprehenders were taught how to make inferences from key "clue" words in deliberately obscure texts (Yuill & Joscelyne, 1988). For example, in one story, the text does not state explicitly that the main character was lying in the bath, but this setting can be inferred from words such as "soap," "towel," and "steamy." The poor comprehenders who received the training were significantly better at answering questions to measure their comprehension of the story than were a control group of poor comprehenders. The effect of instruction was not significant for the skilled comprehenders.

In another study, Yuill and Oakhill (1988) compared the effects of different types of training: one condition involved learning how to generate questions to test understanding—for example, "Why did she do that?"—and generating inferences from specific words, as described above; a second condition involved practice in standard comprehension exercises—for example, question answering; the third condition focused on practice in rapid word decoding (mentioned previously). The poor comprehenders who had received the inference- and question-generation training made the greatest gains on a standardized measure of reading comprehension, compared to the other training groups, and increased their reading comprehension age to within 6 months of that of the skilled comprehenders. McGee and Johnson (2003) tested a similar training program based on Yuill and Oakhill's (1988) study and found that seven out of 10 poor comprehenders could be classified as good comprehenders after the intervention.

One difficulty in our interpretation of the inference-training work is the specificity of any effects. For example, training children to be aware of clues in a text to show them when and where to make an inference involves an element of comprehension monitoring. Despite the interest in poor comprehenders' monitoring skills (e.g., Ehrlich et al., 1999; Oakhill et al., 2005), there has been little work investigating the causal relations between reading comprehension and comprehension monitoring. We know of no work that has used the CAM design in this area and our own attempts to train comprehension monitoring specifically have met with little success (see Yuill & Oakhill, 1991).

Although we have considered comprehension monitoring as a "stand-alone" skill in our discussion so far, it is often considered as one component of metacognition (see also Oakhill & Cain, Chapter 1, this volume). Metacognitive knowledge about reading can include knowledge about the goals and processes of reading, and skill in applying such knowledge, for example, by monitoring one's comprehension and executing a repair strategy such as rereading when a failure to comprehend is detected. Paris and colleagues have developed programs to teach knowledge and use of different reading strategies to typically developing children. Unfortunately, knowledge increments have been modest and the trained groups do not demonstrate superior performance on standardized assessments of comprehension (Paris & Jacobs, 1984; Paris, Saarnio, & Cross, 1986). However, Cain (1999) has shown that poor comprehenders are less able than both good comprehenders and a CAM group to adjust their reading style to meet different goals—for example, reading to study for a later comprehension test versus skim-reading to identify a particular piece of information. Thus, there is evidence that some aspects of metacognition might be causally related to reading comprehension failure.

Another intervention that focuses on teaching children the metacognitive skill of "how to read effectively" was developed by Brown and colleagues. Their approach was to teach comprehension-fostering skills such as summarization of the text so far and self-directed questioning to children identified as poor comprehenders to enhance their interpretation of the text and their prediction of what might happen next (see Brown, Palincsar, & Armbruster, 1984, for a review). They argue that these skills improve monitoring and help to foster comprehension more generally. In their program, the behaviors are modeled, feedback is provided, and the students gradually take control of how to monitor and adapt their reading. This training has been shown to improve the comprehension of poor comprehenders in interventions conducted both by researchers and by classroom teachers. Work with children identified with a specific comprehension deficit is required to examine the efficacy of this procedure further and to identify the key elements of this rather broad-ranging but clearly very effective intervention.

We now turn to the third discourse-level skill area: narrative structure. Our own work, using the comprehension–age match design, has also identified poor narrative structure skills as a causal candidate for comprehension failure. In this work, as described earlier, we manipulated the type of prompt used to elicit oral narratives and classified the narrative productions using a scheme that reflected the level of inter-connectedness and causality between story events (Cain, 2003; Cain & Oakhill, 1996). As also mentioned earlier, the poor comprehenders produced particularly poorly structured stories when provided with only a topic prompt, such as "Pirates," and their stories in this condition were of poorer quality that those produced by a younger CAM group. Importantly, there were no differences in the length of the narratives produced by the groups: it was not simply the case that poor comprehenders lacked the expressive skills necessary to perform the task. Neither were the poor comprehenders less likely to include story conventions—for example, "Once upon a time." Thus, their knowledge about this aspect of stories was comparable to that of the other groups. We found that the poor comprehenders produced more structurally coherent stories when provided with structural support in the form of a sequence of pictures or a goal-directed title. This finding suggests that poor comprehenders lack knowledge about story structure and organization.

Despite the growing recognition that a child's early competence in understanding and structuring narrative is predictive of later reading comprehension success (e.g., van den Broek et al., 2005), we have found no published accounts of narrative structure interventions for children with comprehension difficulties. However, our own longitudinal work concurs with the findings of van den Broek and colleagues that the ability to structure narratives and knowledge about narrative structure is related to later comprehension success. Feagans and Appelbaum's (1986) longitudinal findings that children with weak narrative skills were more likely to experience later comprehension problems than were children with weak vocabulary or syntactic skills also strongly support a causal relation between narrative comprehension and reading comprehension.

Summary

These studies, in conjunction with recent longitudinal investigations of comprehension skills in typically developing children, strongly suggest that good reading and listening comprehension depends on the skills that help us to construct coherent and integrated representations of meaning: inference and integration, comprehension monitoring and metacognitive knowledge about reading and repair strategies, and the ability to impose a causal structure on the events in a narrative. There is increasing evidence that impairments in these skills underpin comprehension failure. More work is needed to explore these issues further. There are surprisingly few published accounts of intervention studies, so it is not possible to identify the most effective components of the training programs reported to date. Longitudinal designs that include adequate controls for initial performance on these skills are lacking, and there are also few prospective studies of comprehension skill. These studies are necessary to identify which of the very many early language skill deficits are *directly* related to a later poor comprehender profile.

CONSEQUENCES

In this final section we consider the wider effects that a reading and listening comprehension deficit might have on language and literacy development in general, and the implications for the prevention and remediation of comprehension difficulties.

Implications for Language and Literacy Development

Few studies have tracked the progress of poor comprehenders over time. This is unfortunate because studies of poor comprehenders are crucial for (at least) two reasons. First, we need to know about the persistence of comprehension deficits. One possibility is that comprehension deficits are transitory: they may arise because of a developmental delay in the growth of a crucial comprehension-related skill. Thus, some children may do poorly on a measure of reading or listening comprehension relative to their chronological or language age at one time point, but "grow out" of their deficit over time without the need for any intervention. Second, we need to consider the wider implications of poor comprehension. How do weak comprehension skills affect the development of other language skills, and what are the later educational implications of being a poor comprehender?

We first consider the persistence of comprehension deficits. The findings from the research tracking poor comprehenders across time are inconclusive. For example, Cornoldi and colleagues (1996) tested a group of poor comprehenders first when they were 11 years old and again 2 years later. Not all of the poor comprehenders had an impairment at the follow-up: Seven of the original 12 children still had a comprehension deficit, but the other five participants did not. This statistic is encouraging because it suggests that around 40% of those with a comprehension problem at 11 years do not have a persistent severe deficit. Levorato et al. (2004) found fewer poor comprehenders in a sample of 10-year-olds than in a sample of 8-year-olds, which led them to propose that the proportion of poor comprehenders in the school-age population will decrease with increasing age. Indeed, they found that 67% of their younger sample of poor comprehenders and 54% of their older sample of poor comprehenders were no longer classed as poor comprehenders when retested 8 months later. Aarnoutse, van Leeuwe, Voeten, and Oud (2001) tracked the reading development of poor, average, and good performers on measures of decoding, reading comprehension, vocabulary, and spelling. The group differences in reading comprehension ability got smaller over time.

The good and poor comprehenders in Levorato et al.'s (2004) study differed not only in their reading comprehension skills, but also in their word-reading accuracy and speed at the start of the study. Thus, improvements in the efficiency of word-reading skills may have led to the improvements in reading comprehension skill because of the strong relationship between word reading and reading comprehension (Perfetti, 1994). Similarly, the groups in Aarnoutse et al.'s (2001) study were not matched for word-reading ability, so this variable may have differed between the groups. It is not possible to determine whether or not the group differences decreased over time because of improvements in other skills, such as word reading, that may have limited initial comprehension.

In contrast to the above studies, our own work shows a greater persistence of reading comprehension deficits. We followed the progress of two groups of 23 children who were classified as either good or poor comprehenders when at age 8 (Cain & Oakhill, 2006a). In contrast to Levorato et al.'s groups, our groups did not differ in their word-reading ability at outset. At 11 years, the remaining children in each group (19 poor comprehenders and 17 good comprehenders) differed on a standardized measure of reading comprehension. When we looked at the individual performance of the children available at the follow-up, only one of the poor comprehenders obtained an age-appropriate reading comprehension score. Obviously, a larger number of longitudinal studies is needed to determine an accurate estimate of the persistence of comprehension problems.

We next consider how individual differences in reading comprehension impact the development of other language and literacy skills. Although we have considered very simple cause-and-effect paths of causality thus far, the situation is likely to be far more complex and probably involves interactions between component skills and also reciprocal relations, where expertise in one component skill leads to gains in reading comprehension, which, in turn, lead to further gains in the component skill.

This type of reciprocity has been considered in detail with regard to reading and vocabulary development. Here we will use the relation between these two skills as an example. Reading ability and vocabulary knowledge are highly correlated skills (Carroll, 1993). However, the relation between the two is far from simple: a relatively high number of rare words in a text is required before comprehension is disrupted (Freebody & Anderson, 1983), many poor comprehenders have age-appropriate vocabulary skills (Cain, Oakhill, et al., 2005), and reading comprehension is more highly correlated with vocabulary knowledge in older than in younger children (de Jong & van der Leij, 2002; Torgesen et al., 1997). Thus, it does not appear to simply be the case that text comprehension follows from word comprehension.

In his discussion of what he called "Matthew effects" in reading, Stanovich (1986) considered the mechanisms that may drive the complex relation between vocabulary knowledge and reading. Some beginner readers may start out with better vocabulary knowledge than others, perhaps because of superior early oral language and literacy experience. The children who are better readers with larger vocabularies at outset may subsequently read more than children with poorer word reading and vocabulary skills because the good readers derive more pleasure from reading. As a result, the better readers have more practice at reading and come across and learn a greater number of words in print, which develops their reading still further and, as a result, the gap between good and poor readers grows over time. There are two primary influences here: the better readers have greater exposure to the printed word over time and they are also more experienced at reading and deriving meaning from print, so they benefit more from exposure to new words (Stanovich, 1986; see also Daneman, 1988; Nagy, Herman, & Anderson, 1985).

There is a considerable body of work from Stanovich and Cunningham suggesting the importance of print exposure to growth in vocabulary and other literacy-related skills, such as spelling, word reading, and reading comprehension (Cunningham & Stanovich, 1997; Stanovich, 1993). Nation and colleagues have found that poor comprehenders have specific knowledge deficits for low-frequency exception words (Nation & Snowling, 1998a) and that poor comprehenders' errors on measures of syntactic production indicate a lack of familiarity with the irregular forms of verbs rather than a linguistic deficit, in contrast to children with specific language impairment (SLI; Nation et al., 2004). There is some indication of differences in out-of-school literacy activities between good and poor comprehenders (Cain, 1994; Cain & Oakhill, 2006b). For these reasons, it is tempting to speculate that poor comprehenders may fall further behind their peers not only in reading comprehension level, but also in other reading-related skills such as word reading, spelling, and vocabulary.

There are three reasons to urge caution in such speculation. First, there are very few studies tracking children with specific comprehension deficits across time, and these studies are crucial to determine the existence and strength of reciprocal relations. Second, the evidence for Matthew effects in other areas of reading development is inconclusive (see Scarborough, 2005, for a review). Third, our own work paints a more complex picture. We have explored whether poor comprehenders with different additional weaknesses differed in their language and literacy development between ages 8 and 11 years (Cain & Oakhill, 2006a). We found that the poor comprehenders with the weakest cognitive abilities at 8 years made less progress in reading comprehension across a 3-year period, but that their word-reading development was comparable to that of their peers. In contrast, the poor comprehenders with weaker vocabulary skills at outset experienced impaired growth in word-reading skills, although their reading comprehension development was comparable to that of peers. Thus, we may need to consider more complex interactive relations between language and literacy skills before we can accurately predict a child's developmental trajectory. Clearly, more longitudinal research is needed.

What Should Be the Aims for Teaching and Remediation?

The population of poor comprehenders that we have considered in this chapter have developed age-appropriate word-reading skills. Thus, it is clear that simply teaching children to read the words on the page will not ensure good reading comprehension. Comprehension of written and spoken language is underpinned by the same skills (see Oakhill & Cain, Chapter 1, this volume, for a fuller discussion of this point). Although there may be differences in the structure and register of language and the context between the two modalities, the aim of the reader or the listener is to derive a coherent representation of the text or discourse. Thus, we need to consider how best to teach poor comprehenders the skills and strategies that will enable them to achieve this goal.

The skills and strategies on which we have focused in this chapter, and which have consistently been found to be deficient in poor comprehenders, all help the reader or listener to construct coherent representations of meaning. *Inferences* are made to maintain coherence within a text, *anaphors* are solved to form cohesive links between successive sentences, *comprehension monitoring* aids the detection of inconsistencies that must be resolved through appropriate repair strategies if a text is to make sense, and an *appreciation of narrative structure* may aid the reader to establish causality between events, which will guide his or her understanding. With so many component skills implicated in good comprehension, which should we teach in our language classes and include in programs of remediation?

Earlier in this chapter, we discussed some recent studies that report different profiles of children with poor comprehension, all of whom have developed age-appropriate word-reading skills: for example, not all poor comprehenders had a deficit in vocabulary, or inference making, or comprehension monitoring. This work suggests that no one skill will be found to be deficient in all children with a poor comprehender profile. Indeed, it would be rather depressing if we were to find that *all* of the skills associated with good comprehension were deficient in *all* poor comprehenders. Thus, we clearly need to teach a range of comprehension-fostering skills if no one skill will ensure comprehension success.

This work also suggests that we should also consider different routes to comprehension difficulties and an individual child's strengths and weaknesses before embarking on a program of remediation. For example, throughout this book we will consider children who experience reading and listening comprehension failure with different fundamental deficits: children with SLI, who experience syntactic and pragmatic language difficulties; children with hearing impairment, who experience difficulties in acquiring good word-reading skills to support comprehension; and children with learning disabilities whose memory appears to limit their comprehension. For other children, initial poor lexical and sentence skills may limit comprehension and, in addition, restrict the development of discourse-level comprehension skills. Thus, some children may require a more comprehensive program of intervention.

CONCLUSIONS

The work reviewed in this chapter demonstrates that children with specific reading comprehension deficits experience difficulties on a range of language and literacy skills. Their difficulties extend to the comprehension of spoken language. We now have a large and fairly comprehensive catalogue of the skills associated with reading comprehension problems. However, although a large number of skills are correlates of poor comprehension, few have been found to be causally implicated in reading and listening comprehension difficulties. This does not mean that deficits in only a few skills lead to poor comprehension; rather, our understanding of the skills that are *causally implicated* in comprehension is still developing. One reason for this is that the studies needed to test theories of causality are expensive in terms of finance and research time and can only be properly designed once a core body of knowledge of skill deficits has been established. We believe that we now have that knowledge, and we hope that future research will strive to develop more comprehensive models of reading and listening comprehension development that will, in turn, lead to more effective interventions to help children with specific comprehension difficulties.

REFERENCES

Aarnoutse, C., van Leeuwe, J., Voeten, M., & Oud, H. (2001). Development of decoding, reading comprehension, vocabulary, and spelling during the elementary school years. *Reading and Writing, 14,* 61–89.

Barnes, M. A., & Dennis, M. (1998). Discourse after early-onset hydrocephalus: Core deficits in children of average intelligence. *Brain and Language, 61,* 309–334.

Bentin, S., Deutsch, A., & Liberman, I. Y. (1990). Syntactic competence and reading ability in children. *Journal of Experimental Child Psychology, 48,* 147–172.

Bishop, D. V. M. (1983). *Test for the Reception of Grammar.* Manchester, UK: Age and Cognitive Performance Research Centre, University of Manchester.

Bowey, J. A. (1994). Grammatical awareness and learning to read: A critique. In E. M. H. Assink (Ed.), *Literacy acquisition and social context* (pp. 122–149). New York: Harvester Wheatsheaf.

Bowyer-Crane, C., & Snowling, M. J. (2005). Assessing children's inference generation: What do tests of reading comprehension measure? *British Journal of Educational Psychology, 75,* 189–201.

Bradley, L., & Bryant, P. E. (1983). Categorising sounds and learning to read: A causal connexion. *Nature, 301,* 419–421.

Brown, A. L., Palincsar, A. S., & Armbruster, B. B. (1984). Instructing comprehension-fostering activities in interactive learning situations. In H. Mandl, N. L. Stein, & T. Trabasso (Eds.), *Learning and comprehension of text* (pp. 255–286). Hillsdale, NJ: Erlbaum.

Bryant, P., & Goswami, U. (1986). Strengths and weaknesses of the reading level design: A comment on Backman, Mamen and Ferguson. *Psychological Bulletin, 100,* 101–103.

Cain, K. (1994). *An investigation into comprehension difficulties in young children.* Sussex, UK: Unpublished PhD dissertation, University of Sussex.

Cain, K. (1996). Story knowledge and comprehension skill. In C. Cornoldi & J. V. Oakhill (Eds.), *Reading comprehension difficulties: Processes and remediation* (pp. 167–192). Mahwah, NJ: Erlbaum.

Cain, K. (1999). Ways of reading: How knowledge and use of strategies are related to reading comprehension. *British Journal of Developmental Psychology, 17,* 295–312.

Cain, K. (2003). Text comprehension and its relation to coherence and cohesion in children's fictional narratives. *British Journal of Developmental Psychology, 21,* 335-351.

Cain, K. (2006a). Children's reading comprehension: The role of working memory in normal and impaired development. In S. Pickering (Ed.), *Working memory and education* (pp. 62-91). San Diego: Academic Press.

Cain, K. (2006b). Individual differences in children's memory and reading comprehension: An investigation of semantic and inhibitory deficits. *Memory, 14,* 553-569.

Cain, K., & Oakhill, J. V. (1996). The nature of the relationship between comprehension skill and the ability to tell a story. *British Journal of Developmental Psychology, 14,* 187-201.

Cain, K., & Oakhill, J. V. (1999). Inference making and its relation to comprehension failure. *Reading and Writing: An Interdisciplinary Journal, 11,* 489-504.

Cain, K., & Oakhill, J. V. (2006a). Profiles of children with specific reading comprehension difficulties. *British Journal of Educational Psychology, 76,* 683-696.

Cain, K., & Oakhill, J. V. (2006b, July). *What happens to poor comprehenders?* Paper presented at the annual meeting of the Society for the Scientific Studies of Reading, Vancouver, British Columbia.

Cain, K., Oakhill, J. V., Barnes, M. A., & Bryant, P. E. (2001). Comprehension skill, inference making ability and their relation to knowledge. *Memory and Cognition, 29,* 850-859.

Cain, K., Oakhill, J. V., & Bryant, P. E. (2000a). Investigating the causes of reading comprehension failure: The comprehension–age match design. *Reading and Writing: An Interdisciplinary Journal, 12,* 31-40.

Cain, K., Oakhill, J. V., & Bryant, P. E. (2000b). Phonological skills and comprehension failure: A test of the phonological processing deficit hypothesis. *Reading and Writing: An Interdisciplinary Journal, 13,* 31-56.

Cain, K., Oakhill, J. V., & Bryant, P. E. (2004). Children's reading comprehension ability: Concurrent prediction by working memory, verbal ability, and component skills. *Journal of Educational Psychology, 96,* 31-42.

Cain, K., Oakhill, J. V., & Elbro, C. (2003). The ability to learn new word meanings from context by school-age children with and without language comprehension difficulties. *Journal of Child Language, 30,* 681-694.

Cain, K., Oakhill, J. V., & Lemmon, K. (2004). Individual differences in the inference of word meanings from context: The influence of reading comprehension, vocabulary knowledge, and memory capacity. *Journal of Educational Psychology, 96,* 671-681.

Cain, K., Oakhill, J. V., & Lemmon, K. (2005). The relation between children's reading comprehension level and their comprehension of idioms. *Journal of Experimental Child Psychology, 90,* 65-87.

Cain, K., Patson, N., & Andrews, L. (2005). Age- and ability-related differences in young readers' use of conjunctions. *Journal of Child Language, 32,* 877-892.

Carroll, J. B. (1993). *Human cognitive abilities: A survey of factor-analytic studies.* New York: Cambridge University Press.

Catts, H. W., Adlof, S. M., & Ellis Weismer, S. (2006). Language deficits in poor comprehenders: A case for the simple view of reading. *Journal of Speech Language and Hearing Research, 49,* 278–293.

Cornoldi, C., de Beni, R., & Pazzaglia, F. (1996). Profiles of reading comprehension difficulties: An analysis of single cases. In C. Cornoldi & J. Oakhill (Eds.), *Reading comprehension difficulties: Processes and interventions* (pp. 113–136). Mahwah, NJ: Erlbaum.

Cragg, L., & Nation, K. (2006). Exploring written narrative in children with poor reading comprehension. *Educational Psychology, 26,* 55–72.

Cunningham, A. E., & Stanovich, K. E. (1997). Early reading acquisition and its relation to reading experience and ability 10 years later. *Developmental Psychology, 33,* 934–945.

Daneman, M. (1988). Word knowledge and reading skill. In M. Daneman, G. MacKinnon, & T. G. Waller (Eds.), *Reading research: Advances in theory and practice* (Vol. 6, pp. 145–175). San Diego: Academic Press.

Daneman, M., & Merikle, P. M. (1996). Working memory and language comprehension: A meta-analysis. *Psychonomic Bulletin and Review, 3,* 422–433.

de Beni, R., & Palladino, P. (2000). Intrusion errors in working memory tasks: Are they related to reading comprehension ability? *Learning and Individual Differences, 12,* 131–143.

de Jong, P. F., & van der Leij, A. (2002). Effects of phonological abilities and linguistic comprehension on the development of reading. *Scientific Studies of Reading, 6,* 51–77.

Ehri, L. C. (1979). Linguistic insight: Threshold of reading acquisition. In T. G. Waller & G. E. MacKinnon (Eds.), *Reading research: Advances in theory and practice* (Vol. 1, pp. 63–114). New York: Academic Press.

Ehrlich, M. F. (1996). Metacognitive monitoring in the processing of anaphoric devices in skilled and less skilled comprehenders. In C. Cornoldi & J. V. Oakhill (Eds.), *Reading comprehension difficulties: Processes and remediation* (pp. 221–249). Mahwah, NJ: Erlbaum.

Ehrlich, M. F., & Rémond, M. (1997). Skilled and less skilled comprehenders: French children's processing of anaphoric devices in written texts. *British Journal of Developmental Psychology, 15,* 291–309.

Ehrlich, M. F., Rémond, M., & Tardieu, H. (1999). Processing of anaphoric devices in young skilled and less skilled comprehenders: Differences in metacognitive monitoring. *Reading and Writing: An Interdisciplinary Journal, 11,* 29–63.

Feagans, L., & Appelbaum, M. I. (1986). Validation of language subtypes in learning disabled children. *Journal of Educational Psychology, 78,* 358–364.

Forrest-Pressley, D. L., & Waller, T. G. (1984). *Cognition, metacognition, and reading.* New York: Springer-Verlag.

Freebody, P., & Anderson, R. C. (1983). Effects on text comprehension of differing proportions and locations of difficult vocabulary. *Journal of Reading Behavior, 15,* 19–39.

Gaux, C., & Gombert, J. E. (1999). Implicit and explicit syntactic knowledge and reading in pre-adolescents. *British Journal of Developmental Psychology, 17,* 169–188.

Hulme, C., & Snowling, M. (1992). Deficits in output phonology: A cause of reading failure? *Cognitive Neuropsychology, 9*, 47–72.

Jetton, T. L., Rupley, W. H., & Willson, V. L. (1995). Comprehension of narrative and expository texts: The role of content, topic, discourse, and strategy knowledge. In K. A. Hinchman, D. J. Leu, & C. K. Kinzer (Eds.), *Perspectives on literacy research and practice: Forty-fourth yearbook of the National Reading Conference* (pp. 197–204). Chicago: National Reading Conference.

Kirby, J. R., & Moore, P. J. (1987). Metacognitive awareness about reading and its relation to reading ability. *Journal of Psychoeducational Learning, 2*, 119–137.

Layton, A., Robinson, J., & Lawson, M. (1998). The relationship between syntactic awareness and reading performance. *Journal of Research in Reading, 21*, 5–23.

Levorato, M. C., & Cacciari, C. (1992). Children's comprehension and production of idioms: The role of context and familiarity. *Journal of Child Language, 19*, 415–433.

Levorato, M. C., Nesi, B., & Cacciari, C. (2004). Reading comprehension and understanding idiomatic expressions: A developmental study. *Brain and Language, 91*, 303–314.

Long, D. L., Oppy, B. J., & Seely, M. R. (1994). Individual differences in the time course of inferential processing. *Journal of Experimental Psychology, 20*, 1456–1470.

Long, D. L., Oppy, B. J., & Seely, M. R. (1997). Individual differences in readers' sentence- and text-level representations. *Journal of Memory and Language, 36*, 129–145.

McGee, A., & Johnson, H. (2003). The effect of inference training on skilled and less skilled comprehenders. *Educational Psychology, 23*, 49–59.

McGregor, K. K. (2004). Developmental dependencies between lexical semantics and reading. In C. A. Stone, E. R. Silliman, B. J. Ehren, & K. Apel (Eds), *Handbook of language and literacy: Development and disorders* (pp. 302–317). New York: Guilford Press.

Mergherbi, H., & Ehrlich, M. F. (2005). Language impairment in less skilled comprehenders: The on-line processing of anaphoric pronouns in a listening situation. *Reading and Writing: An Interdisciplinary Journal, 18*, 715–753.

Nagy, W. E., Herman, P. A., & Anderson, R. C. (1985). Learning words from context. *Reading Research Quarterly, 20*, 233–253.

Nation, K., Adams, J. W., Bowyer-Crane, C. A., & Snowling, M. J. (1999). Working memory deficits in poor comprehenders reflect underlying language impairments. *Journal of Experimental Child Psychology, 73*, 139–158.

Nation, K., Clarke, P., Marshall, C. M., & Durand, M. (2004). Hidden language impairments in children: Parallels between poor reading comprehension and specific language impairment? *Journal of Speech, Language, and Hearing Research, 47*, 199–211.

Nation, K., & Snowling, M. J. (1998a). Individual differences in contextual facilitation: Evidence from dyslexia and poor reading comprehension. *Child Development, 69*, 996–1011.

Nation, K., & Snowling, M. J. (1998b). Semantic processing and the development of word-recognition skills: Evidence from children with reading comprehension difficulties. *Journal of Memory and Language, 39,* 85–101.

Nation, K., & Snowling, M. J. (1999). Developmental differences in sensitivity to semantic relations among good and poor comprehenders: Evidence from semantic priming. *Cognition, 70,* 81–83

Nation, K., & Snowling, M. J. (2000). Factors influencing syntactic awareness in normal readers and poor comprehenders. *Applied Psycholinguistics, 21,* 229–241.

Oakhill, J. V. (1982). Constructive processes in skilled and less-skilled comprehenders' memory for sentences. *British Journal of Psychology, 73,* 13–20.

Oakhill, J. V. (1983). Instantiation in skilled and less-skilled comprehenders. *Quarterly Journal of Experimental Psychology, 35A,* 441–450.

Oakhill, J. V. (1984). Inferential and memory skills in children's comprehension of stories. *British Journal of Educational Psychology, 54,* 31–39.

Oakhill, J. V., Cain, K., & Bryant, P. E. (2003). The dissociation of word reading and text comprehension: Evidence from component skills. *Language and Cognitive Processes, 18,* 443–468.

Oakhill, J. V., Hartt, J., & Samols, D. (2005). Levels of comprehension monitoring and working memory in good and poor comprehenders. *Reading and Writing: An Interdisciplinary Journal, 18,* 657–686.

Oakhill, J. V., & Yuill, N. M. (1986). Pronoun resolution in skilled and less skilled comprehenders: Effects of memory load and inferential complexity. *Language and Speech, 29,* 25–37.

Oakhill, J. V., Yuill, N. M., & Parkin, A. (1986). On the nature of the difference between skilled and less-skilled comprehenders. *Journal of Research in Reading, 9,* 80–91.

Paris, S. G., Carpenter, R. D., Paris, A. H., & Hamilton, E. E. (2005). Spurious and genuine correlates of children's reading comprehension. In S. G. Paris & S. A. Stahl (Eds.), *Children's reading comprehension and assessment* (pp. 131–160). Mahwah, NJ: Erlbaum.

Paris, S. G., & Jacobs, J. E. (1984). The benefits of informed instruction for children's reading awareness and comprehension skills. *Child Development, 55,* 2083–2093.

Paris, S. G., Saarnio, D. A., & Cross, D. R. (1986). A metacognitive curriculum to promote children's reading and learning. *Australian Journal of Psychology, 38,* 107–123.

Perfetti, C. A. (1994). Psycholinguistics and reading ability. In M. A. Gernsbacher (Ed.), *Handbook of psycholinguistics* (pp. 849–894). San Diego: Academic Press.

Scarborough, H. S. (2005). Developmental relations between language and reading: Reconciling a beautiful hypothesis with some ugly facts. In H. W. Catts & A. G. Kamhi (Eds.), *The connections between language and reading disabilities* (pp. 3–24). Mahwah, NJ: Erlbaum.

Shankweiler, D. (1989). How problems of comprehension are related to difficulties in decoding. In D. Shankweiler & I. Y. Liberman (Eds.), *Phonology and reading disability: Solving the reading puzzle* (pp. 35–68). Ann Arbor: University of Michigan Press.

Smith, S. T., Macaruso, P., Shankweiler, D., & Crain, S. (1989). Syntactic comprehension in young poor readers. *Applied Psycholinguistics, 10*, 429–454.

Snyder, L. S., & Downey, D. M. (1991). The language–reading relationship in normal and reading-disabled children. *Journal of Speech and Hearing Research, 34*, 129–140.

Stanovich, K. E. (1986). Matthew effects in reading: Some consequences of individual differences in the acquisition of literacy. *Reading Research Quarterly, 21*, 360–407.

Stanovich, K. E. (1993). Does reading make you smarter?: Literacy and the development of verbal intelligence. In H. Reese (Ed.), *Advances in child development and behavior* (Vol. 24, pp. 133–180). New York: Academic Press.

Stothard, S. E., & Hulme, C. (1992). Reading comprehension difficulties in children: The role of language comprehension and working memory skills. *Reading and Writing: An Interdisciplinary Journal, 4*, 245–256.

Stothard, S. E., & Hulme, C. (1995). A comparison of phonological skills in children with reading comprehension difficulties and children with word reading difficulties. *Journal of Child Psychology and Child Psychiatry, 36*, 399–408.

Swanson, H. L., & Berninger, V. (1995). The role of working memory in skilled and less skilled readers' comprehension. *Intelligence, 21*, 83–108.

Torgesen, J. K., Wagner, R. K., Rashotte, C. A., Burgess, S., & Hecht, S. (1997). Contributions of phonological awareness and rapid automatic naming ability to the growth of word-reading skills in second- to fifth-grade children. *Scientific Studies of Reading, 1*, 161–185.

Trabasso, T., & Nickels, M. (1992). The development of goal plans of action in the narration of a picture story. *Discourse Processes, 15*, 249–276.

van den Broek, P., Kendeou, P., Kermer, K., Lynch, J., Butler, J., White, M. J., et al. (2005). Assessment of comprehension abilities in young children. In S. G. Paris & S. A. Stahl (Eds.), *Children's reading comprehension and assessment* (pp. 107–130), Mahwah, NJ: Erlbaum.

Wagner, R., & Torgesen, J. K. (1987). The nature of phonological processing and its causal role in the acquisition of reading skills. *Psychological Bulletin, 101*, 192–212.

Yuill, N. M., & Joscelyne, T. (1988). Effect of organisational cues and strategies on good and poor comprehenders' story understanding. *Journal of Educational Psychology, 80*, 152–158.

Yuill, N. M., & Oakhill, J. V. (1988). Understanding of anaphoric relations in skilled and less skilled comprehenders. *British Journal of Psychology, 79*, 173–186.

Yuill, N. M., & Oakhill, J. V. (1991). *Children's problems in text comprehension: An experimental investigation.* Cambridge: UK: Cambridge University Press.

Yuill, N. M., Oakhill, J. V., & Parkin, A. J. (1989). Working memory, comprehension ability and the resolution of text anomaly. *British Journal of Psychology, 80*, 351–361.

PART II

Comprehension Impairments in Children with Developmental Disorders

The chapters in this part consider the written and spoken language comprehension difficulties experienced by children with particular developmental disorders: children with specific language impairment (SLI) and pragmatic language impairment (PLI), children with autism spectrum disorders (ASD),[1] children with attention-deficit/hyperactivity disorder (ADHD), and children with learning disabilities (LD). In addition to other language and communication difficulties, these populations often experience problems with skills that are crucial to comprehending extended text and discourse.

In Chapter 3, Botting considers the language profiles of children with SLI and PLI. Both groups are impaired on measures of written and spoken language comprehension that tap, for example, inference generation and understanding of figurative expressions such as idioms. One question raised is the extent to which these language impairments can be considered "specific" and to exist independently of more

---

[1]Please note that the National Autistic Society (United Kingdom) uses the term "autistic spectrum disorders," while the U.S. National Institute of Mental Health uses "autism spectrum disorders." The acronym ASD used in this volume is intended to cover both usages of the term.

general cognitive impairment. Botting reviews the wider cognitive skills of these groups—notably, short-term memory, nonverbal IQ, and social cognition—and finds that children and adolescents with SLI are impaired in all three areas. However, to determine the direction of causality, we need to consider the interaction between these and other skills during the course of typical and atypical development. A key finding is that the diagnosis of SLI is not stable: As Botting states, "receptive abilities may wax and wane over time." Botting's own work suggests that skills once considered to be intact, such as nonverbal IQ, are not necessary spared throughout the course of development and suggests the need for longitudinal studies to map the interaction between nonverbal and receptive language abilities in atypical populations. This work suggests an important role for early and effective intervention.

Children with ASD often experience significant language and comprehension impairments: Indeed, many lack verbal communication skills. In Chapter 4, Leekam reviews the nature of the language difficulties experienced by verbal children with autism and the different cognitive explanations that have been proposed to account for their difficulties. Although children with ASD are noted for their pragmatic language impairments, they can also have language comprehension difficulties similar to those found in children with SLI, most notably structural language impairments. Leekam identifies two problems with cognitive explanations of ASD. First, the cognitive deficits are not specific to children with ASD. Second, rather than providing an explanation for the language deficits experienced by children with ASD, recent research suggests that language impairment might be the causal factor in these deficits. She concludes that we need to consider the similarities that exist between different groups with language problems to develop better focused interventions. We also need to look at the process of development, from early attentional and perceptual abilities to later complex language skills, to understand more fully the origins of the language comprehension difficulties experienced by children with ASD.

Comprehension of written and spoken narratives is often considered a more ecologically valid means to assess language understanding in young children than many more laboratory-style experimental tasks (see, e.g., Botting, Chapter 3). In Chapter 5, Lorch, Berthiaume, Milich, and van den Broek review their innovative approach to the study of narrative comprehension in children with ADHD: the television-viewing methodology. This technique enables the study of processes common to the understanding of both written and spoken text, namely, understanding of the causal relations among story events, use of the goal structure of a story to build a coherent representation of meaning, identification of important information, and generation of inferences and monitoring of ongoing understanding of the story (e.g., van den Broek, 1990). Both visual attention and comprehension and memory for the narrative are recorded. Their experimental work shows that children with attention deficits are not typically impaired in their recall of story facts (see also Cain & Oakhill, Chapter 2, this volume). Their difficulties are related to skills that aid the construction of an integrated representation of meaning, including understanding of the causal relations between story events, use of story goal structure to guide integration, and inference generation. The identification of key skill deficits leads to specific suggestions for interventions, such as strategies that children can be taught to help them to use story structure to guide their comprehension.

In Chapter 6, the final chapter in this part, we turn to the relation between working memory and reading comprehension in children with LD. Adequate memory skills are crucial to support the processing required to extract meaning from text and discourse. In Chapter 6, Swanson, Howard, and Sáez pursue the theory that memory weaknesses underpin specific language comprehension difficulties. Their previous research demonstrates that executive-processing deficits exist in this group independent of their deficits in phonological processing. This profile is in contrast to the well-established phonological-processing difficulties often found in children with developmental dyslexia (e.g., Snowling, 2000). In their recent work, they explore further the specificity of the relations between memory processes and reading comprehension. To disentangle these relations, they compare the performance of three types of reader on a range of memory and memory-related tasks: children with word-reading and reading comprehension deficits, children with adequate word recognition skills but poor comprehension, and children with poor word reading and comprehension in the presence of low verbal intelligence. As one might expect, all of the groups perform poorly relative to a control group of skilled readers. The key findings presented here are the distinct differences between the poor reader groups. For example, storage difficulties appear to be specific to children with both poor word reading and poor comprehension, whereas performance on tasks that tap the executive system discriminate poor comprehenders from skilled readers.

Similar to other populations studied in this volume, the working memory differences that emerge between the skilled and the less skilled readers appear to be related to processes that are nonspecific to reading (see also Cain, 2006, for a review of the working memory impairments of poor comprehenders). They conclude that interventions must focus on strategies that will compensate for these working memory impairments.

Together, these chapters provide a detailed insight into the comprehension problems experienced by these diverse populations. There are common findings: the comprehension difficulties experienced by these populations are not specific to presentation modality and go beyond comprehension of the single word. The research presented in these chapters has, to a large extent, investigated deficits in individual skills and processes that may be necessary to construct meaning—for example, inference, attention, and memory. This focused and meticulous approach is essential to identify which individual skills and processes are specifically related to each population's comprehension difficulties. An emergent theme is the complexity of language comprehension and the need to study the interaction between different language skills and processing systems as comprehension develops over time.

REFERENCES

Cain K. (2006). Children's reading comprehension: the role of working memory in normal and impaired development. In S. Pickering (Ed.), *Working memory and education* (pp. 61–91). San Diego: Academic Press.

Snowling, M. J. (2000). *Dyslexia* (2nd ed.). Oxford, UK: Blackwell.

van den Broek, P. (1990). Causal inferences in the comprehension of narrative texts. In A. C. Graesser & G. H. Bowler (Eds.), *The psychology of learning and motivation: Inferences and text comprehension* (Vol. 25, pp. 175–194). San Diego: Academic Press.

CHAPTER 3

Comprehension Difficulties in Children with Specific Language Impairment and Pragmatic Language Impairment

NICOLA BOTTING

CHILDREN WITH SPECIFIC LANGUAGE IMPAIRMENT: WHO ARE THEY?

Specific language impairment (SLI) is the term currently used to describe children who have significant language difficulties without identifiable cause such as global delay, neurological impairment, physical disability, deafness, or autism spectrum disorders (ASD). The incidence of children who experience language-learning difficulties has been documented for around 100 years. Such children comprise about 7% of the population (Tomblin et al., 1997). SLI is reported to affect this large minority. Indeed, an increasing number of studies document this population.

Despite this, the comprehension skills of children with SLI have perhaps received less attention than their expressive or phonological skills. Key texts such as Bishop (1997) have served to highlight the need for more research in this area. Furthermore, it is now becoming increasingly evident that individuals with SLI have long-term difficulties extending beyond middle childhood (Conti-Ramsden, Botting,

Simkin, & Knox, 2001) and into adulthood (Clegg, Hollis, Mawhood, & Rutter, 2005). The etiology of SLI is still not clear despite many decades of investigations into the area. However, recent studies point toward a genetic influence. The data include increased evidence of familial aggregation (Tallal, Ross & Curtiss, 1989; Choudhury & Benasich, 2003), higher rates of concordance in monozygotic compared to dizygotic twins (Bishop, North, & Donlan, 1995; Tomblin & Buckwalter, 1998), and the identification of specific gene sites in affected individuals (SLI Consortium, 2002). The SLI Consortium (2002) has narrowed the search for a genetic basis for SLI to chromosomes 16 and 19, which are both implicated in language impairment across families using generalized language measures and independent of nonverbal IQ.

SLI is not a unitary disorder: It encompasses a number of different types of language profiles. Several attempts have been made at subgrouping the wider SLI population (e.g., Conti-Ramsden, Crutchley, & Botting, 1997; Rapin, 1996), but in the main, the following terms are used: expressive SLI (which refers to children who only have difficulty *producing* language); receptive SLI (which refers to children who only have difficulties *understanding* language); and mixed expressive-receptive SLI (referring to children with *both* types of difficulty) who make up the largest proportion of those with long-term language challenges (Conti-Ramsden & Botting, 1999). These terms are also those referred to in diagnostic manuals such as DSM-IV (American Psychiatric Association, 1994) and the ICD-10 (World Health Organization, 1992).

WHAT IS PRAGMATIC LANGUAGE IMPAIRMENT?

Children with pragmatic language impairment (PLI) are another subgroup of children with language impairment recognized in both research and clinical practice. These children have social language difficulties, but not autism, and are often referred to as having "semantic pragmatic disorder." These children have been described a number of times in the literature (Bishop, 1998; Bishop & Adams, 1992; Bishop & Norbury, 2002; Bishop & Rosenbloom, 1987; Botting & Conti-Ramsden, 1999; Boucher, 1998; McTear & Conti-Ramsden, 1992). Children with PLI tend to be able to produce complex sentences (although usually not entirely without errors) and are often verbose. However, they have a poor understanding of functional communication including turn taking, poor understanding of roles, limited conversational topics, a lack of sensitivity to social cues, and a tendency to give too much or too little information.

It is not certain if, in fact, these children are individuals with high-functioning autism or Asperger syndrome. Some researchers believe that no separate distinction should be made between PLI and ASD (Brook & Bowler, 1988; Shields, Varley, Broks, & Simpson, 1996). This group may also overlap with those who have pervasive developmental disorder not otherwise specified (PDDNOS), a label used more often in psychiatry. The precise definition of this term is also unclear, but it tends to be used to describe children with autistic symptoms who do not fully meet criteria for this disorder (see Cox et al., 1999). However, some recent studies (Bishop & Norbury, 2002; Botting & Conti-Ramsden, 1999; Conti-Ramsden, Simkin, & Botting, 2006) have found clear cases of children who were experiencing pragmatic difficulties but who could not be described as having PDDNOS or autism using the gold standard measures of the Autism Diagnostic Observation Schedule (ADOS; Lord et al., 1997). Furthermore, those described as PLI and ASD, respectively, show different patterns of difficulty on measures of pragmatic language skills and other psycholinguistic tasks (Botting, 2004; Botting & Conti-Ramsden, 2003).

RESEARCH INTO
THE COMPREHENSION DIFFICULTIES
OF CHILDREN WITH LANGUAGE IMPAIRMENTS

Prevalence of Comprehension Difficulties within SLI and PLI Groups

As this chapter concerns comprehension difficulties, it is important to note how many children with SLI are thought to have such receptive language difficulties. However, this proves not to be an easy question to answer. In a study "mapping out" children attending educational provision that specialized in language disorders, Gina Conti-Ramsden and I found that around one-third had expressive and receptive difficulties when measured on standardized tests at 7 years of age (Conti-Ramsden, Crutchley, & Botting, 1997; Conti-Ramsden & Botting, 1999). The proportion was similar when the children were assessed the following year. However, the individual trajectories of the children were not static. Indeed, regarding children between 7 and 14 years of age, we find that those with SLI move "in and out" of having receptive difficulties. The stability of subgroup membership (i.e., whether children could be described as expressive SLI or mixed expressive–

receptive SLI) is around 50% between any two time points. Interestingly, however, children who had receptive difficulties at age 7 were significantly more likely than those with only expressive difficulties at age 7 to have a mixed expressive–receptive profile at age 14.

For children with PLI, receptive difficulties are a key characteristic of the disorder (Bishop, 1997; McTear & Conti-Ramsden, 1992). However, it is also true that because of the strengths this group may have, they may "appear" not to have receptive difficulties when tested on formal measures of language comprehension. For example, they may have good rote memory or phonological skills (Chiat, 2001) and they may perform well in highly structured testing paradigms. The issue of measurement is discussed in more detail later. However, compared to work on children with the more typical SLI profile, relatively little work has been done to investigate the receptive profiles of children with PLI. Indeed, there is no work to my knowledge on the development of receptive skills in this population. An interesting study recently highlighted the different language profiles using a standardized assessment of receptive and expressive language: a group with SLI, a group with ASD, and a group with "shared symptoms" (similar to a PLI group) all exhibited slightly different profiles of receptive language. In particular, those with shared symptoms looked more similar to peers with ASD in terms of receptive–expressive discrepancy (Lloyd, Paintin, & Botting, 2006).

Different Types of Receptive Difficulties in SLI and PLI

Receptive difficulties can take many different forms and can be assessed in a variety of ways (see Bishop, 1997, for an overview). Receptive vocabulary skills are some of the first language skills to emerge in typically developing children. Thus they are sometimes used by researchers as an index of cognitive ability. But often *difficulties* in this area are not recognized by caregivers and health professionals until later expressive difficulties become apparent. Early measures of receptive vocabulary include parent checklists such as the Macarthur Bates Child Development Inventory (MCDI: UKSF; Dale, Price, Bishop, & Plomin, 2003), on which parents indicate which words their own child can understand. There are also more direct measures like the British Picture Vocabulary Scale II (Dunn, Dunn, Whetton, & Burley, 1998) in which children are asked to point at the correct picture out of four after hearing a spoken word. However, structured test environments are different to real-life comprehension scenarios. Clinicians report that older children sometimes show good receptive vocabulary skills while still having relatively poor comprehension of language.

Children with SLI are well documented as having particular difficulties with expressive morphology and syntax (see Leonard, 1998), and their comprehension of these aspects of language is also affected. Thus judgments of correct or incorrect morphology prove difficult for children with SLI. The Rice–Wexler Test of Early Grammatical Impairment (Rice & Wexler, 2001) assesses this by saying, for example, "Teddy says 'here are two fork'—did he say it right or not so good?" In addition, complex sentences that involve embedded clauses—for example, "The bus, which was running late, arrived outside the house"—or with complex spatial relationships—"The brown dog is under the green table"—are difficult for children with SLI to comprehend.

The Test for Reception of Grammar (TROG; Bishop, 1982), which directly tests the understanding of such structures, is one of the most commonly used tests of receptive syntax. Children with SLI commonly do poorly on this task (see Bishop, 1997, for a review). Furthermore, children with SLI have more difficulty acting on sentences where the morphology and the syntax provide clues to the action. For example, in studies using sentences such as "Big Bird is tickling Elmo," children must use the syntactic and morphological cues to correctly act out the sentence using the characters (Hirsch-Pasek & Golinkoff, 1996). Other tasks included on composite assessments such as the Clinical Evaluation of Language Fundamentals (CELF-3; Semel, Wiig, & Secord, 1995) are also designed to measure difficulties with syntactic complexity, as well as to assess other forms of receptive language ability. However, in a recent study mentioned earlier (Lloyd et al., 2006), the Listening to Paragraphs subtest from the CELF, which is often used as a key measure of receptive ability in clinical practice, was shown to be the strongest subtest relative to others for a "shared symptom" (or PLI) group as well as for the ASD group. This was despite the fact that both groups showed lower overall receptive language scores when compared to expressive language. This study highlights the need for comprehensive assessment across a number of different receptive skills in pragmatically impaired groups.

A difficulty in the comprehension of syntactically complex utterances has substantial implications for whether children with SLI are able to access educational and therapeutic inputs. As children become older, they are increasingly disadvantaged in adult conversation, a large proportion of which tends to consist of complex sentences. For children with PLI, syntactic understanding may appear relatively good compared to those with more typical SLI, especially in the context of a structured test, but some children with PLI have substantial grammatical difficulties even in the expressive form (Botting & Conti-Ramsden, 1999).

In contrast to the wealth of information about syntactic ability in SLI, relatively little is known about SLI and the more subtle impairments of semantic and pragmatic comprehension, such as nonliteral language, idioms, and inference. This is despite the fact that these areas are core skills in early language learning and are essential to competent conversation (Leionen & Kerbel, 1999). The studies that *have* been conducted show that children with SLI are impaired on idiom comprehension tasks (Kerbel & Grunwell, 1998), tests of nonliteral language (Vance & Wells, 1994; Bishop & Adams, 1992), and in understanding inference (Botting & Adams, 2005). In the last of these, children with SLI, children with PLI, and children with typical development were read a picture-book story and subsequently asked to say whether statements about the story were true or false. To answer correctly, children had to infer information from the text and pictures. Figure 3.1 illustrates an example page from the book, the text that was read to the child, and a related response item.

Perhaps surprisingly, these investigations have failed to find the predicted difference between the children with typical SLI and those with PLI, who reportedly show more obvious difficulty with these aspects of language in everyday conversation. There are a number of reasons that studies may not find those differences. It may be that both groups have difficulties in their comprehension of higher-level language, but that for children with PLI this difference is more marked in everyday conversation because these difficulties exist in the context of their verbosity and use of syntactically complex language. Alternatively, heavy verbal-processing loads inherent in many tasks might cause the children with SLI (who are now known to have processing difficulties; see Montgomery, 2003, 2004) to perform especially poorly under

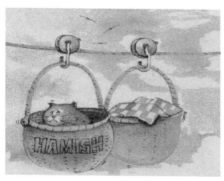

Picture 8: Poor Hamish. His fur stood on end when the basket swayed and he felt much too sick to even notice the seagulls.

Inference item: Hamish liked being in the basket (false).

FIGURE 3.1. An example part of inferencing stimuli used in Botting and Adams (2005).

experimental conditions. Such difficulties may be minimized in natu-ralistic settings by other available strategies (such as the use of visual cues).

Some other work highlights the potential role of narrative to assess receptive difficulties. Naturalistic language samples may provide useful additional qualitative information about the comprehension level of some children. For example, in narrative there is more poten-tial to separate semantic and pragmatic skills, which are intertwined and often considered together. In an analysis of words used in sponta-neous picture narratives (where the target item was obvious from the story and the picture), children with PLI appeared to be substituting words in a qualitatively different way from children with typical SLI, causing more of a *pragmatic* breakdown (Botting & Conti-Ramsden, 1999). Where those with SLI might replace the word *antlers* with another similar word such as *horns* or a nondescriptive word like *things*, children with PLI were more likely to pick unrelated alternatives such as *stunk* for *stuck* or to use neologisms such as *stickfire* for match. Although these are essentially expressive differences, these substitu-tions may provide insight into the understanding of words themselves and of their communicative effect. Furthermore, children with SLI show a weaker relationship between semantic and pragmatic language skills than those with PLI or with typical development (Botting & Adams, 2005), perhaps suggesting that they complete tasks in qualita-tively different ways from those in the other groups. Norbury and Bishop (2002) also found a complex relationship between diagnostic group and narrative comprehension. Although they found no differ-ences between groups of children with SLI, PLI and ASD in the abso-lute number of target inferences made, when the errors were further analyzed, some of the children with PLI and ASD made inferences that were not always relevant to the story. Nevertheless, two-thirds of the PLI group still scored within normal limits.

Another method of assessing some aspects of comprehension, particularly those involving pragmatic skill, is the use of checklists about a child's language understanding (see Adams, 2002, for a com-prehensive review). In particular, Bishop's (1998) Children's Communi-cation Checklist (CCC), which assesses some aspects of comprehension as well as other conversational skills, appears to be very successful. The CCC was designed as a research tool, but is now available as a clinical measure. Bishop (1998) reports that scores on this checklist (when completed by a professional who knows the child) produced good group-level discrimination between those with SLI who did not show more subtle comprehension difficulties and those with marked prag-matic language impairments. The checklist comprises nine subscales of communication and interactive behavior: speech, syntax, inappropriate initiation,* coherence,* stereotyped conversation,* context,* rapport,* social behavior, and interests. A composite "pragmatic impairment score" can be derived from the middle five scales marked "*" above and a score of 132 or below is used as a cutoff for pragmatic language impairment. Each scale consists of a number of behavioral items that professionals are asked to rate as "does not apply," "applies somewhat," or "definitely applies." The interrater reliability for the pragmatic scale has been shown to be very good when used in populations with communication difficulties and produces different ranges of scores between different clinical subgroups as well as between those with atypical and typical development (Bishop & Baird, 2001; Botting, 2004). Although this measure does not directly assess comprehension alone, it may indicate that a checklist is an ecologically valid assessment tool when we consider complex receptive difficulties.

Our understanding of how to assess these more subtle receptive skills is gradually improving. Recent studies have sought to directly compare assessments in groups of children with complex receptive difficulties. Adams and Lloyd (2005), for example, found that a conversational task was superior to a communicative function elicitation task. More recent formal tests, such as the Assessment of Comprehension and Expression (Adams, Cooke, Crutchley, Hesketh, & Reeves, 2000), have begun to include tasks of inference, nonliteral language, and narrative. However, our knowledge is still limited in this respect and the poor sensitivity of available tests may contribute to some of the differential findings reported between production and comprehension.

THE RELATIONSHIP BETWEEN COGNITION AND LANGUAGE IN CHILDREN WITH SLI AND PLI

In typical development, comprehension at the word level is developing throughout childhood. Very young typically developing children cannot always correctly understand semantic roles for agent and patient using novel transitive verbs (e.g., *Minnie is dakking Tigger*; Skipp, Windfuhr, & Conti-Ramsden, 2002). Furthermore, in a series of insightful experiments with 5-year-olds, McGregor (2002) showed that the semantic lexicon includes functional and physical features, and that the risk of semantic retrieval error for a word is related to the degree of semantic *knowledge* about that lexicon. The ability to retrieve the meaning of the word is not just related to whether you know what it means, it is also related to how *much* you know about it. This latter study reveals something about the conceptual element in typical comprehension development that is not always easy to detect.

Specific Cognitive Difficulties in SLI and PLI

One of the interesting aspects of SLI is that it has been used theoretically to represent evidence that language impairment can exist independently of more general cognitive difficulty, hence the term "specific." However, questions have been raised recently about whether the impairments seen in this group of individuals can really be termed "specific" at all. A discussion of the interplay between cognition and language in this widely heterogeneous clinical group forms the basis of much of this chapter.

While the cognitive underpinnings of comprehension difficulties in SLI are not entirely clear, numerous studies have shown that some specific cognitive skills, both verbal and nonverbal, are often affected in those with SLI. For example children with SLI have been shown to be poorer than their peers on tasks measuring phonological memory (Gathercole & Baddeley, 1990), verbal memory (Ellis-Weismer, Evans & Hesketh, 1999), visuospatial memory span (Hick, Botting, & Conti-Ramsden, 2005), symbolic play (Roth & Clark, 1987), and spatial rotation (Johnston & Ellis-Weismer, 1983; see Leonard, 1998, for a full discussion). Thus it appears that SLI cannot be used to argue convincingly for a dissociation between language and cognition. Indeed, many now consider that cognitive models can explain the causes and mechanisms behind SLI (in direct contrast to a modular "innate grammar" theory).

There are different cognitive models under consideration by researchers including the working memory model developed by Baddeley (1986), which posits separate domains for verbal/phonological and visuospatial processing, along with a controlling central executive; and an alternative model of functional working memory or limited capacity models such as that of Just and Carpenter (1992), who describe a domain-general system in which storage and processing of information are directly competing for space. The most frequently explored construct in SLI is that of phonological working memory, which is usually assessed using tests of nonword repetition. A large body of research now shows that children with SLI have difficulties with this task (Conti-Ramsden & Botting, 2001; Gathercole & Baddeley, 1990; Stothard, Snowling, Bishop, Chipchase, & Kaplan, 1998), that it shows heritability (Bishop, North, & Donlan, 1995), and that nonword tasks relate to language development over time and to language status, even when general IQ is controlled for (Botting & Conti-Ramsden,

2001; Walker & Archibald, 2006). However, the direct associations between this deficit and comprehension are rarely studied.

Other researchers have focused on verbal short-term memory in SLI using limited capacity models. Ellis-Weismer and colleagues (1999) found that children with SLI were impaired on "competing language tasks" (in which children must make a judgment about the veracity of a statement while they are also remembering the final word) and that performance on these tasks was related to sentence comprehension. Montgomery (2003) has also conducted a series of studies over the past decade examining the possible cognitive associations with comprehension difficulties in SLI. A number of different factors appeared to predict receptive language ability. In one study, for example, the rate of input of sentences was varied. Comprehension of typically developing children (including a younger group matched for receptive syntax ability) was not affected by input rate. However, for those with SLI, slower presentation rate increased the performance of the group with SLI so that it was in line with that of the younger language-matched children (Montgomery, 2004). In a study comparing children with hearing impairment and language impairment on a number of sentence comprehension and processing tasks, Norbury, Bishop, and Briscoe (2002) also concluded that limited processing capacity was a more likely explanation for the data than a model that posited an innate "grammar module."

However, specific cognitive difficulties in SLI are not restricted to the verbal domain or to memory, but may also include visual short-term memory as well as non-memory spatial abilities (Bavin, Wilson, Maruff, & Sleeman, 2005; Hick et al., 2005). In a recent study by Hick and colleagues (2005) developmental time was shown to be of vital importance when considering the possible dynamics of cognition and language in atypical development. Three groups of children participated: those with typical development, those with Down syndrome, and those with SLI. All were matched on nonverbal mental age at the start of the study, but over the course of a year groups showed different pathways of development on a pattern recall task. Surprisingly, perhaps, it was the children with SLI who showed the flattest trajectory and thus the least improvement in this nonverbal skill. In a study of unaffected siblings of those with SLI that is still in progress (Botting, in preparation), the data suggests that while siblings outperform those with SLI on nonverbal IQ tests, the pattern of strengths and weaknesses on the different subtests is strikingly similar, and statistically different to that of typically developing children matched on overall nonverbal cognitive ability. Bavin and colleagues also reported further evidence of limitations in spatial span, pattern recall, and "associative" learning of patterns and locations, indicating that memory difficulties extend beyond that of phonological short-term memory (Bavin et al., 2005).

If individuals with SLI and PLI experience different aspects of comprehension difficulty (or at least a different balance or profile of weaknesses), it may be interesting to consider how these groups differ cognitively in general terms. It may be important, for instance, that children with PLI tend to have higher nonverbal IQs than non-PLI peers with SLI. It may be that this is an artefact of identification, that only children whose pragmatic skill is clearly out of line with their cognitive skill are recognized and referred. However, even in studies controlling for nonverbal IQ, children with PLI do not seem as susceptible to the phonological memory deficits that are now thought to be characteristic of SLI (Botting & Conti-Ramsden, 2003; Gathercole & Baddeley, 1990). Furthermore, those with PLI may have more difficulty with social cognition (Shields et al., 1996; see also below). In general, there is still a lack of information concerning the detailed cognitive and linguistic profiles of these two groups, particularly over time.

Another potential association between cognition and comprehension difficulties is ability on theory of mind (ToM) tasks. *Theory of mind* refers to the ability to infer the mental states of others, which is thought to be a core deficit in autism. Whether individuals with SLI have difficulties with ToM is still equivocal. A number of studies have shown that children with SLI do not have problems in this area (e.g., Shields et al., 1996; Ziatas, Durkin, & Pratt, 1998). However, others suggest that even social cognition is not a "spared" skill in SLI. Farmer (2000), for example, found that children with SLI had difficulties with ToM tasks compared to peers. Recent analysis in progress from adolescents in the Conti-Ramsden Manchester Language Study also suggests ToM difficulties even in early adulthood.

Importantly, some researchers believe that the understanding of particular types of language structure, namely, the use of mental state verbs and sentence complements, such as "he tried to find it" or "she wanted to swim" are prerequisites for ToM success in both normally developing children and those with SLI (see de Villiers & de Villiers, 2000). In support of this model, a study by Hale and Tager-Flusberg (2003) showed that training on sentential complements improved performance on false-belief ToM tasks, but that the opposite was not true: Those trained in false belief did not improve their comprehension of complement terms. However, cross-linguistic studies do not always support the notion that the linguistic structure provides the mental structure for ToM. For example, Cheung and colleagues (Cheung et al., 2004) found that no relationship remained when general language comprehension was controlled for in English- and Cantonese-speaking children. Questions have also been raised regarding the nature of the tasks used in some of the supporting studies (Ruffman, Slade, Rowlandson, Rumsey, & Garnham, 2003).

Despite the evidence for limitations in short-term memory, ToM, and other specific cognitive difficulties, research continues to attempt to map out the relations between these skills and language development in more detail, taking into account both individual change and also overlapping and dynamic skills. Any model of cognitive deficit in SLI needs to be able to explain why individuals with the disorder are not the same as those with more general learning impairments. I return to the distinction between SLI and nonspecific language difficulties in the next section.

General Cognitive Abilities over Time and within Families

One reason that the term "specific" is used in SLI, despite the cognitive difficulties described above, derives from the fact that overall IQ is not impaired at diagnosis and/or because cognitive delay alone cannot explain the language deficits. However, very few investigations have taken development itself into account. Indeed, overall nonverbal IQ has also been shown to decline over time in those with SLI (e.g., Botting, 2005; Tomblin, Freese, & Records, 1992), suggesting that while limited cognitive skill might not be an obvious cause of language difficulty at a single time point, it may be an associated factor when development over time is considered.

Specifically, I found that around a quarter of the children who had been diagnosed at 7 years with a specific language disorder without global delay showed depressed nonverbal IQ scores of below 70 at 14 years of age (Botting, 2005). The mean drop in IQ over time for the group as a whole was a substantial 23 points. Yet, when we examine these children's IQ profiles at age 14, a significant mean difference between Verbal IQ and Performance IQ of around 6 IQ points is evident, in line with a typical SLI profile. Although at earlier ages our study did not measure Verbal IQ, this may suggest a general decline in cognitive skills, which means that language-based skills are still relatively more impaired than other aspects of functioning. It is important to note that very little is known about the measurement of cognition over time in clinical populations. Ongoing research suggests that there may be an interaction between the type of nonverbal assessment used and perceived changes in development in SLI: While typically developing groups score similarly on different nonverbal test types at different time points, those with SLI appear to perform much better (i.e., are more stable) over time on matrix-type assessments than timed assessments (Julie Dockrell, personal communication). However, the findings still suggest that conceptualizing those with SLI as having "spared" or "intact" cognitive skills is not as appropriate as once imagined. Importantly, the lag found in nonverbal IQ development was found to be associated with receptive language abilities over time, implying that these two skills are dynamic and interactive over time in ways we do not yet fully understand.

Recall that earlier the heterogeneous and also fluid nature of SLI diagnosis was introduced. As part of this longitudinal analysis, it was also interesting to see whether we could identify a group who, despite having severe and persistent SLI, did not appear to show receptive language deficits at any point over the 7-year study period. Compared to those who had experienced receptive difficulties at one or more time points, these children (19% of our sample) showed better nonverbal IQ at 7 and at 14, higher performance on tasks of ToM and social understanding, and different patterns of IQ change over time.

Recently, there have been some interesting investigations into the theoretical divide between children with SLI and those with nonspecific language impairment (NLI). Rice, Tomblin, Hoffman, Richman, and Marquis (2004) found that although general cognitive delay did not necessarily lead to poor syntactic development, the combination of depressed cognitive ability and language difficulties led to the poorest performance on syntactic tasks. However, both NLI and SLI groups showed difficulty with grammatical marking and could be clinically identified on these grounds. These authors call for more longitudinal growth modeling studies to tease out the developmental pathways. Using a different approach, Hayiou-Thomas, Oliver, and Plomin (2005) conducted a genetic twin study on monozygotic and dyzygotic pairs where one twin had SLI and the other had NLI. They found that although multiple genetic and environmental factors were likely to underlie both disorders, only some genetic overlap existed between the groups (i.e., especially when the cognitive impairments were more severe), suggesting that there may be some valid reasons for treating the groups separately.

Are Production and Comprehension Separate Dimensions?

Recent genetic and neurological research has also revealed some interesting findings about the possible dissociations between production and comprehension of language. For example, the SLI consortium

(2001) found genetic linkage for expressive but not receptive language difficulties. In a recent twin study, all the expressive language tasks but neither of the receptive ones showed moderate genetic influence (Kovas et al., 2005). In a different investigation using brain-imaging techniques, Pecini et al. (2005) found that children with expressive language impairment showed less left-hemispheric specialization for language compared to peers. However, children with receptive language difficulties did not show this difference, but instead performed more poorly on tests of working memory.

A dimensional approach, in which children are not described as having a mutually exclusive disorder, but may have different degrees of difficulty in a combination of different areas, has been suggested previously by Rapin and Allen (1987; Rapin, 1996) and Bishop and Rosenbloom (1987) and might therefore prove an increasingly useful model in the way we view developmental language and communication disorders. Clinical populations such as those with SLI might allow the examination of expression and comprehension in separate ways to a greater extent than typically developing groups. Differences in the pathways and associations of different types of language proficiency may also be more "visible" in atypical development.

THE WIDER IMPLICATIONS
OF COMPREHENSION DIFFICULTIES IN SLI

Relationship between Oral and Text Comprehension in Communication Disorders

Elsewhere in this volume, Cain and Oakhill (Chapter 2) consider the group of children referred to as "poor text comprehenders" who have been recruited from mainstream schools. In groups of children with SLI, very high rates of difficulty with reading comprehension are reported. For example, in a longitudinal study of children based at Manchester, more than 80% showed reading comprehension scores outside of the normal range at 11 years of age (Conti-Ramsden et al., 2001). In a subsequent study, we also found that good earlier receptive language (taken at 7 years of age) was the only predictor of reading outcome at 14 once nonverbal IQ was accounted for in the analyses. Although reading comprehension difficulties in this group are almost always combined with poor reading accuracy or poor decoding skills, it was interesting to note that about 10% of those in the Nuffield Foundation Study showed poor text comprehension but normal range decoding skills at 11 years of age. Indeed, while 26% of the sample showed a 10-point discrepancy (where standardization has a population mean of 100 and an SD of 15) between reading accuracy and comprehension with higher accuracy, only 2.5% showed the opposite pattern. Furthermore, oral comprehension and reading comprehension were significantly correlated ($r = 0.6$). While some children in this SLI group had no apparent reading difficulties, the majority (75%) were generally poor readers with depressed decoding *and* reading comprehension scores. This suggests that, even in an SLI population, oral comprehension and reading comprehension are both impaired in associated ways as children enter secondary school. This may in turn lead us to consider that children with SLI have additional qualitatively different impairments from those with a more "dyslexic" pattern (which extend beyond phonological deficits) and that these lead to different developmental pathways despite early similarities (see Bishop & Snowling, 2004, and Nation & Norbury, 2005, for reviews of dyslexia and SLI and reading comprehension and SLI, respectively).

Social and Behavioral Outcomes
Related to Comprehension Problems in SLI

The presence of oral comprehension difficulties appears to be associated with poor outcome in general, not just in language and literacy (Clegg et al., 2005; Lindsay & Dockrell, 2000). For example, a group with mixed-expressive SLI showed increasingly concerning behavioral scores from 7 to 8 years of age while a group with expressive difficulties appeared to improve slightly (Botting & Conti-Ramsden, 2000). On closer analysis, problem behaviors were largely those relating to emotional difficulties and peer relationships, rather than antisocial behaviors. Those with comprehension difficulties at 11 years of age were also significantly more likely to be the victims of bullying (Conti-Ramsden & Botting, 2004). Receptive language difficulties might also predict higher rates of mental health difficulties in later life (Beitchman, Wilson, & Johnson, 2001; Clegg et al., 2005). Higher rates of language impairment have been noted in psychiatric samples (Cohen, Barwick, Horodezky, Vallance, & Im, 1998). However, it is not known whether these associations are causal in either direction, or whether they represent an unrelated comorbid risk. Higher rates of mental health issues in groups with communication difficulties without clear connection to language ability may suggest that the latter is true.

SUMMARY AND IMPLICATIONS

In summary, oral and text comprehension difficulties are common features in children diagnosed as having SLI and PLI. However, for individual children, receptive abilities may wax and wane over time, creating a fluid picture of abilities. Specific cognitive abilities, particularly those involving verbal memory, have recently been heavily implicated in the comprehension abilities of those with SLI (and, to a lesser extent, those with PLI).

In a recent review of studies on intervention for language impairment, Law and colleagues (Law, Boyle, Harris, Harkness, & Nye, 1998) concluded that while expressive language impairments were likely to be ameliorated through the expertise of therapists and educators, interventions for receptive difficulties were far less successful. At the same time, clinicians report a large number of children in specialist language provision with increasingly complex receptive difficulties, but have had little guidance about the underlying cognitive difficulties of these children, or the types of interventions that might be most effective (Adams & Lloyd, 2005). One anecdote from a speech–language therapist stands out. A boy of 11 with PLI had been successfully integrated into a mainstream class and was managing to complete work sheets about the "life cycle" of a frog. However, despite completing the classroom task successfully, when he was asked about the content of his lesson, he replied that it had been about animals and "bikes," clearly revealing a miscomprehension of the word *cycle* at some level. Hence one major challenge for those supporting individuals with comprehension difficulties is that they may be successfully "hidden" behind good or well-controlled expressive language. One possible mode of intervention that could be implemented more frequently in classrooms is the use of typical comprehension role models. Paired classroom activities where children with SLI work alongside and in cooperation with a typically developing peer may be one possibility. Reverse integration in which mainstream children spend time in the language provision may be another. Commonly, children with comprehension difficulties are attending mainstream classrooms with support. While this support is, of course, much needed, it may be important to consider the potential "isolation" from peer role models that may result.

Alternatively, targeting some of the cognitive difficulties reported may in turn enhance language development. Although Lahey (1988) argues against targeting so called prerequisite skills, because of poor generalization to language ability, the current models of U.K. intervention may nevertheless need rethinking for children with severe and persistent SLI. Ninety percent of the children in the Nuffield Foundation

Study scored 1*SD* below the mean on at least one test of language at 14 years of age, despite at least 1 year of early and intensive language therapy (Conti-Ramsden et al., 2001). It may also be possible to be aware of and thus "support" the cognitive weaknesses of children with SLI in educational settings (e.g., by using more visual prompts) in order to maximize their linguistic potential. In addition, assessors need to be aware of the type of cognitive and educational tests they use for children with SLI, how these tests represent their strengths and weaknesses, and what they might reveal about a child's learning.

Finally, while children with SLI and PLI appear to show significant cognitive difficulties, these appear to occur in different measure to younger typically developing children with similar communicative ability and to those from other clinical groups, and indeed, cognitive skills may develop differently over time in these groups. The exploration of individual cognitive and receptive profiles, the relationship between the two, and the development of comprehension and cognition over time will no doubt prove to be vital factors in our future understanding.

ACKNOWLEDGMENTS

I would like to thank the Economic and Social Research Council for Fellowship Grant No. RES-000-27-0003, the Nuffield Foundation for its generous ongoing funding (Grant Nos. AT251/OD and DIR/28), and Gina Conti-Ramsden for her continuous support.

REFERENCES

Adams, C. (2002). The assessment of language pragmatics. *Journal of Child Psychology and Psychiatry, 43,* 973–987.

Adams, C., Cooke, R. E., Crutchley, A., Hesketh, A., & Reeves, D. (2001). *Assessment of Comprehension and Expression.* Windsor, UK: NFER–Nelson.

Adams, C., & Lloyd, J. (2005). Elicited and spontaneous communicative functions and stability of conversational measures with children who have pragmatic language impairments. *International Journal of Language and Communication Disorders, 40,* 333–347.

American Psychiatric Association. (1994). *Diagnostic and statistical manual of mental disorders* (4th ed.). Washington, DC: Author.

Baddeley, A. D. (1986). *Working memory.* Oxford, UK: Oxford University Press.

Bavin, E. L., Wilson, P., Maruff, P., & Sleeman, F. (2005). Spatio-visual memory of children with specific language impairment: Evidence for generalised processing problems. *International Journal of Language and Communication Disorders, 40,* 319–332.

Beitchman, J. H., Wilson, B., & Johnson, C. J. (2001). Fourteen year follow-up of speech/language-impaired and control children: Psychiatric outcome. *Journal of American Academy of Child and Adolescent Psychiatry, 40,* 75–82.

Bishop, D. V. M. (1982). *Test for Reception of Grammar.* Manchester University, Manchester, UK: Author.

Bishop, D. V. M. (1997). *Uncommon understanding.* Hove, UK: Psychology Press.

Bishop, D. V. M. (1998). Development of the Children's Communication Checklist (CCC): A method for assessing qualitative aspects of communicative impairment in children. *Journal of Child Psychology and Psychiatry, 39,* 879–893.

Bishop, D. V. M., & Adams, C. (1992). Comprehension problems in children with specific language impairment: Literal and inferential meaning. *Journal of Speech and Hearing Research, 35,* 119–129.

Bishop, D. V. M., & Baird, G. (2001). Parent and teacher report of pragmatic aspects of communication: Use of the Children's Communication Checklist in a clinical setting. *Developmental Medicine and Child Neurology, 43,* 809–818.

Bishop, D. V. M., & Norbury, C. F. (2002). Exploring the borderlands of autistic disorder and specific language impairment: A study using standardised diagnostic instruments. *Journal of Child Psychology and Psychiatry, 43,* 917–930.

Bishop, D. V. M., North, T., & Donlan, C. (1995). Genetic basis of specific language impairment: Evidence from a twin study. *Developmental Medicine and Child Neurology, 37,* 56–71.

Bishop, D. V. M., & Rosenbloom, L. (1987). Classification of childhood language disorders. In W. Yule & M. Rutter (Eds.), *Language development and disorders* (pp. 16–41). *Clinics in Developmental Medicine* (double issue), Nos. 101–102. London: MacKeith Press.

Bishop, D. V. M., & Snowling, M. J. (2004). Developmental dyslexia and specific language impairment: Same or different? *Psychological Bulletin, 130,* 858–886.

Botting, N. (2004). Child Communication Checklist (CCC) scores and children with communication impairments at 11 years. *International Journal of Language and Communication Disorders, 39,* 215–227.

Botting, N. (2005). Non-verbal cognitive development and language impairment. *Journal of Child Psychology and Psychiatry, 46,* 317–326.

Botting, N., & Adams, C. (2005). Semantic and inferencing abilities in children with communication disorders. *International Journal of Language and Communication Disorders, 40,* 49–66.

Botting, N., & Conti-Ramsden, G. (1999). Pragmatic language impairment without autism: The children in question. *Autism, 3,* 371–396.

Botting, N., & Conti-Ramsden, G. (2000). Social and behavioural difficulties in children with language impairment. *Child Language, Teaching and Therapy, 16,* 105–120.

Botting, N., & Conti-Ramsden, G. (2001). Non-word repetition and language development in children with language impairments. *International Journal of Language and Communication Disorders, 36,* 421–432.

Botting, N., & Conti-Ramsden, G. (2003). Autism, primary pragmatic difficulties and specific language impairment: Can we distinguish them using psycholinguistic markers? *Developmental Medicine and Child Neurology, 45,* 515–545.

Botting, N., & Conti-Ramsden, G. (submitted). *Subgroups of children with SLI: from childhood to adolescence.*

Boucher, J. (1998). SPD as a distinct diagnostic entity: Logical considerations and directions for future research. *International Journal of Language and Communication Disorders, 33,* 71–81.

Brook, S., & Bowler, D. (1992). Autism by another name?: Semantic and pragmatic impairments in children. *Journal of Autism and Developmental Disorders, 22,* 61–81.

Cheung, H., Hsuan-Chih, c., Creed, N., Ng, L., Ping Wang, S., & Mo, L. (2004). Relative roles of general and complementation language in theory-of-mind development: Evidence from Cantonese and English. *Child Development, 75,* 1111–1155.

Chiat, S. (2001). Mapping theories of developmental language impairment: Premises, predictions and evidence. *Language and Cognitive Processes, 16,* 113–142.

Choudhury, N., & Benasich, A. (2003). A family aggregation study: The influence of family history and other risk factors on language development. *Journal of Speech, Language and Hearing Research, 46,* 261–272.

Clegg, J., Hollis, C., Mawhood, L., & Rutter, M. (2005). Developmental language disorders—A follow-up in later adult life: Cognitive, language and psychosocial outcomes. *Journal of Child Psychology and Psychiatry, 46,* 128–149.

Cohen, N. J., Barwick, M., Horodezky, N., Vallance, D. D., & Im, N. (1998). Language, achievement, and cognitive processing in psychiatrically disturbed children with previously identified and unsuspected language impairments. *Journal of Child Psychology and Psychiatry, 36,* 865–878.

Conti-Ramsden, G., & Botting, N. (1999). Classification of children with specific language impairment. *Journal of Speech, Language and Hearing Research, 42,* 1195–1204.

Conti-Ramsden, G., & Botting, N. (2004). Social difficulties and victimization in children with SLI at 11 years of age. *Journal of Speech, Language and Hearing Research, 47,* 145–161.

Conti-Ramsden, G., Botting, N., Simkin, Z., & Knox, E. (2001). Follow-up of children attending infant language units: Outcomes at 11 years of age. *International Journal of Language and Communication Disorders, 36,* 207–220.

Conti-Ramsden, G., Crutchley, A., & Botting, N. (1997). The extent to which psychometric tests differentiate subgroups of children with specific language impairment *Journal of Speech, Language and Hearing Research, 40,* 765–777.

Conti-Ramsden, G., Simkin, Z., & Botting, N. (2006). The prevalence of ASD in adolescents with a history of SLI. *Journal of Child Psychology and Psychiatry and Allied Disciplines, 47*(6), 621–628.

Cox, A., Klein, T., Charman, T., Baird, G., Baron-Cohen, S., Swettenham, J., et al. (1999). Autism spectrum disorders at 20 and 42 months of age: Stability of clinical and ADI-R diagnosis. *Journal of Child Psychology and Psychiatry, 40,* 719–732.

Dale, P., Price, T., Bishop, D., & Plomin, R. (2003). Outcomes of early language delay: I. Predicting persistent and transient language difficulties at 3 and 4 years. *Journal of Speech, Language and Hearing Research,46,* 544–560.

de Villiers, J. G., & de Villiers, P. A. (2000). Linguistic determinism and the understanding of false beliefs. In P. Mitchell & K. J. Riggs (Eds.), *Children's reasoning and the mind* (pp. 191–228). Hove, UK: Psychology Press/Taylor & Francis.

Dunn, L., Dunn, L., Whetton, C., & Burley, J. (1998) *British Picture Vocabulary Scale II.* Windsor, UK: NFER–Nelson.

Ellis-Weismer, S., Evans, J., & Hesketh, L. J. (1999). An examination of verbal working memory capacity in children with specific language impairment. *Journal of Speech, Language and Hearing Research, 42,* 1249–1260.

Farmer, M. (2000). Language and social cognition in children with specific language impairment. *Journal of Child Psychology and Psychiatry, 41,* 627–636.

Gathercole, S. E., & Baddeley, A. D. (1990). Phonological memory deficits in language disordered children: Is there a causal connection? *Journal of Memory and Language, 29,* 336–360.

Hale, M., & Tager-Flusberg, H. (2003). The influence of language on theory of mind. *Developmental Science, 6,* 346–359.

Hayiou-Thomas, M., Oliver, B., & Plomin, R. (2005). Genetic influences on specific versus non-specific language impairment in 4-year-old twins. *Journal of Learning Disabilities, 38,* 222–232.

Hick, R., Botting, N., & Conti-Ramsden, G. (2005). Short-term memory and vocabulary development in children with Down syndrome and children with specific language impairment. *Developmental Medicine and Child Neurology, 47,* 532–538.

Hirsch-Pasek, K., & Golinkoff, R. M. (1996). *The origins of grammar: Evidence from early language comprehension.* Cambridge, MA: MIT Press.

Johnston, J., & Ellis-Weismer, S. (1983). Mental rotation abilities in language-disordered children. *Journal of Speech and Hearing Research, 26,* 397–403.

Just, M., & Carpenter, P. (1992). A capacity theory of comprehension: Individual differences in working memory. *Psychological Review, 99,* 122–149.

Kerbel, D., & Grunwell, P. (1998). A study of idiom comprehension in children with semantic–pragmatic difficulties: Part II. Between group results and discussion. *International Journal of Language and Communication Disorders, 33,* 23–44.

Kovas, Y., Hayiou-Thomas, M. E., Oliver, B., Dale, P., Bishop, D. V. M., & Plomin, R. (2005). Genetic influences in different aspects of language development: The etiology of language skills in 4.5 year old twins. *Child Development, 76,* 632–651.

Lahey, M., (1988). *Language disorders and language development.* New York: Macmillan.

Law, J., Boyle, J., Harris, F., Harkness, A., & Nye, C. (1998). Screening for speech and language delay: A systematic review of the literature. *Health Technology Assessment, 2*(9) 184.

Leinonen, E., & Kerbel, D. (1999). Relevance theory and pragmatic impairment. *International Journal of Language and Communication Disorders, 34,* 367–390.

Leonard, L. B. (1998). *Children with specific language impairment.* Cambridge, MA: MIT Press.

Lloyd, H., Paintin, K., & Botting, N. (2006). Performance of children with different types of communication impairment on the Clinical Evaluation of Language Fundamentals (CELF). *Child Language Teaching and Therapy, 22*(1), 47–67.

Lord, C., Pickles, A., McLennan, J., Rutter, M., Bregman, J., Folstein, S., et al. (1997). Diagnosing autism: Analyses of data from the Autism Diagnostic Interview. *Journal of Autism and Developmental Disorders, 27,* 501–517.

McGregor, K. (1997). The nature of word-finding errors of preschoolers with and without word-finding deficits. *Journal of Speech, Language and Hearing Research, 40,* 1232–1244.

McTear, M., & Conti-Ramsden, G. (1992). *Pragmatic disability in children.* London: Whurr.

Montgomery, J. (2003). Working memory and comprehension in children with SLI: What we know so far. *Journal of Communication Disorders, 36,* 221–231.

Montgomery, J. (2004). Sentence comprehension in children with SLI: Effects of input rate and phonological working memory. *International Journal of Language and Communication Disorders, 39,* 115–133.

Nation, K., & Norbury, C. F. (2005). Why reading comprehension fails: Insights from children with developmental disorders. *Topics in Language Disorders, 25,* 21–32.

Norbury, C. F., & Bishop, D. V. M. (2002). Inferential processing and story recall in children with communication problems: A comparison of specific language impairment, pragmatic language impairment and high-functioning autism. *International Journal of Language and Communication Disorders, 37,* 227–251.

Norbury, C. F., Bishop, D. V. M., & Briscoe, J. (2002). Does impaired grammatical comprehension provide evidence for an innate grammar module? *Applied Psycholinguistics, 23,* 247–268.

Pecini, C., Casalini, C., Brizzolara, D., Cipriani, P., Pfanner, L., & Chilosi, A. (2005). Hemispheric specialization for language in children with different types of specific language impairment. *Cortex, 41,* 157–167.

Rapin, I. (1996). Developmental language disorders: A clinical update. *Journal of Child Psychology and Psychiatry, 37,* 643–656.

Rapin, I., & Allen, D. (1987). Developmental dysphasia and autism and preschool children: Characteristics and subtypes. In *Proceedings of the First International Symposium on Specific Speech and Language Disorders in Children* (pp. 20–35). Brentford, UK: Association for All Speech Impaired Children.

Rice, M. L., Tomblin, J. B., Hoffman, L., Richman, W. A., & Marquis, J. (2004). Grammatical tense deficits in children with SLI and non specific language impairment: Relationships with nonverbal IQ over time. *Journal of Speech, Language, and Hearing Research, 47,* 816–834.

Rice, M., & Wexler, K. (2001). *Test of Early Grammatical Impairment.* San Antonio, TX: Psychological Corporation.

Roth, F., & Clark, D. (1987). Symbolic play and social participation abilities of language-impaired and normally-developing children. *Journal of Speech and Hearing Disorders, 52,* 17–29.

Ruffinan, T., Slade, L., Rowlandson, K., Rumsey, C., & Garnham, A. (2003). How language relates to belief, desire, and emotion understanding. *Cognitive Development, 18,* 139–158.

Semel, E., Wiig, E., & Secord, W. (1995). *Clinical Evaluation of Language Fundamentals III.* San Antonio, TX: Psychological Corporation.

Shields, J., Varley, R., Broks, P., & Simpson, A. (1996). Social cognition in developmental language disorders and high level autism. *Developmental Medicine and Child Neurology, 38,* 487–495.

Skipp, A., Windfuhr, K., & Conti-Ramsden, G. (2002) Children's grammatical categories of verb and noun: A comparative look at children with specific language impairment (SLI) and normal language (NL). *International Journal of Language and Communication Disorders, 37,* 253–272.

SLI Consortium. (2002). A genome wide scan identifies two novel loci involved in specific language impairment. *American Journal of Human Genetics, 70,* 384–398.

Stothard, S. E., Snowling, M. J., Bishop, D. V. M., Chipchase, B. B., & Kaplan, C. A. (1998). Language impaired preschoolers: A follow up into adolescence. *Journal of Speech, Language and Hearing Research, 41,* 407–418.

Tallal, P., Ross, R., & Curtiss, S. (1989). Familial aggregation in specific language impairment. *Journal of Speech and Hearing Disorders, 54,* 167–173.

Tomblin, J. B., & Buckwalter, P. (1998). Heritability of poor language achievement among twins. *Journal of Speech, Language and Hearing Research, 41,* 188–199.

Tomblin, J. B., Freese, P., & Records, N.(1992). Diagnosing specific language impairment in adults for the purpose of pedigree analysis. *Journal of Speech, Language and Hearing Research, 35,* 832–843.

Tomblin, J. B., Records, N., Buckwalter, P., Zhang, X., Smith, E., & O'Brien, M. (1997). Prevalence of specific language impairment in kindergarten children. *Journal of Speech, Language and Hearing Research, 40,* 1245–1260.

Vance, M., & Wells, B. (1994). The wrong end of the stick: Language-impaired children's understanding of non-literal language. *Child Language, Teaching and Therapy, 10,* 23–46.

Viding, E., Price, T. S., Spinath, F. M., Bishop, D. V. M., Dale, P. S., & Plomin, R. (2003). Genetic and environmental mediation of the relationship between language and nonverbal impairment in 4–year-old twins. *Journal of Speech, Language and Hearing Research, 46,* 1271–1282.

Walker, J., & Archibald, L. (2006). Articulation rate in preschool children:

A 3 year longitudinal study. *International Journal of Language and Communication Disorders, 41*(5), 541–566.

World Health Organization. (1993). *The ICD-10 classification of mental and behavioural disorders: Diagnostic criteria for research.* Geneva, Switzerland: Author.

Ziatas, K., Durkin, K., & Pratt, C. (1998). Belief term development in children with autism, Asperger syndrome, specific language impairment, and normal development: Links to theory of mind development. *Journal of Child Psychology and Psychiatry, 39,* 755–763.

CHAPTER 4

Language Comprehension Difficulties in Children with Autism Spectrum Disorders

SUSAN LEEKAM

The term "autism spectrum" captures a broad range of developmental disorders that are seen on a continuum of severity. The term as used by Wing (1997) includes, but is wider than, the subgroups in the category of pervasive developmental disorders as defined in DSM-IV (American Psychiatric Association, 1994) and ICD-10 (World Health Organization, 1993). All disorders that are within this spectrum of autism (ASD) are characterized by the presence of a "triad" of impairment in language and communication, impairment in social interaction, and repetitive behavior that is associated with impaired imagination.

Children with ASD have severe language comprehension impairments. This chapter outlines the nature of these difficulties and the traditional cognitive explanations that account for them and concludes that we need to rethink the cognitive basis of language comprehension deficits in children with ASD. First, we need to rethink the nature of the language comprehension difficulties, especially in relation to the language impairments seen in children with ASD compared with other disorders such as specific language impairment (SLI) and specific reading comprehension disorder. Second, we need to rethink the cause-and-effect relationship between language difficulties and the cognitive impairments that appear to underlie them. Such rethinking will have implications for the way that clinicians and teachers work with language impairments, a topic considered at the end of this chapter.

WHAT IS IMPAIRED?

What Are the Language Difficulties in Children with ASD ?

When you first meet a child with an ASD, his or her language impairments are often immediately apparent. It is common for a child with autism to have no verbal language at all. This lack of verbal ability will be accompanied by poor use of nonverbal communication, such as eye contact or gestures. Children who lack language will either show little attempt to communicate or else communicate only to obtain their needs, perhaps taking your hand to an object, rather than looking at you to convey a request. Even a verbal child with autism will probably have poor nonverbal communication, and his or her prosody and conversation skills will also be impaired. He or she may greet you in a strange way, talk in a loud voice, have flat or high intonation, or talk repetitively on the same theme. Although this child may communicate, he or she will do so in a one-sided manner. All children with ASD, whether verbal or nonverbal, lack reciprocity in their communication.

The communication and language difficulties in children with autism need to be seen against a background of developmental delay and in terms of a graded degree of impairment. The majority of children with ASD have language delays and comprehension difficulties that go far beyond difficulties of language expression. Even older children with some degree of language may be delayed in engaging in joint attention acts that are seen in normal infants by 12–18 months. That is, they fail to follow another's gaze and fail to show or to point to objects in order to share interest. When language does develop, it tends to show immaturity of function and it is repetitive and inflexible. For example, children with ASD tend to use *echolalia*–they echo or repeat the words or phrases spoken to them by others. They also have difficulty with pronouns–for example, by using the word *she* to refer to herself, and with deictic terms such as *here* and *there*). In addition they may be confused by words that have multiple meanings and they may attach meanings to words or phrases in a restricted or unusual way.

Language difficulties do improve to some extent, however. As they get older, many children with ASD develop good comprehension of vocabulary and grammar. However, they will continue to have difficulties with the comprehension of discourse. Even the highest functioning children may have residual problems. In conversations with others, these children may show turn-taking rules and conversation skills to some degree, but are still one-sided in their communication, failing to take account of their partner's needs as a listener. Similar difficulties apply to both spoken and written language. Children with autism have difficulty grasping intended meanings that are indirect or implicit. They have difficulty using verbal and written narratives, understanding nonliteral language, and recognizing meaning in its context. Difficulties in understanding subtle alternative meanings in language may remain, even in adulthood.

Regardless of a child's developmental level or the mildness of his or her autism, the most prominent language problems of children with ASD relate to the domain of pragmatics. These impairments are listed among the diagnostic criteria for autism and are noticeable during social interactions. These problems have also guided researchers in their attempts to explain the cognitive difficulties of children with ASD. Research in the last 30 years has confirmed that these impairments are distinctive in comparison with impairments in phonology, vocabulary, syntax, morphology, and semantics that are more commonly found in other language disorders (Bartak, Rutter, & Cox, 1975; Tager-Flusberg, 1989). However, when considering the traditional linguistic distinctions of phonology, grammar, semantics, and pragmatics, it is not correct to assume that the language impairments of children with ASD are restricted to selective impairments in pragmatic aspects of language. While pragmatic and related semantic impairments may be necessary conditions for a diagnosis of ASD, they are frequently accompanied by other general and specific language impairments even in children who are verbal and high functioning. Likewise, pragmatic impairments may be found in children who do not have a diagnosis of ASD.

To elaborate on these points further, it may be helpful to look, on the one hand, at the variability in language skills seen within children who have ASD, and, on the other hand, at the similarity of language skills between children with ASD and children with other language disorders.

Language and Cognitive Profiles

It is important to bear in mind the great variability of language and cognitive abilities in children with ASD. About half of these children never acquire language. Three-quarters have cognitive abilities below the normal range (i.e., mental retardation). Only a small minority of

children with ASD develop language to an age-appropriate level. For
the rest, language problems are profound and pervasive. An uneven
profile of language and cognitive skills, characterized by impaired language skills and good nonverbal cognitive skills, is often the picture
that is most associated with ASD. However, this is not the only profile
found. Joseph, Tager-Flusberg, and Lord (2002) found that although
two-thirds of their population of children with ASD had this profile,
others have a profile of verbal ability greater than nonverbal ability
and some show equal ability on both verbal and nonverbal tests. Interestingly, they also found that the higher the child's nonverbal IQ relative to his or her Verbal IQ, the greater his or her diagnostic impairment in reciprocal social interaction.

At the mild end of the autism spectrum we see children with
Asperger syndrome. Since the mid-1990s when DSM-IV (American Psychiatric Association, 1994) and ICD-10 (World Health Organization,
1993) introduced separate diagnoses for Asperger syndrome and
autism, these subgroupings came to be considered to be distinct from
each other. According to both sets of international diagnostic criteria,
children with autism and those with Asperger syndrome have an identical profile in terms of their qualitative abnormalities in reciprocal
social interaction and the presence of restricted, repetitive activities
and/or circumscribed interests. What distinguishes them is the presence of developmental delay in language, cognitive development, and
adaptive skills. Another crucial distinction is that the criterion for current communication impairment in children with childhood autism is
not included for children with Asperger syndrome. As ICD-10 and
DSM-IV are silent about the presence of a communication impairment,
it is therefore, technically speaking, possible to receive a diagnosis of
Asperger syndrome by having impairments in reciprocal social interaction only, without any language impairments. In practice, of course,
the social interaction problems experienced by individuals with Asperger syndrome will translate into a range of pragmatic language
impairments that will affect both the comprehension and the expression of communication and language.

Our own research using the ICD-10 algorithms from the Diagnostic Interview for Social and Communication Disorders and the algo-
rithm for Gillberg's Asperger syndrome (Leekam, Libby, Wing, Gould,
& Gillberg, 2000) shows that the ICD-10 diagnostic criteria for Asperger syndrome do not work in practice when distinguishing a child
with Asperger syndrome from a child with a diagnosis of childhood
autism. Instead, we found that when applied literally, the ICD-10 criteria identify hardly any children with Asperger syndrome. The reason is
because it is extremely unusual to find the particular profile of cogni-

tive and language skills defined by the ICD-10 Asperger syndrome alongside the social and repetitive symptoms of ASD. In other words, language delays and delays in cognitive and adaptive skills are common in all children who have the behavioral criteria of impaired sociability and repetitive behavior. When DSM-IV criteria have been applied, which are very similar to ICD-10 criteria, the same conclusions have been reached (Mayes & Calhoun, 2003).

In the research study described above we also examined the profiles of children diagnosed using Gillberg's diagnostic criteria (Gillberg, 1991). Unlike ICD-10, Gillberg's criteria includes a list of specific speech and language impairments found in Asperger syndrome including nonreciprocal communication, lack of appreciation of humor, literal interpretation of language, long-winded speech, odd tone of voice, or use of different voices. We found that Gillberg's criteria identified a group that more closely resembled Asperger's original description. However, neither Gillberg's criteria nor clinical judgment were completely successful in discriminating between these Asperger syndrome and ASD groupings on the basis of language delay or current language ability (Eisenmajer et al., 1996). We found that although the majority had age-appropriate language levels, more than one-third had language abilities markedly below their chronological age. Therefore, although clinicians do tend to distinguish between Asperger syndrome and autism on the basis of language level, this is by no means an absolute distinction. If we need to separate ASD into subgroups according to language ability, as has been advocated recently (Reitzel & Szatmari, 2003), it be best not to rely on existing diagnostic distinctions between autism and Asperger syndrome as the basis for this. Instead, it might be better to use the broader concept of the autism spectrum. This broader concept should allow for the possibility of identifying children with language impairments in relation to their different degrees of impairment within each part of the triad of autistic impairments.

Similarities and Differences between ASD and SLI

So far I have been talking about language abilities in autism in terms of language delay and general language level. What specific aspects of structural language are impaired in autism? Surprisingly, there has been limited research on this topic in recent years. Although it has long been known that children with autism have impairments in the comprehension and production of vocabulary, semantics, syntax, and morphology (Bartak et al., 1975), the research focus has tended to be directed away from the lexical, phonological, or grammatical impairments and has instead concentrated on the more unique impairments in pragmatics in line with prevailing research concerns with theory of mind impairments in autism. The consequence of this shift of research focus is that there is very little documented evidence on the patterns of structural language impairment in children with autism compared with children with SLI.

In recent years, Tager-Flusberg and colleagues (Kjelgaard & Tager-Flusberg, 2001; Tager-Flusberg & Joseph, 2003) have conducted a major set of studies examining a wide range of language impairments of a large group of children with ASD who have a history of language impairment (see Tager-Flusberg, 2003, for a review). This research shows that a significant proportion of children with ASD have specific structural impairments and that these children also meet the criteria for SLI. The profile of the children identified in these studies included intact articulation skills but impaired higher order language ability as tested by the CELF (Clinical Evaluation of Language Fundamentals; Semel, Wiig, & Secord, 1995), a test that includes measures of semantics, syntax, morphology, and working memory for language. This subgroup of children also had relatively good lexical knowledge compared with their higher order language problems. However, they had impaired phonological processing as measured by a nonword repetition task taken from the NEPSY developmental neuropsychological assessment (Korkman, Kirk, & Kemp, 1998). Further testing revealed difficulties for this subgroup in the marking of grammatical tense and showed that impairments in grammatical morphology correlated with phonological-processing difficulties.

These studies show that structural language impairments, once uniquely associated with SLI, may be found for some children alongside their pragmatic language impairments. What about the other side of the coin? Are the pragmatic impairments that were once thought to be unique to autism also found in children who do not have the full triad of autism impairments? Several studies have documented the language impairments of children with semantic-pragmatic disorder. These children have exactly the same difficulties in conversation and nonverbal communication as seen in children with ASD, yet they have a diagnosis of SLI rather than ASD.

The status of semantic-pragmatic disorder as either a form of SLI or as an ASD has been the subject of debate (Bishop, 2000). While some researchers suggest that semantic-pragmatic disorder should be incorporated into the description of ASD, others argue that children with semantic-pragmatic disorder do not have all the other symptoms that would qualify them for a diagnosis of autism or Asperger syndrome. Yet if we think about SLI and semantic-pragmatic disorder as being overlapping populations, as Bishop (2000) and Tager-Flusberg (2003) propose, the debate is dissipated. It is possible to consider pragmatic-impairments in children with SLI without a full diagnosis of ASD and SLI in children with ASD.

Bishop's (2000) model shows how these clinical categories might map onto overlapping impairments in language structure and use. The model suggests that the DSM-IV diagnoses of ASD and Asperger syndrome might map onto semantic-pragmatic disorder in rather different ways, with Asperger syndrome overlapping in areas of social use of language and autism disorder overlapping in areas of language structure as well as language function. However, on the basis of our observations of the language differences of children with autism and Asperger syndrome outlined above, we would suggest a different picture, without separate mappings for each group. We think that it is best to think of these two groups, those with Asperger syndrome and those with autism, as one spectrum in which some children have structural language impairments together with pragmatic impairments.

Given that children with ASD have specific and general impairments in language comprehension, it is not surprising to find that their reading comprehension and reading accuracy is also affected. Comprehension problems may show themselves in difficulties with integrating information, understanding anaphors, and monitoring one's own comprehension (O'Connor & Klein, 2004). In a recent study, Nation, Clarke, Wright, and Williams (2006) found poor reading comprehension in the majority of children with ASD. Although many of these children had generally poor reading skills, about one-quarter of the sample had specific comprehension skills that resembled specific reading comprehension impairment, an impairment that is characterized by accuracy in decoding alongside impairment in drawing inferences from text (Oakhill & Yuill, 1996). Nation et al. (2006) also found associations between reading and oral language comprehension problems in the ASD population.

Summary

Children with ASD have crucial difficulties with the comprehension of language. These difficulties relate to pragmatics and discourse and also go beyond these problems, affecting the structural aspects of language. Structural language impairments in both the use and comprehension of language may be found across the autistic spectrum, not only in children with autism but also in children with Asperger syndrome. While these structural impairments in language have been recognized for a long time, it is becoming increasingly clear that it is important to take account of these problems as well as functional language impairments in order to fully understand the language and cognitive impairments in children with ASD.

In addition to an increased awareness of the great variability in the language profiles of people with ASD, greater attention to the form of SLI known as semantic-pragmatic disorder has made it clear that pragmatic impairments may not always accompany the classic syndrome of autism identified by the international classification systems. Furthermore, other impairments that are normally seen in specific rather than in pervasive disorders (e.g., specific phonological impairments and specific reading comprehension difficulties) are also found in children with ASD. As discussed below, these changes in thinking about the nature of the language impairments in autism have important implications for whether we understand the cognitive basis of these difficulties as either specific or nonspecific to autism.

COGNITIVE THEORIES
OF LANGUAGE COMPREHENSION IMPAIRMENTS

Cognitive Theories of Autism

Autism was not recognized as a distinct disorder until Kanner's case studies were published in 1943. At that point Kanner explained the social and communication impairments he observed in terms of a central social-affective problem with a biological origin. After a period in which environmental, psychogenetic accounts were accepted and subsequently rejected during the 1960s, cognitive explanations of autism began to gain influence in the 1970s and 1980s. These explanations suggested that perceptual, attentional, and cognitive impairments might be central to autism, and these impairments were linked in turn to neurobiological and genetic deficits.

Cognitive and neurobiological theories of autism have continued to remain strong within an explanatory framework that attempts to explain the cause of autism. However, there has been much controversy since the 1980s about the role of cognitive processes in understanding the central impairments in autism. In the last 20 years, theories have tended to focus primarily on either the specific social impairments of the disorder or on its nonsocial cognitive aspects. Both groups of theories have relevance for our understanding of the cognitive basis of language difficulty.

Theories that focus primarily on social-communication impairments can be broadly divided into those that explain these impairments in terms of an impaired representational mechanism—that is, the theory of mind account of autism—and those that explain these problems as arising from low-level sensory-perceptual or affective origins. Historically, the more prominent of these explanations, the theory of mind hypothesis, originally proposed the presence of a single cognitive mechanism that would explain the social and communicative impairments in autism. This cognitive mechanism was a mentalizing or mind-reading capacity that enabled children to decouple the primary representation of an object (a thought about an object or an event) from a secondary representation of that object (a representation of the thought), and therefore to form propositional constructions such as "A thinks that . . . " (Leslie, 1987). The autistic child's difficulty with these constructions was demonstrated by their very poor performance on false-belief tasks in which children are required to predict or explain another person's actions on the basis of that person's false belief (Baron-Cohen, Leslie, & Frith, 1985). Subsequent research showed that this problem was not simply due to a decoupling problem since children with autism had no problem in decoupling when given similar tasks that involved nonmental representations such as photographs (Leekam & Perner, 1991). The theory of mind impairment was therefore considered to be a cognitive impairment that specifically affected the ability to form propositional attitudes of mental states, that is, the ability to represent embedded structures of the form "He thinks that . . . " This problem created difficulty in mentalizing and mind reading in children with ASD.

Communication difficulties in autism have also been linked to low-level cognitive impairments in social perception and social attention. According to many theoretical accounts, these impairments are part of a larger theory of mind system and structurally and developmentally related to higher forms of mentalizing (Baron-Cohen, 1995). Other more recent accounts of the social perceptual and social attention difficulties in autism do not specify direct links between representational theory of mind difficulties and these low-level capacities (Dawson et al., 2004; Klin, Jones, Schultz, & Volkmar, 2003). These alternative accounts tend to emphasize the affective nature of early social perception or else the dynamic properties of attention in social interactive contexts. Both theory of mind and social attentional explanations consider social-cognitive impairments in autism to be primarily connected to the social-communication symptoms of autism (see Leekam & Moore, 2001, and Leekam, 2005, for reviews).

Non–social-cognitive theories attempt to account for the nonsocial symptoms of autism in terms of impairments in cognitive processes. These explanations focus on difficulties in information processing across cognitive domains and highlight difficulties in mental flexibility, cognitive style, and perceptual organization. These accounts also relate to both high-level and low-level cognitive processes.

Weak central coherence theory (Frith, 2003) proposes that individuals with autism have difficulty making meaningful connections between different pieces of information due to impairment in a central drive for coherence. Weakness in this drive for coherence is found at higher levels of cognitive functioning that require different elements of semantic information to be integrated (Frith, 2003) and at lower levels of perception and attention that require the processing of global or configural information (Happé, 1996). A robust finding thought to reflect a lack of central coherence is the bias found in people with autism for detecting details in visual-processing tasks. Originally this was thought to be due to an impairment in global and contextual processing, but more recent evidence has challenged this claim and has suggested that, while children with ASD have a bias for detailed, piecemeal information processing, this may not be at the expense of global or contextual processing (López & Leekam, 2003; Mottron, Burack, Iarocci, Belleville, & Enns, 2003; Ropar & Mitchell, 2001).

More recently, alternative explanations have been proposed for the bias in detailed processing that occurs at lower levels of perception and attention. These explanations include the proposal that children with autism have enhanced capacity to discriminate between stimuli (Mottron et al., 2003) and a proposal that children with autism have reduced capacity to generalize across stimuli (Plaisted, 2001). Plaisted (2001) has also applied this explanation to problems in semantic organization.

The executive dysfunction theory proposes that executive functions that regulate and control behavior are compromised in autism (Pennington & Ozonoff, 1996). These functions include a broad range of mental operations including planning, inhibition of prepotent responses, self-monitoring, shifting of mental set and attention, and the use of working memory. While early studies provided evidence for impairments in many of these functions, methodological confounds and the use of multiple different measures made it difficult to gain consistent evidence of which functions are impaired. Recent research using more systematic research designs shows that not all of these functions may be equally impaired. It has been proposed that the functions related to mental flexibility including impairments in planning and shifting mental set and attention are particularly impaired in autism relative to the functions of either inhibitory control or working memory (see Ozonoff, 2006, for a review). However, there is also substantial evidence that when working memory and inhibitory control functions are tested together in tasks that tap both functions simultaneously, children with ASD do have difficulties (Hughes, 1996; Tager-Flusberg & Joseph, 2005a).

Cognitive Theories and Language Impairments

How do cognitive theories account for language impairments in ASD? Theories that focus on the social impairments in autism offer several different explanations of how cognitive processes operating in the social domain are related to language. Taking first the theory of mind hypothesis, the original claim was that theory of mind ability is required for many aspects of communication (Baron-Cohen, 1988). Abundant evidence has been gathered that supports this view. There is evidence, for example, that pragmatic ability in general (Eisenmajer & Prior, 1991), and listener-adapted conversational ability in particular (Capps, Kehres, & Sigman, 1998), is correlated to performance with theory of mind ability in children with autism. Experimental research also shows that unlike typical children of 2–3 years, children with autism do not adjust the content of their communication to their listener's knowledge state (Perner, Frith, Leslie, & Leekam, 1989). Furthermore, studies that attempted to separate out aspects of communication and language in terms of those that did or did not require theory of mind showed that it was the communication difficulties associated with taking account of another's mental state that were most impaired in autism. For example, individuals with ASD have more difficulties with mental state verbs rather than non-mental state verbs (Tager-Flusberg, 1992) and with nonliteral language that require awareness of others' intention and beliefs than with similes and idioms that are standard parts of speech (Happé, 1993).

Social-perceptual or social-attentional explanations that view low-level social perception as part of a larger theory of mind system are also consistent with the view that normal language development is rooted in the earliest forms of theory of mind (Bloom, 2000; Tomasello, 1999). Children therefore fail to use early forms of joint attention to share attention with others because of an impaired theory of mind, and this impairment affects their ability to learn language (Baron-Cohen, Baldwin, & Crowson, 1997).

Early studies investigating the relationship between pragmatic impairments and theory of mind assumed that language impairments should be seen as a consequence of impaired theory of mind. However, a growing literature documenting a strong association between theory of mind ability and vocabulary comprehension and syntactic comprehension challenged that view and led to different ideas about the causal relationship between theory of mind and language. An obvious alternative proposal was that an impaired theory of mind is a consequence of language impairment (e.g., de Villiers, 2000; Peterson & Siegal, 1995). Another proposal is that language abilities tend to develop independently of theory of mind for children with ASD. Those children with ASD who develop language skills, particularly skills in understanding sentential complementation, are able to use their language knowledge to solve theory of mind tasks (Happé, 1995; Tager-Flusberg & Joseph, 2005b). These views and alternative accounts are discussed further below.

Nonsocial theories of autism rely less on establishing an integral link between communication and cognitive impairments in autism. However, language does take an important part in the discussion of these theories. One proposal is that executive function impairments are due to difficulties in the ability to use language to regulate one's thinking and behavior (Hughes, 1996). There is also extensive evidence that a Verbal IQ and vocabulary comprehension impairment is associated with executive dysfunction (Liss et al., 2001; Tager-Flusberg & Joseph, 2005a). Some language impairments that are explained by executive function theory, such as pronoun reversals involving shifts in perspective, are also explained by the theory of mind hypothesis, while other impairments—for example, verbal rituals, repetition and rigidity in topic use (perseveration) that involves restricted focusing—are also explained by weak central coherence theory.

Both weak central coherence theory and executive dysfunction theories can account for a specific linguistic impairment in the processing of semantic information in sentence contexts. High-functioning individuals with autism fail to adapt the pronunciation of a homograph like "tear" according to the context of the sentence (Happé, 1997; Jolliffe & Baron-Cohen, 1999). Weak central coherence theory explains this impairment in terms of a deficit in contextual processing, a failure to draw together information, while executive function theory may also explain the same effect as a failure to inhibit irrelevant associations (Gernsbacher, 1990). A recent study by Norbury (2005) examined both of these explanations using a modified version of Gernsbacher's method (Gernsbacher, Varner, & Faust 1990; Gernsbacher & Faust, 1991) with children with ASD children who had SLI. Norbury (2005) found that impairments in the use of context could be accounted for by individual differences in structural language ability in both children with ASD and in children with SLI. The finding was not specific to autism, as might be predicted by weak central coherence theory, but related to structural language impairments in semantic knowledge and sentence processing across both groups. Furthermore, although difficulty in suppression of irrelevant information appeared to be seen in these language-impaired children, as predicted by executive function theory, this might simply be explained by their poor contextual processing, which in turn could be explained by language impairments.

Challenges for Cognitive Explanations of Autism

Although the cognitive theories above provide powerful explanatory frameworks for our understanding of the cognitive basis of autism, a number of critical problems need to be addressed when trying to evaluate how well these theories explain the language difficulties of children with autism. First is the problem of specificity. The cognitive impairments that are proposed to underlie language difficulties in autism are not specific to children with autism. Instead, other clinical groups have also been shown to have the same difficulties, including children with SLI (Miller, 2001; Norbury, 2005) and language-delayed children with hearing impairments (Peterson & Siegal, 1995). Similarly, not all children with ASD show either the cognitive impairments or the language impairments predicted by these theories.

The second related issue is the question of causality. Until recently, it was assumed that an impairment in either mentalizing, executive functioning, or central coherence was a primary underlying factor that could explain the language impairments that were thought to be unique to autism and would be seen independently of other language impairments. Recent research, however, seems to be showing that language impairments might themselves be the driving factor leading to these cognitive difficulties.

While this problem of causality applies to all cognitive theories of autism, it has particularly been a focus of debate within the study of theory of mind. While it was previously assumed that theory of mind leads to communication difficulties, an opposing view is that communication difficulties themselves lead to impaired theory of mind (Garfield, Peterson, & Perry, 2001). According to this view, both children with autism and hearing-impaired children who have early language delays have impairments in forming and maintaining conversational exchanges with others. Thus, their restricted involvement in communications that involve talk of mental states leads to an impairment in acquiring an understanding of mental states (Peterson & Siegal, 1995).

Another view is that nonunique language impairments lead to theory of mind problems. In recent research de Villiers (2000) has shown that syntactic knowledge is particularly important for conveying the propositional attitudes that are intrinsic to false-belief understanding. For both late-signing deaf children and typically developing children, the use of sentential complementation is the strongest predictor of false-belief understanding, over and above the effects of general language, nonverbal IQ, and hearing loss.

Can the original proposal that theory of mind impairments lead to communication impairments be sustained in the face of these apparently competing views of the causal relationship? The answer is yes, but only when a broader concept of theory of mind is applied. The broader concept consists of two levels, a social-perceptual level involving attention to social stimuli that provides very basic awareness about intentional actions, and a representational level that enables understanding of false belief. In typical development, the social-perceptual level is first seen in early infancy and the representational level is seen at age 3–4 years. If both of these levels are thought of as "theory of mind," then it is reasonable to argue, as Tager-Flusberg and Joseph (2005b) do, that the influence of language is different at each of these levels of development.

Tager-Flusberg and Joseph (2005b) propose that low-level theory of mind directly leads to both language ability and to high-level theory of mind in typical children. But as language, particularly syntactic skills, and low-level theory of mind develop, they each influence high-level representational theory of mind (false-belief understanding). For children with ASD the relationship is different. Rather than rely on both low-level theory of mind skills and language knowledge, children with ASD use their knowledge of syntactic complementation skills in a more exclusive way to deal with representational theory of mind tasks that involve complement structures. However, instead of relying on knowledge of complements for cognitive verbs ("He thinks that . . . "), they rely on complements for communication verbs ("He says that . . . "), suggesting a different route than might be predicted for typical children.

Tager-Flusberg and Joseph's (2005b) account seems to answer both the alternative causal accounts described above. That is, the view that theory of mind impairments lead to communication and language impairments and the reverse position, that knowledge of language leads to theory of mind. Yet there are still inherent problems in tracing the direction of influence between theory of mind and language. While evidence shows that syntactic language ability is the strongest predictor of false-belief understanding, and that the use of this ability to convey mentalistic sentence constructions might differ for children with autism, little is known about other parts of the model that propose a link between low-level and high-level theory of mind. The developmental connection between social-perceptual theory of mind and representational theory of mind, for example, has been virtually untested by longitudinal studies in either typical children or children with ASD. The connections between different impairments in social-perceptual ability (as opposed to dynamic social-interactional skills, such as joint attention) and language are also not well understood. Mostly, though, we need to know more about how developmental change affects the relationship between these factors.

Summary

Cognitive theories of autism initially explained language impairments as an outcome of a specific cognitive impairment. Recent research highlighting structural as well as pragmatic impairments in ASD has shown that neither the cognitive impairments nor the language impairments are specific to autism. Increasingly, research is also showing that cognitive deficits might be explained by language ability, suggesting that we need to reconsider the direction of causality by which cognitive impairment determines language impairment. The only hypothesized cognitive ability that seems to developmentally precede language impairments in ASD is a low-level theory of mind ability. However, the cognitive status of this ability and its links with either language ability or high-level representational theory of mind are not clear.

RETHINKING THE COGNITIVE BASIS OF LANGUAGE COMPREHENSION DIFFICULTIES IN AUTISM

In recent years, novel research findings, alternative theoretical ideas, and nontraditional methodological approaches are forcing us to re-think the language impairments in children with developmental disorders and their relationship with cognitive impairments. In this final section we look at these new ways of thinking about the relation between cognitive impairments and language.

Rethinking the Language Impairments in Autism

Up until now, the diagnostic boundaries of ASD imposed by the international classification systems have led us to think about language impairments as being either distinctive (e.g., pragmatic difficulties) or nondistinctive (e.g., lexical or syntactic difficulties). It may be more helpful to think first about the particular types of language impairments that children have, and second about whether they co-occur with the diagnosed triad of impairments for ASD.

To better understand the nature of the language impairments of children with autism and how they relate to the language impairments of other groups, we need to consider ASD against the spectrum of language disorders that extend beyond autism. Rapin (2006) provides a classification scheme that helps to identify not only language impairments in autism, but also in the full range of developmental language disorders (DLD).

Rapin (2006) divides language disorders into two groupings according to whether or not children have intact or impaired phonology and then again according to their receptive and expressive difficulties. For example, Rapin's subgrouping of higher order processing disorders describes two disorders in which the problem tends to relate to comprehension of rather than to expression of language. In this group, children with semantic-pragmatic disorder may have apparently intact good comprehension at both the single-word and the sentence level but be impaired in discourse, narrative, and conversation. Children with lexical-syntactic disorder also have intact comprehension at the single-word level but have impaired comprehension for multiword phrases or sentences and may also have difficulties with phonology, syntax, and semantics early in development—although these problems may resolve in time.

While Rapin's classification may not capture all the distinctions between different language abilities of children with ASD, it provides the opportunity to link language impairments to different language profiles regardless of whether the child has a diagnostic label of ASD, SLI, or some other diagnosis. Of particular interest is the recognition within this scheme that phonological and grammatical language disorders can be found in children with autism as well as those with DLD (Rapin & Dunn, 2003). This is particularly significant given recent research by Kjelgaard and Tager-Flusberg (2001) that shows specific phonological impairments and profiles of SLI in children with autism. Rapin's (2006) scheme may allow us to look at the relationship between different types of language problems and different kinds of cognitive problems. It may also help us to chart changes in language subtypes from preschool to the school-age years alongside changes in the social impairments seen in children with these different subtypes.

Rethinking the Cognitive Basis of Language Impairments

A different approach to the cognitive basis of language impairments may help us to address the problems of specificity and causality. Traditional views of the cognitive basis of autism have been heavily influenced by theories in adult cognitive psychology. These theories posit the existence of mechanisms and systems that exist within a larger cognitive architecture. Assumptions about the specificity of these mechanisms, the separateness of component systems, and the unidirectional nature of causal links connecting them have been challenged by recent researchers investigating impairments in cognitive development (Bishop, 1997; Karmiloff-Smith, 1998). New ideas in cognitive development have inspired the development of new theories and theoretical frameworks such as connectionism, dynamic systems theory, and transactional theory, reflecting similar theoretical changes within the field of developmental biology and genetics.

These new approaches highlight the importance of the developmental process as central to the study of typical and atypical development and challenge the traditional notion of causality. The view is that the early form of a problem in language, cognitive, or social functioning may not be the same as a later form of that problem, and therefore developmental outcomes are best seen as probabilistic and emergent rather than as deterministic. Impairments may begin as a general difficulty but become more specific in time, depending on the type of experience that the child has. Causes of impairment are also multidimensional and interact with each other in complex, nonlinear ways. The upshot of this view is that it may not be helpful to look for simple causal explanations of development in ASD. Instead, it is important to focus on the process of development.

The relevance of this view of the study of language impairments is suggested by Bates (2004). In commenting on similarities in language impairment across different clinical groups, Bates suggests that language impairments might emerge from abilities that lie outside of the language system, initially from a range of different early attentional and perceptual "starter skills" that include cross-modal perception, sensorimotor skills, computational skills, and attentional orientating to either objects or people. All these are skills that are present at birth or emerge soon after. She argues that none of these capacities is unique to the acquisition of language, but that a defect in one or more of them may have consequences for language learning. Recent social-orienting explanations of autism fit with Bates's suggestion by proposing way in which very early perceptual-cognitive capacities and social-emotional capacities might interact with each other (Dawson et al., 2004; Leekam & Moore, 2001; Mundy & Neal, 2001). These transactional models also represent an attempt to specify some of the ways in which perceptual-cognitive abilities are both triggered and changed by social experience.

Once we think less compartmentally, and extend our understanding of language impairments in ASD to incorporate a wider range of phonological and syntactic difficulties that also affect children with SLI, it also makes sense to link these to either low-level perceptual or higher-level cognitive impairments that are known to be associated with SLI. Hence recent proposals that low-level auditory processing might be an underlying factor in autism are consistent with recent proposals about the origins of SLI and dyslexia (Siegal & Blades, 2003). Further research may also be needed to reexamine higher-level cognitive impairments, such as working memory, that are strongly associated with SLI and other disorders (Gathercole & Alloway, 2006) but to date have been less associated with ASD.

Implications for Practice

Practitioners who identify autism should be aware that a broad range of language impairments can accompany the pragmatic impairments seen in children, whether or not a child has an autism spectrum deficit. Co-occuring phonological, lexical, and syntactic language impairments may be seen even if the child is high functioning with a diagnosis of Asperger syndrome.

As early language comprehension ability is an important predictor not only of later language ability but also of social skills and overall function in later life in people with ASD (Mawhood, Howlin, & Rutter, 2000), practitioners need to be especially alert to the possibilities of language comprehension difficulties early in development. However, language comprehension difficulties may be difficult to detect when expressive language is apparently functioning normally, a profile that is often found in autism. Comprehension problems tend to be detected when the child is asked questions that refer to concepts outside of the immediate visible situation, but it is important to remember that some children may have difficulties in comprehending sentences or discourse but not in comprehending vocabulary. Where comprehension is impaired at any level, Rapin (2006) suggests that the use of a visual referent while speaking may help to enhance comprehension.

Recent research described in this chapter seems to suggest that for highly verbal children, intervention into syntactic aspects of language may help to facilitate the use of propositional attitude constructions that are integral to the understanding of false beliefs. For less verbal children who lack joint attention skills, it is important to promote motivating contexts in which children may learn to look at the face of a conversational partner, since we know that orienting to another's voice is related not only to joint attention ability but also to language ability (Leekam, López, & Moore, 2000; Leekam & Ramsden, 2006).

More generally, practitioners (and researchers) need to look for multiple, rather than single, reasons for a child's language impairment. Early forms of language impairments may be general rather than specific and may originate from outside of the language system. Depending on which symptoms of autism are found alongside which language impairments and how severe these symptoms are, it is possible to expect to see change in some areas of language but not in others depending on the individual profile of the child and the social and language experience available to that child.

Conclusion

Research on language comprehension in autism is moving forward in an exciting way. New empirical findings that force us to reconsider the distinctions between language impairments in different groups have been joined by new theoretical approaches that encourage us to rethink the cognitive basis of language difficulties in ASD. These new developments in the field are likely to have far-reaching implications. An increasing emphasis on developmental change and on the similarity of early impairments across different groups, as well as their differences, will hopefully have implications for research and practice across both SLI and autism groups. At a practical level, greater recognition of problems that are common to as well as independent from different groups will lead to more focused intervention strategies that are influenced less by the diagnostic label and more by the language problem. At a theoretical level, greater consideration of the developmental link between particular types of early impairments and particular kinds of later outcomes will help to clarify why the developmental pathway for some children with early language problems leads to autism while for others it does not. In summary, rethinking the cognitive basis of language comprehension difficulties in autism means that we need to move between ideas of specificity and generality, challenge traditional category distinctions, and prioritize the study of developmental change.

REFERENCES

American Psychiatric Association. (1994). *Diagnostic and statistical manual of mental disorders* (4th ed.). Washington, DC: Author.

Baron-Cohen, S. (1988). Social and pragmatic deficits in autism: Cognitive or affective? *Journal of Autism and Developmental Disorders, 18,* 379–402.

Baron-Cohen, S. (1995). *Mindblindness: An essay on autism and theory of mind.* Cambridge, MA: MIT Press.

Baron-Cohen, S., Baldwin, D.A., & Crowson, M. (1997). Do children with autism use the speaker's direction of gaze strategy to crack the code of language? *Child Development, 68,* 48–57.

Baron-Cohen, S., Leslie, A., & Frith, U. (1985). Does the autistic child have a "theory of mind"? *Cognition, 21,* 37–46.

Bartak, L., Rutter, M., & Cox, A. (1975). A comparative study of infantile autism and specific developmental receptive language disorder. *British Journal of Psychiatry, 126,* 127–145.

Bates, E. (2004). Explaining and interpreting deficits in language development across clinical groups: Where do we go from here? *Brain and Language, 88,* 248–253.

Bishop, D. V. M. (1997). *Uncommon understanding: Development and disorders of language comprehension.* Hove, UK: Psychology Press.

Bishop, D. V. M. (2000). Pragmatic language impairment: A correlate of SLI, a distinct subgroup or part of the autistic continuum? In D. V. M. Bishop & L. B. Leonard (Eds.), *Speech and language impairments in children: Causes, characteristics, intervention and outcome* (pp. 99–113). Hove, UK: Psychology Press.

Bloom, P. (2000). *How children learn the meanings of words.* Cambridge, MA: MIT Press.

Capps, L., Kehres, J., & Sigman, M. (1998). Conversational abilities among children with autism and children with developmental delays. *Autism, 2,* 325–344.

Dawson, G., Toth, K., Abbott, R., Osterling, J., Munson, J., Estes, A., et al. (2004). Social attention impairments in young children with autism: Social orienting, joint attention and attention to distress. *Developmental Psychology, 40,* 271–283.

de Villiers, J. (2000). Language and theory of mind: What are the developmental relationships? In S. Baron-Cohen, H. Tager-Flusberg, & D. Cohen (Eds.), *Understanding other minds: Perspectives from developmental cognitive neuroscience* (pp. 83–123). Oxford, UK: Oxford University Press.

Eisenmajer, R., & Prior, M. (1991). Cognitive linguistic correlates of "theory of mind" ability in autistic children. *British Journal of Developmental Psychology, 9,* 351–364.

Eisenmajer, R., Prior, M., Leekam, S., Wing, L., Gould, J., Welham, M., et al. (1996). Comparison of clinical symptoms in autism and Asperger's disorder. *Journal of American Academy of Child and Adolescent Psychiatry, 35,* 1523–1531.

Frith, U. (2003). *Autism: Explaining the enigma* (2nd ed.). Oxford, UK: Blackwell.

Garfield, J. L., Peterson, C. C., & Perry, T. (2001). Social cognition, language acquisition and the development of theory of mind. *Mind and Language, 16,* 494–541.

Gathercole, S. E., & Alloway, T. P. (2006). Practitioner report: Short term and working memory impairment in neurodevelopmental disorders: Diagnosis and remedial support. *Journal of Child Psychology and Psychiatry, 4*, 4–15.

Gernsbacher, M. A. (1990). *Language comprehension as structure building*. Hillsdale, NJ: Erlbaum.

Gernsbacher, M. A., & Faust, M. (1991). The mechanism of suppression: A component of general comprehension skill. *Journal of Experimental Psychology: Memory and Cognition, 17*, 245–262.

Gernsbacher, M. A., Varner, K. R., & Faust, M. (1990). Investigating differences in general comprehension skill. *Journal of Experimental Psychology: Learning, Memory and Cognition, 16*, 430–445.

Gillberg, C. (1991). Clinical and neurobiological aspects of Asperger syndrome in six family studies. In U. Frith (Ed.), *Autism and Asperger syndrome* (pp. 122–146). New York: Cambridge University Press.

Happé, F. (1993). Communicative competence and theory of mind in autism: A test of relevance theory. *Cognition, 48*, 101–119.

Happé, F. (1995). The role of age and verbal ability in the theory of mind performance of subjects with autism. *Child Development, 66*, 843–855.

Happé, F. (1996). Studying weak central coherence at low levels: Children with autism do not succumb to visual illusions: A research note. *Journal of Child Psychology and Psychiatry, 37*, 873–877.

Happé, F. (1997). Central coherence and theory of mind: Reading homographs in context. *British Journal of Developmental Psychology, 15*, 1–12.

Hughes, C. (1996). Control of action and thought: Normal development and dysfunction in autism: A research note. *Journal of Child Psychology and Psychiatry, 37*, 229–236.

Jolliffe, T., & Baron-Cohen, S. (1999). A test of central coherence theory: Linguistic processing in high-functioning adults with autism or Asperger syndrome: Is local coherence impaired? *Cognition, 71*, 149–185.

Joseph, R. M., Tager-Flusberg, H., & Lord, C. (2002). Cognitive profiles and social-communicative functioning in language and learning impaired children. *Journal of Child Psychology and Psychiatry, 6*, 807–881.

Kanner, L. (1943). Autistic disturbances of affective contact. *Nervous Child, 2*, 217–250.

Karmiloff-Smith, A. (1998). Development itself is the key to understanding developmental disorders. *Trends in Cognitive Sciences, 2*, 389–398.

Kjelgaard, M., & Tager-Flusberg, H. (2001). An investigation of language impairment in autism: Implications for genetic subgroups. *Language and Cognitive Processes, 16*, 287–308.

Klin, A., Jones, W., Schultz, R., & Volkmar, F. (2003). The enactive mind, or from actions to cognition; Lessons from autism. *Philosophical Transactions of the Royal Society of London, B, 358*, 345–360.

Korkman, M., Kirk, U., & Kemp, S. (1998). *NEPSY: A developmental neuropsychological assessment*. San Antonio. TX: Psychological Corporation/Harcourt Brace & Co.

Leekam, S. R. (2005). Why do children with autism have a joint attention impairment? In N. Eilan, C. Hoerl, T. McCormack, & J. Roessler (Eds.),

Joint attention: Communication and other minds (pp. 205–229). Oxford, UK: Oxford University Press.

Leekam, S. R., Libby, S., Wing, L., Gould, J., & Gillberg, C. (2000). Comparison of ICD-10 and Gillberg criteria for Asperger syndrome. *Autism, 4,* 11–28.

Leekam, S. R., López, B., & Moore, C. (2000). Attention and joint attention in preschool children with autism. *Developmental Psychology, 36,* 261–273.

Leekam, S. R., & Moore, C. (2001). The development of attention and joint attention in children with autism. In J. Burack, T. Charman, N. Yirmiya, & P. Zelazo (Eds.), *The development of autism: Perspectives from theory and research* (pp. 105–129). Mahwah, NJ: Erlbaum.

Leekam, S. R., & Perner, J. (1991). Does the autistic child have a meta-representational deficit? *Cognition, 40,* 203–218.

Leekam, S. R., & Ramsden, C. A. (2006). Dyadic orienting and joint attention in preschool children with autism. *Journal of Autism and Developmental Disorders, 36,* 185–197.

Leslie, A. (1987). Pretense and representation: The origins of "theory of mind." *Psychological Review, 94,* 412–426.

Liss, M., Fein, D., Allen, D., Dunn, M., Feinstein, C., Morris, R., et al. (2001). Executive functioning in high-functioning children with autism. *Journal of Child Psychology and Psychiatry, 42,* 261–270.

López, B., & Leekam, S. (2003). Do children with autism fail to process information in context? *Journal of Child Psychology and Psychiatry, 44,* 285–300.

Mawhood, L., Howlin, P., & Rutter, M. (2000). Autism and developmental receptive language disorder—A comparative follow-up in early adult life. *Journal of Child Psychology and Psychiatry, 41,* 547–559.

Mayes, S. D., & Calhoun, S. L. (2003). Relationship between Asperger syndrome and high functioning autism. In M. Prior (Ed.), *Learning and behavior problems in Asperger syndrome* (pp. 15–34). New York: Guilford Press.

Miller, C. (2001). False belief understanding in children with specific language impairment. *Journal of Communication Disorders, 34,* 73–86.

Mottron, L., Burack, J., Iarocci, G., Bellville, S., & Enns, J. T. (2003). Locally oriented perception with intact global processing among adolescents with high-functioning autism: Evidence from multiple paradigms. *Journal of Child Psychology and Psychiatry, 44,* 904–913.

Mundy, P., & Neal, R. (2001). Neural plasticity, joint attention and a transactional social-orienting model of autism. *International Review of Research in Mental Retardation, 23,* 139–168.

Nation, K., Clarke, P., Wright, B. J., & Williams, C. (2006). Patterns of reading ability in children with autism spectrum disorders. *Journal of Autism and Developmental Disorders, 36,* 911–919.

Norbury, C. F. (2005). Barking up the wrong tree?: Lexical ambiguity resolution in children with language impairments and autistic spectrum disorders. *Journal of Experimental Child Psychology, 90,* 142–171.

Oakhill, J. V., & Yuill, N. (1996). Higher order factors in comprehension disability: Processes and remediation. In C. Cornoldi & J. V. Oakhill (Eds.), *Reading comprehension difficulties* (pp. 69–92). Mahwah, NJ: Erlbaum.

O'Connor, I. M., & Klein, N. (2004). Exploration of strategies for facilitating the reading comprehension of high-functioning students with autistic spectrum disorders. *Journal of Autism and Developmental Disorders, 34,* 115–127.

Ozonoff, S. (2006). Executive functions. In J. Pérez, P. M. Gonzalez, M. Llorente Comi, & C. Nieto (Eds.), *New developments in autism: The future is now* (pp. 185–213). London: Kingsley.

Pennington, B. F., & Ozonoff, S. (1996). Executive functions and developmental psychopathology. *Journal of Child Psychology and Psychiatry, 37,* 51–87.

Perner, J., Frith, U., Leslie, A.M., & Leekam, S. R. (1989). Exploration of the autistic child's theory of mind: Knowledge, belief and communication. *Child Development, 60,* 688–700.

Peterson, C. C., & Siegal, M. (1995). Deafness, conversation and theory of mind. *Journal of Child Psychology and Psychiatry, 36,* 459–474.

Plaisted, K. C. (2001). Reduced generalization in autism: An alternative to weak central coherence. In J. A. Burack, T. Charman, N. Yirmiya, & P. R. Zelazo (Eds.), *The development of autism* (pp. 149–172). Mahwah, NJ: Erlbaum.

Rapin, I. (2006). Language and its development in the autistic spectrum disorders. In J. Pérez, P. M. Gonzalez, M. Llorente Comi, & C. Nieto (Eds.), *New developments in autism: The future is now* (pp. 214–236). London: Kingsley.

Rapin, I., & Dunn, M. (2003). Update on the language disorders of individuals on the autistic spectrum. *Brain and Development, 25,* 166–172.

Reitzel, J.-A., & Szatmari, P. (2003) Cognitive and academic problems. In M. Prior (Ed.), *Learning and behavior problems in Asperger syndrome* (pp. 35–54). New York: Guilford Press.

Ropar, D., & Mitchell, P. (2001). Susceptibility to illusions and performance on visuo-spatial tasks in individuals with autism. *Journal of Child Psychology and Psychiatry, 42,* 539–549.

Semel, E., Wiig, E. H., & Secord, W. A. (1995). *Clinical evaluation of language fundamentals* (3rd ed.). San Antonio, TX: Psychological Corporation/Harcourt Brace & Co.

Siegal, M., & Blades, M. (2003). Language and auditory processing in autism. *Trends in Cognitive Sciences, 7,* 373–380.

Tager-Flusberg, H. (1989). A psycholinguistic perspective on language development in the autistic child. In G. Dawson (Ed.), *Autism: Nature, diagnosis, and treatment* (pp. 92–115). New York: Guilford Press.

Tager-Flusberg, H. (1992). Autistic children talk about psychological states: Deficits in the early acquisition of a theory of mind. *Child Development, 63,* 161–172.

Tager-Flusberg, H. (2003). Language impairments in children with complex neurodevelopmental disorders: The case of autism. In Y. Levy & J. Schaeffer (Eds.), *Language competence across populations: Toward a definition of specific language impairment* (pp. 297–321). Mahwah, NJ: Erlbaum.

Tager-Flusberg, H., & Joseph, R. M. (2003). Identifying neurocognitive phenotypes in autism. *Philosophical transactions of the Royal Society of London, B,* 303–314.

Tager-Flusberg, H., & Joseph, R. M. (2005a). Theory of mind, language and executive functions in autism: A longitudinal perspective. In W. Schneider, R. Schumann-Hegsteler, & B. Sodian (Eds.), *Young children's cognitive development: Interrelationships among executive functioning, working memory, verbal ability and theory of mind* (pp. 239–257). Mahwah NJ: Erlbaum.

Tager-Flusberg, H., & Joseph, R. M. (2005b). How language facilitates the acquisition of false belief in children with autism. In J. Astington & J. Baird (Eds.), *Why language matters for theory of mind* (pp. 298–318). New York: Oxford University Press.

Tomasello, M. (1999). *The cultural origins of human cognition.* Cambridge, MA: Harvard University Press.

Wing, L. (1997). Syndromes of autism and atypical development. In D. Cohen & F. Volkmar (Eds.), *Handbook of autism and pervasive developmental disorders* (2nd ed., pp. 148–172). New York: Wiley.

World Health Organization. (1993). *The ICD-10 classification of mental and behavioral disorders: Diagnostic criteria for research.* Geneva, Switzerland: Author.

CHAPTER 5

Story Comprehension Impairments in Children with Attention-Deficit/Hyperactivity Disorder

ELIZABETH P. LORCH
KRISTEN S. BERTHIAUME
RICHARD MILICH
PAUL VAN DEN BROEK

Attention-deficit/hyperactivity disorder (ADHD) is one of the most prevalent childhood behavior disorders (American Psychiatric Association, 1994). In addition, it may well be the most widely investigated childhood disorder, with literally thousands of studies examining its etiology, symptom patterns, treatment, and long-term outcomes. Despite this wealth of information, there are still many important questions to be answered. One of the most intriguing questions concerns how the deficits in cognitive processing associated with ADHD may contribute to the well-documented academic difficulties experienced by these children. The goals of this chapter are to review a series of studies that attempt to identify specific story comprehension impairments evident in children with ADHD, and to offer both research and treatment recommendations that arise from the results of these studies.

ADHD is believed to affect between 5 and 10% of school-age children, which translates into an average of one or two children per classroom. Boys are more likely than girls to be diagnosed with ADHD, with the boy-to-girl ratio ranging from 2.5:1 to 5:1 (Barkley, 1998). The primary symptoms of the disorder are developmentally inappropriate levels of inattention, overactivity, and impulsivity (American Psychiatric Association, 1994). Translated into everyday behaviors, this means that these children are more often off-task and complete less school work than their classmates; they are more likely to be fidgety or actually out of their seats during class; and they engage in disruptive behaviors such as calling out in class or cutting in line. These problematic, age-inappropriate behaviors result in significant impairment in many aspects of daily functioning. For example, these children are often actively rejected by their peers, even after relatively brief interactions with an unfamiliar peer (Diener & Milich, 1997). Children with ADHD have similar aversive interactions with the adults in their lives, especially parents and teachers. Additionally, ADHD is noted to produce long-term negative outcomes in that when children with ADHD grow up they are at increased risk for substance use/abuse, psychiatric disorders including depression and personality disorders, and traffic violations and car accidents (Barkley, 1998).

Although the symptoms of ADHD adversely affect many areas of a child's functioning, perhaps the domain that is most impaired is academic functioning. No matter which outcome measure is examined, children with ADHD perform more poorly than their classmates. For example, they are more likely to fail classes, to be held back, and to drop out of school. In addition, they earn lower grades than their classmates and score more poorly on standardized achievement tests. Associated with these academic difficulties are problems during adulthood, including being less likely to enter or complete college, having lower than expected occupational status, and having more frequent changes in occupation (Barkley, 1998).

It is easy to document the fact that children with ADHD have significant academic impairment. It is less clear how the symptoms associated with ADHD contribute to these academic difficulties. Certainly, there are a number of potential "suspects." Children with ADHD are at increased risk for having a comorbid learning disability (LD), with comorbidity estimates ranging anywhere from 20 to 70% (Barkley, 1998). Researchers have attempted to disentangle which aspects of the academic impairment may be due to ADHD versus LD (see Douglas, 1999; Pennington, Groisser, & Welsh, 1993; Purvis & Tannock, 1997). For example, Pennington et al. (1993) found that ADHD alone was associated with deficits in executive functioning, LD alone was associated with phonological deficits, and the functioning of children with comorbid ADHD/LD was more similar to that of the LD alone group. In a similar vein, Purvis and Tannock (1997) found that children with ADHD had difficulty organizing their recall of a story, whereas children with LD performed similarly to comparison children. These findings suggest that there are clear differences between children with ADHD and children with LD, and that the academic difficulties of the former cannot be explained entirely by their comorbid LD status.

In accounting for the academic difficulties of children with ADHD, considerable focus has been given to the role of their attentional problems. Investigators have consistently shown that children with ADHD are off-task at much higher rates than their classmates, and that they produce less academic work. Academic productivity is an important indicator of school performance: Decreased levels of productivity will certainly impair performance.

Despite the large number of studies examining the academic performance of children with ADHD, there is a major gap in the present literature. Although there is research examining how the core symptoms of ADHD (e.g., inattention, impulsivity) may relate to performance on standardized achievement tests, little is known about the higher-order cognitive-processing skills (e.g., applying, analyzing, synthesizing, and evaluating information) that are required for many academic tasks, such as understanding texts and lectures. One approach to understanding the higher-order cognitive-processing skills of children with ADHD is to investigate their comprehension of complex stories. Story comprehension tasks make up a significant component of school performance (e.g., reading and writing tasks) and involve many cognitive skills in addition to simple visual attention (Lorch et al., 1999; Sanchez, Lorch, & Milich, 1999). Investigating story comprehension skills allows us to obtain insight into many aspects of children's cognitive functioning including the strategic allocation of attention; the selection, encoding, and interpretation of important information; the use of story structure; the retrieval of relevant background information; the generation of inferences that allow interpretation of presented information; the monitoring of comprehension; and the use of retrieval skills (Milich, Lorch, & Berthiaume, 2005).

The present chapter reviews a series of studies focused specifically on the story comprehension impairments of children with ADHD that may contribute to their academic problems. Four specific areas of impairment among these children have been identified: (1) difficulty understanding the causal relations among story events, which appear to be related to problems in sustaining cognitive engagement; (2) difficulty using the goal structure of a story to build a coherent story representation; (3) difficulty recognizing the important information in a story and using this information to guide recall; and (4) difficulty making inferences about story information and monitoring ongoing understanding of the story. After reviewing the literature documenting these difficulties among children with ADHD, we identify educational interventions that may directly target the specific deficits exhibited by these children.

DIFFICULTIES UNDERSTANDING CAUSAL RELATIONS AMONG STORY EVENTS

In the story comprehension literature, many theories emphasize the importance of causal relations among story events (Ackerman, Silver, & Glickman, 1990; Graesser & Clark, 1985; Trabasso & Nickels, 1992). To achieve a coherent understanding of a story, individuals must determine the *causes* of a given event and the *effects* of that event on subsequent events. A *network model* has been proposed to represent different kinds of story events, the types of *causal relations* among events, and the overall *structure* of causal relations (Trabasso & van den Broek, 1985; Trabasso, van den Broek, & Suh, 1989; van den Broek, 1990).

In a network representation of a story, one important property of events concerns the number of *causal connections* that an event has to other events in the story. If an event is connected to many other events in a story through antecedents and/or consequences, it plays an important role in maintaining the coherence of the story. To illustrate this point, an example story is presented in Appendix 5.1. The story is divided into individual events, and the number of causal connections associated with each event is listed. For example, event # 13 ("and challenging the Dragon to a fight") has a relatively large number of causal connections, with two immediate antecedent events (#s 11 and 12) and both immediate (#s 14, 16, and 17) and long-term consequences (#s 30 and 71). In contrast, event #15 has only one immediate antecedent (# 14) and no consequences, making it a "dead-end" event. Thus, event # 13 is important to the coherence of the story and relatively likely to be recalled, whereas event # 15 is incidental to the plot of the story and unlikely to be recalled. More detailed examples of network representations of stories appear in Trabasso and Sperry (1985) and van den Broek, Lorch, and Thurlow (1996).

Even young children's story comprehension is influenced by causal connections. Children as young as age 4 years recall events with many causal connections more often than events with few causal connections (van den Broek et al., 1996). In addition, as children develop, they become better able both to identify causal relations in a story and to use them to guide their recall (Ackerman, Paine, & Silver, 1991; van den Broek, 1989).

To examine story comprehension and attention among children with ADHD, we have conducted a series of studies employing a television-viewing methodology (Landau, Lorch, & Milich, 1992; Lorch et al., 2000; Lorch et al., 2004). In this approach, children watch two television programs, one in the presence of toys and one in their absence. Visual attention to the television is recorded throughout each program. At the end of each program children are asked questions assessing their recall of factual (i.e., "what" questions) and causal relations (i.e., "why" questions) information. The results of these studies reveal that in the absence of toys there are no significant differences in visual attention or story recall between 7- to 11-year-old children with ADHD and comparison children. In contrast, in the presence of toys, children with ADHD show a steeper decrease in visual attention than do comparison children. In terms of story recall, children with ADHD again show no deficit in the recall of factual information, but exhibit significantly poorer performance than comparison children on questions testing causal relations. In fact, comparison children show no drop in recall of causal relations information when toys are present, despite a significant decrease in their visual attention. Thus, in three studies (Landau et al., 1992; Lorch et al., 2000, Studies 1 and 2), differences in story comprehension between ADHD and comparison groups emerged when tasks tapped the understanding of specific causal relations between story events, but only in the presence of toys. This indicates that children with ADHD do not necessarily have a generalized deficit in understanding causal relations. Instead, their ability to understand how story events are connected is more easily disrupted by distractors than is that of comparison children.

How might the attentional problems of children with ADHD impair their understanding of causal relations, but not factual events, in the presence of toys? To answer this question we need to look more closely at differences in the patterns of attention for comparison children and for children with ADHD. One possibility is that children with ADHD shift their visual attention more frequently, thus disrupting the continuity of their story processing. However, studies consistently have failed to find group differences in the number of looks at the television in the toys-present condition (Landau et al., 1992; Lorch et al., 2000). A second possibility is that children with ADHD engage in shorter looks at the television during the toys-present condition, thus impeding their construction of a coherent story representation. Indeed, these same studies consistently found that the average length of looks at the television is significantly shorter for children with ADHD than for comparison children. The question thus becomes how the group differences in look lengths might account for the problems children with ADHD have in understanding causal relations. One viable explanation stems from evidence that long looks at the television reflect greater cognitive engagement (Anderson, Choi, & Lorch, 1987).

A link between look length and cognitive engagement is suggested by studies of a phenomenon known as "attentional inertia." *Attentional inertia* is defined as an increasing probability of a look continuing the longer the look already has been in progress (Anderson, Alwitt, Lorch, & Levin, 1979). That is, a look at the television is most likely to be terminated early in the look (within the first 3 seconds), with an increasing probability of the look being maintained until around 15 seconds, when the probability begins to level off (Anderson & Lorch, 1983). Research also suggests that long looks (i.e., $\geq$ 15 seconds) are indicative of increased cognitive engagement and deeper processing, for both adults (Burns & Anderson, 1993; Hawkins, Tapper, Bruce, & Pingree,1995) and children (Anderson et al., 1987; Lorch & Castle, 1997).

Although several studies suggest a relation between long looks and cognitive engagement, no studies had investigated whether differences in look length are linked to differences in story recall between children with ADHD and comparison children. One possible explanation for the difficulties children with ADHD have in answering causal relations questions when their attention is divided is that these children spend less time engaged in long looks at the television. If long looks are indicative of increased cognitive engagement, these children would be less engaged with the material and thereby less likely to make connections among events.

Lorch et al. (2004) specifically investigated, among a sample of boys and girls ranging in age from 7 to 11, whether time spent in long looks, but not short looks, accounts for the differences between children with ADHD and comparison children in performance on causal relations questions when toys are present during viewing. Employing the same procedures as in the earlier studies, they replicated the basic visual attention and factual and causal recall findings for both viewing conditions from Landau et al. (1992) and Lorch et al. (2000). In addition, there were no group differences in terms of number of looks the children made to the television, but in the toys-present condition the comparison children spent more time in long looks (i.e., $\geq$ 15 seconds) than did the children with ADHD.

The primary purpose of the Lorch et al. (2004) study was to test the hypothesis that differences in cognitive engagement accounted for group differences in recall of causal relations in the toys-present condition. Three different analytic strategies focused on how patterns of attention in the toys-present condition related to recall. The first analyses tested whether time spent in long looks, but not time spent in short (i.e., < 15 seconds) looks, significantly mediated group differences in recall of causal relations. The second set of analyses compared the groups in their distributions of long looks, short looks, and looks away during presentation of information necessary to answer causal relations questions. The third set of analyses compared the groups' performance on the causal relations questions for long looks, short looks, and looks away during presentation of the relevant information.

The results of these three analytic strategies converged to offer compelling support for the hypothesis that greater cognitive engagement enables the comparison children to form a more coherent representation of the relations among story events, thereby accounting for group differences when toys are present. The first set of analyses revealed that total time spent in long looks, but not total time spent in short looks, was a significant mediator of group differences in recall of causal relations. The second set of analyses demonstrated that comparison children were engaged in long looks during presentation of information relevant to causal relations questions significantly more often than were children with ADHD. In contrast, children with ADHD were found to be looking away during presentation of information relevant to causal relations questions significantly more often than were comparison children. Finally, the third set of analyses indicated that children with ADHD and the comparison children performed comparably on causal relations questions when both groups of children were looking away during presentation of information needed to answer the questions. In contrast, the comparison group significantly outperformed the children with ADHD on these questions when the children were engaged in short looks during presentation of the relevant information. Most importantly, the two groups did not differ significantly when the participants were engaged in long looks during the presentation of information necessary to answer the causal relations questions.

Taken together, the findings from Lorch et al. (2004) are consistent with the literature on attentional inertia and provide further support for the interpretation that long looks lead to deeper cognitive processing (Burns & Anderson, 1993; Hawkins et al., 1995). Of greater significance, these findings constitute the first evidence that the amount of time spent in long looks helps explain the differential patterns of recall in children with ADHD and comparison children. The most likely explanation for this relation is that long looks are an external indicator of deeper cognitive processing. Further, the similar performance on causal relations questions by the two groups of children when toys are absent can be explained by the fact that in this condition both groups engage primarily in long looks. In contrast, the deficiency in the recall of causal relations shown by children with ADHD in the toys-present condition is attributable to the fact that they spend significantly less time engaged in long looks than comparison children. The most compelling support for this interpretation is that when toys are present, children with ADHD do process information more deeply during long looks, as shown by their improved performance on causal relations questions testing information presented while they are engaged in long looks.

Two intriguing questions arise from these findings. First, why is it that children with ADHD spend less time in long looks in the presence of toys than comparison children? Second, why is it that time spent in long looks is associated with better recall of causal relations? Regarding the first question, the results of Lorch et al. (2004) are consistent with observations that the attention of children with ADHD is especially susceptible to disruption by salient distractors (Barkley, 1997). As the contrasting results of the toys-absent and toys-present conditions revealed, the problem these children have is not specifically sustaining attention, but sustaining attention in the presence of salient distractors. Comparison children, relative to children with ADHD, may be able to divide their attention more systematically between the ongoing story and their toy play so that they are more likely to be engaged in a long look when information relevant to understanding causal relations is presented.

The second question raised is why time spent in long looks is associated with better recall of causal relations. A possible explanation is that construction of coherent story representations requires periods of uninterrupted attention so that children can hold relevant information in working memory, detect connections among events, and store these connections in the developing story representation. According to this interpretation, children who spend more time in long looks then can use their more coherent emerging representations to guide further processing and thereby make additional causal connections. This perspective also could explain why the greater time in long looks among comparison children might enhance their comprehension of causal relation information presented during short looks. First, by developing a more coherent story representation, comparison children may monitor more systematically their ongoing understanding of the story than do children with ADHD, which enables the comparison children to use short looks to fill in missing information. Second, more coherent story representations among comparison children may provide a structure for connecting incoming information, even that obtained during short looks. Finally, more coherent story representations may enable more effective retrieval strategies. Specifically, comparison children may use these story representations to make inferences about the connections among events during cued recall testing, even if short looks did not allow for deeper processing at the time of viewing.

DIFFICULTIES USING THE GOAL STRUCTURE OF A STORY

In addition to the central role of causal relations, a second feature of the network model of story comprehension is a focus on the *goals* arising from certain story events that in turn motivate other actions and outcomes (Mandler & Johnson, 1977; Stein & Glenn, 1979). The goals of a character in a story may be stated explicitly, or they may need to be inferred from other events that suggest the character's motivations. A given goal may motivate a number of subsequent action sequences. For example, in the story in Appendix 5.1, the goal of protecting the people of the kingdom motivates the Knight's intention to challenge the Dragon and in turn many of the Knight's subsequent actions. Thus, understanding a character's goals is an important influence on overall story comprehension. Young children show considerable difficulty in using goal information to enhance their story comprehension. This is true regardless of whether the task involves memory demands (i.e., recalling a story) or minimizes such demands (i.e., narrating a story from a sequence of pictures) (Trabasso & Stein, 1997). With increasing age, goals take on added importance, to the point where they become a dominant feature in older children's story representations (Goldman & Varnhagen, 1986; Trabasso & Nickels, 1992; Trabasso, Secco, & van den Broek, 1984; van den Broek et al., 1996).

Renz et al. (2003) used an online story narration procedure to examine the use of goal structure among children with ADHD. The story used by Renz et al. (2003), *Frog, Where Are You?*, by Mercer Mayer (1969), contains 24 pictures and includes a hierarchical goal structure. The story begins with a frog escaping from its owner, a little boy. The overall goal that can be inferred from the pictures is for the boy to find the frog and bring it back home. The story then progresses with a number of unsuccessful attempts to meet this goal, creating subgoals. Ultimately, the boy does find the frog, and to his surprise, the frog's family. The boy is then allowed to take a baby frog home, thus resolving his overall goal of bringing a frog back home.

In the Renz et al. (2003) study, 9- to 11-year-old boys with or without ADHD were asked to tell a story based on the pictures, and these narratives were then coded using story grammar categories (Stein & Glenn, 1979). The establishment of the overall goal, the subsequent subgoal attempts and outcomes, and the resolution of the overall goal were the most important story grammar categories coded. The subgoal attempts were classified into unlinked attempts (i.e., not explicitly related to finding the frog), linked attempts (i.e., specifying the overall goal of finding the frog), and specific linked attempts (i.e., when the boy searched specific locations for the frog). Linked attempts suggest an understanding of both goal structure and causal connections because the child restates the boy's goal of searching to recover the frog, which was established at the beginning of the story.

The results indicated that the two groups of children told stories of similar length. However, comparison children included the resolution of the overall goal significantly more often than children with ADHD, suggesting that comparison children are better able to maintain a goal plan throughout the narration of a story. Children with ADHD also used fewer specific linked attempts than did comparison children. This suggests that children with ADHD have a less developed understanding of goal plans than their comparison peers.

Although the Renz et al. (2003) study is important to understanding the organization of narratives of children with ADHD, the age range of children within the study may not have captured major developmental changes in story comprehension. According to Trabasso et al. (1992), the most important ages for the development of the understanding of causal structure and goal plan are between age 3 and age 9. Thus, in a subsequent study (Flory et al., 2006), the methodology of Renz et al. (2003) was replicated using 7- to 9-year-old boys and girls with and without ADHD. Similar to the results of Renz et al., the two groups of children did not differ in the lengths of stories they narrated. However, there were group differences on several of the story grammar categories related to the causal structure of the stories. Specifically, comparison children were significantly more likely to mention the initiating event (e.g., the boy discovers that the frog is missing from the jar) than were the children with ADHD. The former were also more likely to include goal–attempt–outcome (GAO) sequences in their narratives, and to state the completion of the overall goal.

The results of the Renz et al. (2003) and Flory et al. (2006) online story narration studies both revealed problems that children with ADHD have in narrating a coherent, goal-based story. To create a coherent story representation, children need to recognize events that motivate the overall goal, actions and outcomes that result from the goal, and subgoals that may follow from actions and outcomes. Although the results of Renz et al. and Flory et al. are not identical, both studies point to goal-based story events as a major area in which children with ADHD are deficient in their story narrations. Further, these deficiencies are evident even when memory and attentional demands are relatively low, as is the case for online narrations.

DIFFICULTIES RECOGNIZING
IMPORTANT INFORMATION IN A STORY

Theories of story comprehension emphasize the importance of causal relations among events, and the special role that goals play as the linchpin of story representation. Because goals motivate so many story events, they almost invariably have many causal relations with other events. Goals and other events with many causal connections are likely to represent the information in a story judged to be most important by mature comprehenders (Trabasso & Sperry, 1985). Thus, in order to demonstrate effective story comprehension, children's recall must focus on these important events with many causal connections. As noted earlier, children as young as age 4 recall events with many causal connections more often than events with few causal connections (van den Broek et al., 1996), and this effect becomes more pronounced as children develop (Ackerman et al., 1991; van den Broek, 1989).

Lorch et al. (1999) examined the role of causal relations, as well as perceived importance, in predicting the recall of children with ADHD and their comparison classmates. The boys and girls, ranging in age from 7 to 11, listened to audiotape presentations of two relatively brief (e.g., 4 minutes) folktales, used previously by Brown and Smiley (1977). After hearing each story, the children were asked to retell the stories. Importance ratings and causal network analyses of the folktales were available, and regression analyses were used to predict recall of each story unit from the number of causal connections and importance of each story unit for the two groups of children.

Consistent with the story comprehension literature (van den Broek et al., 1996), as the number of causal connections and their importance increased, recall increased for both groups, but these relations were stronger for comparison children than for children with ADHD. Further examination revealed that the number of causal connections was the only predictor variable to make a unique contribution to the interaction. Thus, as the number of causal connections to a story event increased, the increase in recall was steeper for comparison children than for children with ADHD.

Lorch, O'Neil, et al. (2004) replicated and extended the findings of Lorch et al. (1999) by evaluating recall immediately after hearing the story and then following an opportunity to study the story among a sample of boys and girls, ranging in age from 7 through 11. Consistent with Lorch et al. (1999), the number of causal connections predicted recall, and also interacted significantly with diagnostic group in predicting recall, such that children with ADHD benefited less than comparison children in their recalls as the number of causal connections increased. After studying, comparison children added more new story events to their recalls than children with ADHD, but this difference only occurred for events with the highest number of causal connections. Thus, studying appears to be more effective for the comparison children in helping them add the information that is the most important for a coherent understanding of the story.

These two studies indicate that children with ADHD are less likely than comparison children to remember the most important information in a story. One factor that may contribute to such a difference is the ability to recognize variations in importance among story events. Lorch, Milich, Astrin, and Berthiaume (2006) investigated this issue by having boys and girls, ranging in age from 4 through 10, watch one of two television programs and then sort selected events from the program into categories reflecting high, medium, or low importance to the story. The 12 selected events were designated as high, medium, or low in importance based on causal network analyses and adult importance ratings. Relative to this ideal categorization, children with ADHD made more sorting errors than comparison children. Further, sorting errors significantly predicted cued recall performance. In fact, a group difference obtained in cued recall performance was eliminated when the number of sorting errors was accounted for in the analysis. These findings support the hypothesis that the recall of children with ADHD may show less sensitivity to the importance of story events because these children have difficulty differentiating the degree to which events matter to the plot of a story.

DIFFICULTIES IN MAKING INFERENCES
AND MONITORING COMPREHENSION

Two related skills important for effective story comprehension are the abilities to make appropriate inferences and to monitor ongoing comprehension (Berthiaume, Lorch, & Milich, 2005). Inference making requires the use of relevant general knowledge to make sense of information implied in a text or story (van den Broek et al., 2005). Once generated, inferences must be continually monitored and modified as new information is encountered. Inferential processing has been identified as an academic skill critical to success in listening and reading comprehension tasks (Pearson, Dole, Duffy, & Roehler, 1992). Inference making in preschool has been found to strongly predict later reading comprehension, over and above the effects of basic literacy skills like word identification and phonemic awareness (van den Broek et al., 2005). Inferential processing helps not only with understanding of text, but also with recall of text information (Yuill & Oakhill, 1991), and is highly important for connecting events in stories and integrating story information to form a mental representation (van den Broek et al., 2005). The process of connecting prior knowledge and story events to create inferences propels the student forward by facilitating comprehension and making the story more meaningful (Yuill & Oakhill, 1991). Finally, young children and those classified as "poor" comprehenders make fewer inferences from texts and are less able than older and more skilled readers to integrate ideas from different parts of a story to create accurate mental representations (Cain & Oakhill, 1999; Schmidt & Paris, 1983).

Comprehension monitoring is a second, related skill that children need to use in order to comprehend stories effectively. The term "comprehension monitoring" generally applies to both the process of monitoring understanding of text and to the strategy of taking corrective action when comprehension deficits are detected. Thus, comprehension monitoring refers both to the metacognitive strategy by which comprehension is evaluated and to the methods through which the reader regulates it (Wagoner, 1983). Monitoring comprehension of stories is essential for identifying gaps in understanding. If a student fails to recognize these gaps and take corrective action toward filling these gaps, important connections among story events may be missed and comprehension and recall will be compromised. Not surprisingly, levels of reading comprehension and comprehension monitoring are significantly related in groups of both low- and high-achieving students (Kinnunen & Varras, 1998). Specifically, poorer comprehenders have more difficulty detecting inconsistencies in stories and texts than more skilled comprehenders (Grabe & Mann, 1984; Walczyk & Hall, 1989).

Only one study has examined inference making and comprehension monitoring among children with ADHD (Berthiaume et al., 2005). Three tasks were employed to measure how 7- to 12-year-old boys with ADHD and their comparison peers create and evaluate inferences, distinguish between consistent and inconsistent story information, and verbally represent their understanding of a story as it is ongoing (via a think-aloud task). Relative to the comparison group, boys with ADHD had more difficulty making accurate inferences about an ambiguous premise, regardless of how many clues they were given to constrain the inference. In addition, these boys indicated higher confidence in their answers, even when they had very little information on which to base them. On the comprehension-monitoring task, boys with ADHD had more difficulty than comparison boys identifying internally inconsistent stories. On the think-aloud task, boys with ADHD made more implausible explanatory inferences for story events than comparison boys. Further, during the think-aloud task the boys with ADHD had more difficulty thinking of things to say, expressed more uncertainty about what the task required, and offered more irrelevant comments.

Because causal connections among story events often are implicit, difficulty understanding, creating, and monitoring inferences will certainly lead children with ADHD to miss some important connections among story events. Failing to make these connections or to notice gaps in understanding could cause these children to form incomplete mental representations of stories, resulting in poorer understanding of the underlying causal structure. Thus, to the extent children with ADHD have difficulty with aspects of inferential processing and comprehension monitoring, they may show deficits in their understanding of implied causal relations among events (Berthiaume et al., 2005).

TREATMENT IMPLICATIONS

Although a good deal of research has demonstrated the positive impact of training in comprehension strategies for less-skilled readers, very few strategies have been studied specifically for use with an ADHD population (Berthiaume, 2006). The current empirically validated treatments for children with ADHD are stimulant medication, parent training, and behavior modification (Pelham, Wheeler, & Chronis, 1998). Such interventions have demonstrated efficacy for improving some of the academic problems these children experience. For example, these treatments have been found to decrease disruptive behavior and increase the quantity of academic work produced (DuPaul & Eckert, 1997). However, the impact of medication on performance of higher order academic tasks such as comprehension of complex texts and skill acquisition has not been established. Further, emerging evidence strongly suggests that long-term treatment with stimulant medication has no long-term positive effects on the children's academic performance (Fabiano & Pelham, 2002). More specifically, related to story comprehension, Francis, Fine, and Tannock (2001) asked 50 children with a confirmed diagnosis of ADHD/combined type to retell stories they had both heard via audiotape and seen as wordless picture books, both on and off stimulant medication. Findings revealed that although children more often reported story characters' internal responses and attempts when on methylphenidate (Ritalin), the medication had no effect on their inferential comprehension performance.

Stimulant medications and behavioral modification programs may *prime* children with ADHD to perform complex cognitive tasks by helping them focus and attend. However, there is research to suggest that children with ADHD exhibit academic and story comprehension deficits that are not remedied by these treatments. As Rabiner and Coie (2000) hypothesized in their study of reading achievement, children with attentional problems may have trouble acquiring new reading skills and catching up on the reading skills they have failed to acquire. This may be the case even when visual attention and on-task behavior have improved.

Based on the review of story comprehension impairments we offered earlier, we propose that effective academic interventions for children with ADHD may need to go beyond simply increasing their rates of on-task behavior. Although treatment approaches aimed at improving the attending and studying behaviors of children with ADHD might prime them to better understand and remember stories, these methods may not be sufficient to address the higher order deficits in story comprehension discussed earlier. Instead, effective interventions might need to assist these children in making connections among events and in using those connections to form coherent representations of lectures and texts. Many of the comprehension strategies employed successfully for children who experience academic difficulty emphasize integrating information from text and from previous knowledge into mental representations of story and text events. Unfortunately, despite the obvious academic difficulties exhibited by children with ADHD, very little research has examined the use of interventions with this group that are supported by the educational research literature.

This chapter has reviewed four key problems that children with ADHD have in comprehending stories: (1) difficulty sustaining cognitive engagement, which leads to decreased understanding of causal relations; (2) difficulty using a story's goal structure to help build a coherent story representation; (3) difficulty recognizing story-important information and using it to guide recall; and (4) difficulty making inferences and monitoring their own comprehension. Although in this chapter we have presented these as four distinct deficits, in some ways all four of these reflect difficulties in recognizing and utilizing the structure of stories to guide comprehension. Thus, successful academic interventions for children with ADHD should somehow incorporate training that increases these children's sensitivity to key elements of story structure.

A review of the educational literature reveals a number of intervention techniques that have been used successfully with children identified as poor comprehenders. Many of these strategies place emphasis on the interrelated areas of difficulty we have identified for children with ADHD (Berthiaume, 2006). In the remainder of this section, we review some of these techniques, the evidence supporting their use, and the manner in which these interventions could target the specific deficits exhibited by children with ADHD.

Academic interventions that place emphasis on how story events are related to each other and that require connections to be made among events as the story is ongoing may help children with ADHD better sustain their cognitive engagement with important story information. Daily instruction of elementary school-age children too often focuses primarily on helping children gain factual information from lectures or stories, ignoring the importance of how story events are related to one another (Pressley, 2002). Instruction emphasizing causal relations among events might help sensitize children with ADHD to the organizing structure of stories and lectures, and assist them in building more effective representations to guide understanding and recall. One approach might be for teachers to systematically ask students *why* story events occur as information is being presented. These causal relations questions should help students with ADHD appreciate story events as having an underlying coherence, rather than viewing them as a series of discrete facts.

Results suggest that simply encouraging children with ADHD to "study more" or relying solely on interventions that facilitate study behaviors (e.g., behavior modification procedures) may not sufficiently increase the effectiveness of their studying for identifying and remembering causal relations among events (Lorch, O'Neil, et al., 2004). A more effective strategy might be to teach children with ADHD to study the *connections* among story events. Study aids could be created that require students to outline the material to be learned in such a fashion that causal connections are highlighted. For example, a guide like a *story map* (Swanson & De La Paz, 1998) that requires the student to fill in major events in sequence could assist him or her in connecting the events and solidifying the overall causal structure of the story. (See Appendix 5.1 for an example of a story and the story map associated with it.) Given that the studying behavior of children with ADHD was similar to that of their comparison peers in the Lorch et al. (2004) study, examining group differences in cognitive processing while the study period is ongoing might be another fruitful avenue of future research.

Character goals and subgoals have special importance in understanding causal relations among events. Research has found that children need to comprehend how goals and subgoals lead to actions and story outcomes in order to develop a coherent narrative representation (Trabasso & Stein, 1997). Renz et al. (2003) and Flory et al. (2006) demonstrated that children with ADHD have difficulty maintaining focus on characters' goals as they build a story representation. To help children with ADHD better understand the goal structure of stories, instruction should focus on helping these children relate ongoing events to what characters are attempting to accomplish and how characters must change their behavior in response to outcomes that result from unsuccessful attempts to achieve goals. Story maps and similar tools help children understand goals by identifying precipitating events, character goals and actions, and resulting outcomes. Teachers can help students focus on goals by asking questions about character goals, attempts to reach those goals, and the outcomes of those attempts. Students should also be asked to predict character actions and eventual outcomes based on goals and other relevant story events. Teachers might work with students to reexamine and modify implausible or incorrect predictions. When an event is not predicted accurately, the causal chain leading up to it should be graphically mapped to help students understand the preceding events and how those events might have been used to predict the eventual outcome.

It is unclear why children with ADHD have difficulty engaging with, identifying, and recalling central story material. One possibility is that they are unable to filter story information quickly enough to determine what is important in time to increase their engagement with it. Another explanation is that these children do not pick up on cues that signal the significance of an event. Either way, intervention should focus on helping children with ADHD learn what makes an event central versus incidental to a story. Teachers might discuss with students the kinds of events that are generally important in stories (e.g., goals, character attempts to reach goals, outcomes of those attempts) and what signifies that an event is important (e.g., it causes or is caused by other events in the story, its absence would make the story less understandable). A possible tool to give students the opportunity to practice classifying story events into importance categories might follow the structure of the sorting task employed by Lorch et al. (2006). Teachers might review evidence with students that a given event belongs in a given category based on the number of connections it has to other events and its role in the overall causal structure of the story.

Training students with ADHD to use inference-making and self-questioning strategies may be a way to help remedy the story comprehension difficulties they experience. These two approaches appear to directly target many of the complex cognitive processes involved in reading comprehension because they focus on causal connections among story events and the overall causal structure of stories. McGee and Johnson (2003) examined the effects of training 75 6- to 9-year-old children classified as "skilled" versus "less-skilled" comprehenders in inference-making techniques. Findings revealed that training in inference making was superior to standard comprehension strategies for helping less-skilled comprehenders understand the story. This study and others suggest that, given appropriate instruction, children with deficits in understanding connections among story events may learn how to use context and prior knowledge to improve their comprehension and recall skills.

One method of helping students with ADHD improve their skills in inference making might be to provide them with the opportunity to practice drawing inferences as a story is ongoing. Berthiaume et al. (2005) found that children with ADHD are considerably more likely than their comparison peers to make inaccurate or implausible explanatory inferences for story events. Training should teach these children how to constrain their explanations to *plausible* ones based on relevant information. Focusing only on that general knowledge and story information that will most directly help with story understanding can help children with ADHD better solidify their understanding of the relation between precipitating events and outcomes. To train students with ADHD in metacognitive awareness about explanatory inferences, teachers could engage them in evidence-gathering processes. Following the formation of an explanation, teachers might ask students to list the evidence based on previous events and prior knowledge that the inference is plausible. If the inference is shown to be incorrect, students should reexamine their evidence to determine why their explanation was unfounded.

Skilled readers ask themselves questions about texts and about their own understanding of texts. Answering these questions helps the reader develop a richer, more in-depth understanding of story events and the connections among them. In addition, self-questioning assists the reader in identifying where comprehension has failed, allowing him or her to remedy the difficulties before more confusion occurs. Research has supported the use of self-questioning strategies to improve the reading comprehension of school-age children classified as poor comprehenders (Hansen, 1981). A meta-analysis of 68 studies found that interventions including a self-questioning component resulted in greater improvement than instructional approaches that did not include self-questioning (Mastropieri, Scruggs, Bakken, & Whedon, 1996). Consequently, Mastropieri and Scruggs (1997) identified self-questioning strategies as among the best practices for facilitating the reading comprehension of students with learning difficulties.

Learning to use effective comprehension-monitoring strategies might help children with ADHD recognize the gaps in their understanding of how text and lecture events are connected to one another. Explicit training in strategies for filling in those gaps, once identified, will further aid these children in creating more complete story representations. Self-questioning about comprehension is one strategy found to be effective at promoting comprehension monitoring. Teacher modeling of simple, comprehension-related questions might help students with ADHD learn to recognize when comprehension failures occur. Training in strategies like rereading, note taking, and summarizing will assist children in repairing gaps in comprehension.

Unfortunately, the treatment literature rarely, if ever, recommends interventions that focus on training children with ADHD to enhance their representation of story information (Berthiaume, 2006). This omission is explained by the fact that very little research has examined how the cognitive-processing skills of children with ADHD differ from those of their classmates or how children with ADHD might benefit from receiving strategy instruction that focuses on helping children understand and infer connections among story events. Studies suggesting that current empirically validated treatments for children with ADHD fail to improve some aspects of academic performance (Francis et al., 2001; The MTA Cooperative Group, 1999) indicate that a move toward use of strategies that target deficits in understanding connections among events is crucial. Educational intervention will work best in conjunction with the treatments currently recommended for children with ADHD, as the core symptoms (e.g., inattention, impulsivity) of the disorder are likely to interfere with children's ability to attend to, retain, and practice techniques for improving their comprehension skills.

Given that many children with ADHD experience low frustration tolerance and motivational difficulties, applying a reinforcement system for promoting the use of educational intervention strategies is a necessary step (Berthiaume, 2006). In addition, several researchers suggest that children will be more motivated to improve their performance *outcomes* (e.g., test scores) if teachers praise them for engaging in learning *processes* like metacognitive strategies (Gaskins & Gaskins, 1997). For example, a student who asks himself *why* a story event occurred following strategy training should be reinforced for attempting to make connections between events. Similarly, a student who looks back to an earlier part of a story in order to understand something she has just read should be reinforced for using effective comprehension-monitoring skills. Thus, students with ADHD should be reinforced for both improvements in performance and for effectively *engaging* in strategy training (Berthiaume, 2006). Explaining to students the purpose of a task may be a key step toward increasing motivation and task persistence. Students will be more likely to put effort into comprehending texts that are relevant to their lives and interests, and will be better able to understand texts when they already hold some relevant knowledge.

Throughout this section we have discussed strategies and training procedures that can be undertaken regardless of whether children are fluent readers. This is particularly important because basic reading problems are common among children with ADHD. Obviously, teachers need to work to improve decoding skills and other basic reading processes. There are empirically validated interventions that address deficiencies in these areas (Torgesen et al., 2001). However, our findings in story comprehension tasks that do not require reading indicate that interventions must address these higher order processing deficits as well. There are several reasons why employing interventions that target higher order skills but do not require reading may be particularly effective in engaging children with ADHD. First, based on parental reports, children with ADHD enjoy being read to as much as their comparison peers, although they experience less enjoyment than their peers in independent reading (Acevedo-Polakovich, Lorch, & Milich, in press). Second, because teachers are not limited to what the child can read, they can employ more complex and entertaining stories, and they can use presentation modalities (e.g., films) and intervention procedures that are more likely to engage the children. For example, to train children to make appropriate inferences, teachers can incorporate predictive inferences into building excitement about the outcome of a story. Similarly, some children's television programs (e.g., *Ghostwriter, Blue's Clues*) employ a mystery-solving format to motivate children to connect events. As these examples illustrate, even for children who have significant reading problems, interventions targeting these higher order cognitive processes can proceed in parallel with basic reading instruction.

CLOSING COMMENTS

In this review we have identified four broad areas of impairment in story comprehension among children with ADHD. Future research needs to further develop our understanding of these story comprehension problems, and to explore the possibility of other areas of difficulty. Based on the deficits identified to date, we offered preliminary suggestions for potentially beneficial remedial strategies that are consistent with findings from the educational research literature. Systematic research is necessary to evaluate the efficacy of the suggested strategies in ameliorating the story comprehension problems found among children with ADHD. We hope that this chapter will stimulate research necessary to better understand these children's story comprehension difficulties and the most effective intervention strategies to improve their academic outcomes.

ACKNOWLEDGMENTS

Preparation of this chapter was supported by National Institute of Mental Health Grant No. MH47386. We thank Chandra N. Strange and Sara Lonnemann for creating the story included in Appendix 5.1.

REFERENCES

Acevedo-Polakovich, D., Lorch, E. P., & Milich, R. (in press). Comparing television use and reading in children with ADHD and non-referred children across two age groups. *Media Psychology*.

Ackerman, B. P., Paine, J., & Silver, D. (1991). Building a story representation: The effects of early concepts on later causal inferences by children. *Developmental Psychology, 27*, 370–380.

Ackerman, B. P., Silver, D., & Glickman, I. (1990). Concept availability in the causal inferences by children and adults. *Child Development, 61*, 230–246.

American Psychiatric Association. (1994). *Diagnostic and statistical manual of mental disorders* (4th ed.). Washington, DC: Author.

Anderson, D. R., Alwitt, L., Lorch, E., & Levin, S. (1979). Watching children watch television. In G. Hale & M. Lewis (Eds.), *Attention and cognitive development* (pp. 331–361). New York: Plenum Press.

Anderson, D. R., Choi, H. P., & Lorch, E. P. (1987). Attentional inertia reduces distractibility in young children's television viewing. *Child Development, 58*, 798–806.

Anderson, D. R., & Lorch, E. P. (1983). Looking at television: Action or reaction? In J. Bryant & D. R. Anderson (Eds.), *Children's understanding of television: Research on attention and comprehension* (pp. 1–33). New York: Academic Press.

Barkley, R. A. (1997). Behavioral inhibition, sustained attention, and executive functioning: Constructing a unified theory of ADHD. *Psychological Bulletin, 121*, 65–94.

Barkley, R. A. (1998). *Attention-deficit hyperactivity disorder: A handbook for diagnosis and treatment* (2nd ed.). New York: Guilford Press.

Berthiaume, K. S. (2006). Story comprehension and academic deficits in children with ADHD: What is the connection? *School Psychology Review, 35,* 309–323.

Berthiaume, K. S., Lorch, E. P., & Milich, R. (2006). *Getting clued in: Inferential processing and comprehension monitoring in children with ADHD.* Manuscript submitted for publication.

Brown, A. L., & Smiley, S. S. (1977). Rating the importance of structural units of prose passages: A problem of metacognitive development. *Child Development, 48,* 1–8.

Burns, J. J., & Anderson, D. R. (1993). Attentional inertia and recognition memory in adult television viewing. *Communication Research, 20,* 777–799.

Cain, K., & Oakhill, J. V. (1999). Inference making and its relation to comprehension failure. *Reading and Writing, 11,* 489–503.

Diener, M. B., & Milich, R. (1997). The effects of positive feedback on the social interactions of boys with ADHD: A test of the self-protective hypothesis. *Journal of Clinical Child Psychology, 26,* 256–265.

Douglas, V. I. (1999). Cognitive control processes in attention-deficit/hyperactivity disorder. In H. C. Quay & A. E. Hogan (Eds.), *Handbook of disruptive behavior disorders* (pp. 105–138). New York: Kluwer Academic.

DuPaul, G. J., & Eckert, T. L. (1997). The effects of school-based interventions for attention deficit hyperactivity disorder: A meta-analysis. *School Psychology Review, 26,* 5–27.

Fabiano, G. A., & Pelham, W. E. Jr. (2002). Comprehensive treatment for attention-deficit/hyperactivity disorder. In M. Fristad & D. T. Marsh (Eds.), *Handbook of serious emotional disturbance in children and adolescents* (pp. 149–174): New York: Wiley.

Flory, K., Hayden, A. N., Milich, R., Lorch, E. P., Strange, C., & Welsh, R. (2006). Online story comprehension among children with ADHD: Which core deficits are involved? *Journal of Abnormal Child Psychology, 34,* 850–862.

Francis, S., Fine, J., & Tannock, R. (2001). Methylphenidate selectively improves storytelling in children with attention deficit hyperactivity disorder. *Journal of Child and Adolescent Psychopharmacology, 11*(3), 217–228.

Gaskins, R. W., & Gaskins, I. W. (1997). Creating readers who read for meaning and love to read: Benchmark School Reading Program. In S. A. Stahl & D. A. Hayes (Eds.), *Instructional models in reading.* Mahwah, NJ: Erlbaum.

Goldman, S. R., & Varnhagen, C. K. (1986). Memory for embedded and sequential story structures. *Journal of Memory and Language, 25,* 401–418.

Grabe, M., & Mann, S. (1984). A technique for the assessment and training of comprehension monitoring skills. *Journal of Reading Behavior, 16*(2), 131–144.

Graesser, A. C., & Clark, L. F. (1985). *Structures and procedures of implicit knowledge.* Norwood, NJ: Ablex.

Hansen, J. (1981). The effects of inference training and practice on young children's reading comprehension. *Reading Research Quarterly, 3,* 391–417.

Hawkins, R. P., Tapper, J., Bruce, L., & Pingree, S. (1995). Strategic and non-strategic explanations for attentional inertia. *Communication Research, 22,* 188–206.

Kinnunen, R., & Vauras, M. (1998). Comprehension-monitoring in beginning readers. *Scientific Studies of Reading, 2,* 353–375.

Landau, S., Lorch, E. P., & Milich, R. (1992). Visual attention to and comprehension of television in attention-deficit hyperactivity disordered and normal boys. *Child Development, 63,* 928–937.

Lorch, E. P., & Castle, V. J. (1997). Preschool children's attention to television: Visual attention and probe response times. *Journal of Experimental Child Psychology, 66,* 111–127.

Lorch, E. P., Diener, M. B., Sanchez, R. P., Milich, R., van den Broek, P., & Welsh, R. (1999). The effects of story structure on the recall of stories in children with attention deficit hyperactivity disorder. *Journal of Educational Psychology, 92,* 273–283.

Lorch, E. P., Eastham, D., Milich, R., Lemberger, C. C., Sanchez, R. P., Welsh, R., et al. (2004). Difficulties in comprehending causal relations among children with ADHD: The role of cognitive engagement. *Journal of Abnormal Psychology, 113,* 56–63.

Lorch, E. P., Milich, R., Astrin, C. C.,& Berthiaume, K. S. (2006). Cognitive engagement and story comprehension in typically developing children and children with ADHD from preschool through elementary school. *Developmental Psychology, 42,* 1206–1219.

Lorch, E. P., Milich, R., Sanchez, R. P., van den Broek, P., Baer, S., Hooks, K., et al. (2000). Comprehension of televised stories in attention deficit hyperactivity disordered and nonreferred boys. *Journal of Abnormal Psychology, 109,* 321–330.

Lorch, E. P., O'Neil, K., Berthiaume, K. S., Milich, R., Eastham, D., & Brooks, T. (2004). Study time and story recall by children with ADHD and nonreferred children. *Journal of Clinical Child and Adolescent Psychiatry, 33,* 506–515.

Mandler, J. M., & Johnson, N.S. (1977). Remembrance of things parsed: Story structure and recall. *Cognitive Psychology, 9,* 111–151.

Mastropieri, M. A., & Scruggs, T. E. (1997). Best practices in promoting reading comprehension in students with learning disabilities. *Remedial and Special Education, 18,* 197–216.

Mastropieri, M. A., Scruggs, T. E., Bakken, J. P., & Whedon, C. (1996). Reading comprehension: A synthesis of research in learning disabilities. In T. E. Scruggs & M. A. Mastropieri (Eds.), *Advances in learning and behavioral disabilities* (pp. 201–227). Greenwich, CT: JAI Press.

Mayer, M. (1969). *Frog, where are you?* New York: Dial Press.

McGee, A., & Johnson, T. H. (1978–1979). The development and evaluation of a self-questioning study technique. *Reading Research Quarterly, 14,* 605–623.

McGee, A., & Johnson, T. H. (2003). The effect of inference training on skilled and less-skilled comprehenders. *Educational Psychology, 23,* 49–59.

Milich, R., Lorch, E. P., & Berthiaume, K. S. (2005). Story comprehension in children with ADHD: Research findings and treatment implications. In

M. P. Larimer (Ed.), *Attention/deficit hyperactivity disorder research* (pp. 111–138). Hauppauge, NY: Nova Science.

The MTA Cooperative Group. (1999). A 14–month randomized clinical trial of treatment strategies for attention-deficit/hyperactivity disorder. *Archives of General Psychiatry, 56,* 1073–1086.

Oakhill, J. V., & Patel, S. (1991). Can imagery training help children who have comprehension problems? *Journal of Research in Reading, 14,* 106–115.

Pearson, P. D., Roehler, L. R., Dole, J. S., & Duffy, G. G. (1992). Developing expertise in reading comprehension: What should be taught and how should it be taught? In S. J. Samuels & A. E. Farstup (Eds.), *What research has to say about reading instruction* (2nd ed., pp. 145–199). Newark, DE: International Reading Association.

Pelham, W. E. Jr., Wheeler, T., & Chronis, A. (1998). Empirically supported psychosocial treatments for attention deficit hyperactivity disorder. *Journal of Clinical Child Psychology, 27,* 190–205.

Pennington, B. F., Groisser, D., & Welsh, M. C. (1993). Contrasting cognitive deficits in attention deficit hyperactivity disorder versus reading disability. *Developmental Psychology, 29,* 511–523.

Pressley, M. (2002). Comprehension strategies instruction: A turn-of-the-century status report. In C. C. Block & M. Pressley (Eds.), *Comprehension instruction: Research-based best practices* (pp. 11–27). New York: Guilford Press.

Purvis, K. L., & Tannock, R. (1997). Language abilities in children with attention deficit hyperactivity disorder, reading disabilities, and normal controls. *Journal of Abnormal Child Psychology, 25,* 133–144.

Rabiner, D., & Coie, J. D. (2000). Early attention problems and children's reading achievement: A longitudinal investigation. *Journal of the American Academy of Child and Adolescent Psychiatry, 39,* 859–867.

Renz, K., Lorch, E. P., Milich, R., Lemberger, C., Bodner, A., & Welsh, R. (2003). Online story representation in boys with attention deficit hyperactivity disorder. *Journal of Abnormal Child Psychology, 31,* 93–104.

Sanchez, R. P., Lorch, E. P., & Milich, R. (1999). Comprehension of televised stories by preschool children with ADHD. *Journal of Clinical Child Psychology, 28,* 376–385.

Schmidt, C. R., & Paris, S. G. (1983). Children's use of successive clues to generate and monitor inferences. *Child Development, 54,* 742–759.

Stein, N. L., & Glenn, C. G. (1979). An analysis of story comprehension in elementary school children. In R. Freedble (Ed.), *Multidisciplinary approaches to discourse comprehension* (pp. 53–120). Hillsdale, NJ: Erlbaum.

Swanson, P. N., & De La Paz, S. (1998). Teaching effective comprehension strategies to students with learning and reading disabilities. *Intervention in School and Clinic, 33,* 209–218.

Torgesen, J. K., Alexander, A. W., Wagner, R. K., Rashotte, C. A., Voeller, K. S., & Conway, T. (2001). Intensive remedial instruction for children with severe reading disabilities: Immediate and long-term outcomes from two instructional approaches. *Journal of Learning Disabilities, 34,* 33–58.

Trabasso, T., & Nickels, M. (1992). The development of goal plans of action in the narration of a picture story. *Discourse Processes, 15,* 249–275.

Trabasso, T., Secco, T., & van den Broek, P. W. (1984). Causal cohesion and story coherence. In H. Mandler, N. L. Stein, & T. Trabasso (Eds.), *Learning and comprehension of text* (pp. 83–111). Hillsdale, NJ: Erlbaum.

Trabasso, T., & Sperry, L. L. (1985). Causal relatedness and importance of story events. *Journal of Memory and Language, 24,* 595–611.

Trabasso, T., & Stein, N. L. (1997). Narrating, representing and remembering event sequences. In P. W. van den Broek, P. J. Baur, & T. Bourg (Eds.), *Developmental spans in event comprehension and representation: Bridging fictional and actual events* (pp. 237–270). Mahwah, NJ: Erlbaum.

Trabasso, T., & van den Broek, P. W. (1985). Causal thinking and the representation of narrative events. *Journal of Memory and Language, 24,* 612–630.

Trabasso, T., van den Broek, P. W., & Suh, S. Y. (1989). Logical necessity and transitivity of causal relations in stories. *Discourse Processes, 21,* 1–25.

van den Broek, P. (1989). Causal reasoning and inference-making in judging the importance of story statements. *Child Development, 60,* 286–297.

van den Broek, P. (1990). Causal inferences in the comprehension of narrative texts. In A. C. Graesser & G. H. Bowler (Eds.), *The psychology of learning and motivation: Inferences and text comprehension* (Vol. 25, pp. 175–194). San Diego: Academic Press.

van den Broek, P., Kendeou, P., Kremer, K., Lynch, J. S., Butler, J., White, M. J., et al. (2005). Assessment of comprehension abilities in young children. In S. Stahl & S. Paris (Eds.), *Reading comprehension assessment* (pp. 107–130). Hillsdale, NJ: Erlbaum.

van den Broek, P., Lorch, E. P., & Thurlow, R. (1996). Children's and adults' memory for television stories: The role of causal factors, story-grammar categories and hierarchical level. *Child Development, 67,* 3010–3028.

Wagoner, G. A. (1983). Comprehension-monitoring: What it is and what we know about it. *Reading Research Quarterly, 43,* 328–346.

Walcyzk, J. J., & Hall, V. C. (1989). Is the failure to monitor comprehension an instance of cognitive impulsivity? *Journal of Educational Psychology, 81,* 294–298.

Yuill, N. M., & Oakhill, J. V. (1991). *Children's problems in text comprehension.* New York: Cambridge University Press.

APPENDIX 5.1. THE KNIGHT AND THE DRAGON

Story event	Connections	
	Antecedents	Consequences
1. A long, long time ago (Setting)	0	0
2. There was a kingdom (Setting)	0	1
3. high in the mountains (Setting)	0	1
4. called Castle Kingdom. (Setting)	0	1
5. The people of the kingdom were afraid	2	6
6. of a large, scary Dragon (Setting)	0	2
7. who lived on the highest mountain peak. (Setting)	0	1
8. "We're in danger," the King said.	2	1
9. "I must get our finest Knight	1	2
10. to protect us from the Dragon."	2	2
11. The Knight said, "I will protect the people of the kingdom.	2	2
12. I will go to the Dragon's cave	1	1
13. and challenge him to a fight."	2	5
14. First, the Knight got out his finest armor	2	1
15. and began to shine it.	1	0
16. He gathered his sword and shield	1	1
17. and went off to challenge the Dragon.	2	1
18. The Knight began to climb the Dragon's mountain,	2	1
19. but just as he got to the top,	1	1
20. it started to rain.	1	3
21. "Rain can't hurt me," said the Knight.	1	0
22. But then he realized it was getting hard to move his arms and legs.	1	2
23. "What is happening?" cried the Knight.	1	1
24. He looked down and realized his suit of armor had begun to rust!	1	1
25. So he took off his armor	2	3
26. and dropped it on the side of the mountain.	1	0
27. Then he continued on his way	1	1
28. towards the Dragon's cave.	1	1
29. The Knight marched right into the Dragon's cave,	1	4
30. prepared to do battle.	2	0
31. But it was very dark in the cave,	1	2
32. and the Knight couldn't see the Dragon.	1	1
33. As a matter of fact, he couldn't see anything.	1	2

(continued)

Story event	Connections	
	Antecedents	Consequences
34. "I wish I'd brought a lantern," thought the Knight.	2	0
35. But he kept right on walking into the cave,	1	1
36. and the next thing he knew he was falling!	2	1
37. The Knight had fallen into a giant hole in the cave!	1	4
38. There was no way to escape!	2	1
39. The hole was very deep,	1	2
40. and the rain had made it muddy	1	1
41. and the sides too slippery to climb.	1	2
42. The Knight was stuck!	2	4
43. "What will I do?" he thought.	2	0
44. "I'm stuck in this hole with no escape!	1	2
45. Surely the Dragon will eat me now!"	1	3
46. All of the sudden, the Knight saw a light.	2	0
47. It was fire!	1	1
48. Then, over the edge of the hole, the Knight saw a face appear.	0	1
49. It was the Dragon!	1	2
50. The Dragon smiled.	1	1
51. He said, "I am so sorry, Mr. Knight.	4	1
52. I've been meaning to fix that hole for months,	1	1
53. but haven't gotten around to it.	1	1
54. I forget that it's dangerous for the people.	2	1
55. I am so large it doesn't bother me that much,	0	1
56. and no one comes up to see me very often.	0	1
57. Here, let me give you a tail out."	2	3
58. And with that the Dragon flopped his big tail into the hole,	1	1
59. and it became a very sturdy stairway.	1	2
60. The Knight was worried.	2	2
61. "This Dragon acts nothing like the dangerous monster I've heard about in the kingdom.	2	2
62. Should I trust him?	2	2
63. He could still eat me."	2	0
64. But the Knight didn't really have a choice.	3	0
65. He could stay in the hole forever	1	1
66. or trust the Dragon and climb out.	2	2
67. The Knight slowly began to climb.	2	1
68. When he finally reached the top,	1	1
69. the Knight smiled at the Dragon.	2	1

(continued)

| | Connections | |
Story event	Antecedents	Consequences
70. "Well Dragon," he said. "I guess you're not the mean, scary Dragon that we all thought you were.	3	3
71. I'm sorry that I came to fight you.	2	1
72. I would really like it if you would come back to Castle Kingdom	2	1
73. and meet the rest of our townspeople."	3	1
74. I'm sorry that I scared you," the Dragon replied.	2	2
75. "I would love to meet everyone	2	1
76. and show them that I'm actually very friendly."	2	5
77. So the Knight climbed onto the Dragon's back,	1	1
78. and they flew all the way back to Castle Kingdom.	2	1
79. All of the townspeople gathered in the center of the kingdom	1	1
80. to greet the new friend.	2	0
81. Because he didn't need his armor any more,	2	1
82. the Knight turned it into a grill	1	1
83. and the Dragon used his fire to light the grill.	2	1
84. Together they cooked lots of delicious hamburgers, 1	1	
85. and the entire kingdom celebrated with their new friend.	3	0

THE END

(continued)

STORY MAP

Title: The Knight and the Dragon

Setting: A long, long time ago; Castle Kingdom high in the mountains

Characters: The Knight

The Dragon

The King

Problem: | There was a scary dragon |

Goal: | To protect the people of the kingdom so they will feel safe |

Cause:		Attempt:		Outcome:
To help people feel safe	→	He decided to fight Dragon	→	Knight prepared to fight
Needed to fight Dragon	→	Prepared his armor	→	Ready to fight
Needed to fight Dragon	→	Climbed mountain	→	It rained and armor got rusted
Needed to fight Dragon	→	Entered cave	→	Fell into very dark hole
Needed to fight Dragon	→	Can't climb out of hole	→	Dragon saved Knight
Needed to help people feel safe	→	Knight and Dragon cooked for kingdom	→	Dragon became people's friend

Solution: | People feel safe because Dragon is friendly |

CHAPTER 6

Reading Comprehension and Working Memory in Children with Learning Disabilities in Reading

H. Lee Swanson
Crystal B. Howard
Leilani Sáez

The purpose of this chapter is to selectively review some recent research on reading comprehension and working memory (WM) in children with learning disabilities (LD) in reading (referred to as "reading-disabled" [RD]). We provide a brief overview of the field and potential intervention strategies. However, primary emphasis is given to reviewing our studies suggesting that executive-processing deficits exist in children with RD independent of their deficits in phonological processing. We also review recent work investigating the degree to which the phonological and executive system of WM underlies one of three different types of reading deficits: children with RD who experience both word recognition and comprehension deficits, children with RD who experience comprehension-only deficits, and children with RD who have low verbal intelligence as well as word recognition and comprehension deficits (referred to as "poor readers").

Prior to our discussion, however, we provide an overview of the concept of LD itself. Several definitions refer to LD as reflecting a heterogeneous group of individuals with "intrinsic" disorders that are manifested by specific difficulties in the acquisition and use of listening, speaking, reading, writing, reasoning, or mathematical abilities (e.g., Hammill, 1990). Most of these definitions assume that the learning difficulties of such individuals are:

1. *Not* due to inadequate opportunity to learn, or to low general intelligence, or to significant physical or emotional disorders, but are due to *basic* disorders in specific psychological processes (e.g., remembering the association between sounds and letters).
2. *Not* due to poor instruction, but are due to specific psychological-processing problems that have a neurological, constitutional, and/or biological base.
3. *Not* manifested in all aspects of learning. Such individuals' psychological-processing deficits depress only a limited aspect of academic behavior. For example, such individuals may suffer problems in reading, but not in arithmetic.

Thus for the researcher, as well as the practitioner, children labeled as LD are individuals of normal intelligence, but who suffer mental information-processing difficulties that underlie poor academic performance (Swanson, 1989). Depending on the definition, the incidence of children with LD is conservatively estimated to be 2% of the public school population (e.g., Shaywitz et al., 1999). Children with LD also comprise the largest category of children served in special education. Because of the heterogeneity of children classified as LD, several subtypes of LD have been discussed in the literature. Few of these subtypes have been considered valid, however, because (1) the particular subtypes do not respond differently to instructional programs when compared to other subtypes and/or (2) the skills deficient in a particular subtype are not relevant to the academic areas important in a school context (see Swanson, Hoskyn, & Lee, 1999, pp. 134–145, for a review). Two subtypes do have some consensus in the research, however, and are therefore relevant to the school context: reading disabilities (e.g., Siegel, 2003) and mathematical disabilities (e.g., Geary, 2003). These subtypes are defined by standardized (norm-referenced) and reliable measures of intelligence and achievement. The most commonly used intelligence tests are the Wechsler measures and common achievement tests that include measures of word recognition or arithmetic calculation (e.g., Wide Range Achievement Test, Woodcock Reading Mastery Test, Kaufman Test of Educational Achievement, Peabody Individual Achievement Test). In general, individuals with Full Scale IQ scores equal to or above a standard score of 85 and reading subtest scores equal to or below the 25th percentile and/or arithmetic subtest scores equal to or below the 25th percentile reflect two high-incidence disorders within LD: reading (word recognition) and arithmetic (computation, written work) (see Fletcher, Francis, Rourke, Shaywitz, & Shaywitz, 1992; Siegel, 1992, 2003; Siegel & Ryan, 1989, for reviews). By far, the subtype that has received the most research attention is reading disabilities (Geary, 1993).

Because the focus of this chapter is our work on reading comprehension, we focus on children with RD. We assume that children with RD can be distinguished to some degree from children with specific language impairments (SLI; Bishop & Snowling, 2004). Although children with RD and children with SLI share common problems in language (e.g., in terms of oral language, phonological awareness, semantic skills, and syntax), children with SLI are viewed as primarily suffering "a double deficit in which both phonological and non-phonological language processes are impaired" (Bishop & Snowling, 2004, p. 878). In contrast, we assume that because children with RD suffer problems in both word recognition and comprehension, they have primary deficits in phonological processing and WM.

No doubt, our focus on reading comprehension is considered by some to be a secondary issue compared to such children's more fundamental problems in word recognition. For example, Siegel (2003) argues that fundamental to evaluating children with RD is a focus on word recognition because it captures more basic processes and responses than reading comprehension. Her research indicates that children with RD show a remarkable homogeneity in cognitive profiles. For example, her work and the work of others (e.g., see Bishop & Snowling, 2004, comparing children with RD and children with specific language disorders) find that there are three processes critical in analysis of RD: those related to phonological processing (the ability to segment sounds), those related to syntactical processing, and those related to WM (combination of transient memory and long-term memory). In contrast to focusing on processes primarily related to word recognition, however, we would like to broaden the topic of reading to include comprehension. Within this context, we would like to consider children with RD as it applies to difficulties in reading comprehension and WM. Although reading comprehension difficulties are an inevitable consequence of poor word recognition, comprehension difficulties are also related to processes other than those identified with reading recognition. Further, comprehension difficulties can persist in this sample even when basic word skills have been mastered (e.g., Ransby & Swanson, 2003). Thus, although poor phonological processing may underlie such children's word recognition difficulties, we assume that WM plays a major role in their comprehension of text.

READING COMPREHENSION AND WM

Like several authors (e.g., Cain, Oakhill, & Bryant, 2004; Engle, Cantor, & Carrillo, 1992), we find that reading comprehension depends on WM (Swanson, 1999a), which not only takes into account the storage of items for later retrieval, but also the partial storage of information demands related to several levels of text processing (e.g., Cain, Oakhill, & Lemmon, 2004; Haarmann, Davelaar, & Usher, 2003; Nation, Adams, Bowyer-Crane, & Snowling, 1999; Palladino, Cornoldi, De Beni, & Pazzaglia, 2001). Several of these studies suggest that WM plays a critical role in integrating information during the task of comprehending text. WM plays a major role because (1) it holds recently processed information to make connections to the latest input, and (2) it maintains the gist of information for the construction of an overall representation of the text. Additional studies (e.g., Cain, Oakhill, & Lemmon, 2004; Seigneuric, Ehrlich, Oakhill, & Yuill, 2000) have suggested that individual differences in inference making and comprehension monitoring are related to (although not fully determined by) children's WM. Some of the research on WM and reading comprehension has been based on a component view of WM. One such component view, Baddeley's (1986, 1996, 2000) multicomponent model, describes WM as a limited central executive system that interacts with a set of two passive storage systems used for temporary storage of different classes of information: the speech-based phonological loop and the visual–spatial sketchpad. The *phonological loop* is responsible for the temporary storage of verbal information; items are held within a phonological store of limited duration, and the items are maintained within the store via the process of articulation. The *visual–spatial sketchpad* is responsible for the storage of visual–spatial information over brief periods and plays a key role in the generation and manipulation of mental images. Both storage systems are in direct contact with the central executive system. The *central executive system* is considered to be primarily responsible for coordinating activity within the cognitive system, but also devotes some of its resources to increasing the amount of information that can be held in the two subsystems (Baddeley & Logie, 1999). A recent formulation of the model (Baddeley, 2000) also includes a temporary multimodal storage component called the "episodic buffer."

DISTINCTIONS BETWEEN SHORT-TERM MEMORY AND WM

We have argued elsewhere (Swanson & Howell, 2001; Swanson & Siegel, 2001) that the distinctions made between the central executive system and a passive storage system (i.e., the phonological loop) in Baddeley and Logie's model in some ways parallel the distinctions made between WM and short-term memory (STM). WM is referred to as a processing resource of limited capacity involved in the preservation of information while simultaneously processing the same or other information (e.g., Baddeley & Logie, 1999; Engle, Tuholski, Laughlin, & Conway, 1999; Just, Carpenter, & Keller, 1996; Oberauer, Sub, Wilhelm, & Wittman, 2003). To illustrate what we mean by this, consider the following example of a WM task we use to test children adapted from an earlier study by Daneman and Carpenter (1980). The examiner reads sentences arranged into sets of two, three, four, or five to a child. An example of a sentence at the three-sentence level might include:

1. We waited in line for a *ticket*.
2. Sally thinks we should give the bird its *food*.
3. My mother said she would write a *letter*.

After the presentation of sentences in a set, the child is asked a question by the examiner ("Where did we wait?") and then asked to recall the last words in each sentence. Thus, the WM task engages the child in at least two activities after initial encoding: (1) response to a question or questions about the material or related material to be retrieved, and (2) the retrieval of item information of increasing difficulty. The first part of the task is a distractor of the initial encoding of items, whereas the second part tests storage.

In contrast, STM typically involves situations where small amounts of material are held passively (i.e., minimal resources from long-term memory are activated to interpret the task—e.g., digit- or word-span tasks) and then reproduced in a sequential fashion. That is, participants are asked only to reproduce the sequence of items in the order they were presented (e.g., Engle et al., 1999; Daneman & Carpenter, 1980; Dempster, 1985). Although STM and WM share a close relationship (i.e., transient memory; e.g., Engle et al., 1999, reported a correlation of .70), WM tasks are assumed to place heavy demands on an executive system and therefore to tap mental resources not relied upon when performing STM tasks (e.g., Daneman & Carpenter, 1980; Engle et al., 1999). In contrast, the phonological loop is associated with STM

because it involves two major components discussed in the STM literature: a speech-based phonological input store and a rehearsal process
(see Baddeley, 1986, and Gathercole, 1998, for reviews).

In some studies, both STM and WM have been found to make contributions to reading comprehension in children with RD (e.g., de
Jong, 1998; Passolunghi & Siegel, 2001; Siegel, 1994; Stanovich &
Siegel, 1994; Swanson & Ashbaker, 2000). In these studies, children
with RD are defined as having normal intelligence, but word recognition performance below the 25th percentile on a norm-referenced
reading test. As expected, the selection of children with word recognition problems invariably leads to the selection of children with difficulties in reading comprehension. In regards to WM, several studies suggest that children with RD have deficits in at least one component of
WM, the utilization and/or operation of their phonological loop (see
Stanovich & Siegel, 1994, for a comprehensive review). For example,
children with RD (who have combined deficits in word recognition and
comprehension) are less able to generate pronunciations for unfamiliar
or nonsense words than skilled readers (Stanovich & Siegel, 1994), suggesting a deficient utilization or operation of the phonological loop.
There is also evidence that a central feature of RD is a failure to
develop adequate word recognition skills (e.g., Stanovich & Siegel,
1994), even into adulthood (see Ransby & Swanson, 2003, for a review),
skills partially dependent on the phonological system. Because children with RD have small digit spans for item and order information on
STM tasks (see O'Shaughnessy & Swanson, 1998, for a comprehensive
review), some authors have argued that they have basic structural deficiencies in the storage of phonological input that impair higher level
processing, such as reading comprehension (e.g., Crain & Shankweiler,
1990; Shankweiler & Crain, 1986). This bottom-up processing approach views lower level linguistic and cognitive analyses as subserving
or influencing comprehension processing in an "upstream" manner
(Shankweiler, 1990). Much of this research assumes that phonological
processing can explain how readers of English make use of verbal WM.

However, given that the phonological loop is partially controlled
by the central executive (i.e., the executive system shares some variance
with the phonological loop; Baddeley, 1986), deficits in reading comprehension in children with RD may be due to some deficiencies in the
controlling functions of the central executive itself. Although some
studies suggest that limitations in WM for children with RD are primarily attributed to an isolated storage system that holds and maintains
phonological codes (e.g., Shankweiler & Crain, 1986; Siegel, 1994;
Stanovich & Siegel, 1994), other studies (e.g., Bull, Johnston, & Roy,
1999; de Jong, 1998; Passolunghi & Siegel, 2001; Swanson, 2003) sug-

gest that difficulties in executive processing also contribute important variance to the poor reading performance of children with RD above and beyond their deficits in phonological processing (e.g., see Swanson & Ashbaker, 2000). For example, Cain et al. (2000) showed that good and poor reading comprehenders performed comparably in a number of phonological-processing tasks but differed in WM. Thus, it cannot be concluded with certainty that only a bottom-up kind of influence (i.e., problems in the phonological loop) plays the primary role in the comprehension difficulties of children with RD.

EARLIER STUDIES

Before discussing our recent work, we briefly review previous work on the relationship between WM and reading comprehension in children with RD. In one of our earlier studies, Swanson and Alexander (1997) examined the interrelationship among cognitive processes in predicting the word recognition and reading comprehension performance of children with RD. The correlations among phonological, orthographic, semantic, metacognitive, and verbal/visual–spatial WM measures and reading performance were examined in children with RD and skilled readers, ages 7–12. We tested a hypothesis that a general resource WM system interacts with several cognitive processes, and this general system accounts for individual differences in reading performance. The study yielded the following important results: (1) readers with RD were deficient in all cognitive processes when compared to skilled readers, but these differences were not a reflection of IQ scores; (2) readers with RD were deficient compared to skilled readers in a general factor primarily composed of verbal and visual–spatial WM measures, and unique components, suggesting that reading-ability group differences emerge on both general and specific (modular) processes; (3) the general WM factor best predicts reading comprehension for both skilled readers and readers with RD; and (4) phonological awareness best predicts skilled readers' pseudoword reading, whereas the general WM factor best predicts pseudoword performance of readers with RD. Overall, Swanson and Alexander's (1997) study showed that verbal and visual–spatial WM tasks draw from (i.e., share variance with) a common (executive) system, but also have some unique variance related to a specific (phonological) system. Further, both the general WM system and the specific phonological WM system predicted reading comprehension.

Additional studies have shown that processes related to the executive system and the phonological loop account for significant variance in reading comprehension performance of children with RD (e.g., Swanson, 1999a; Swanson & Sachse-Lee, 2001). We select one earlier study (Swanson, 1999a) that identified those components of WM that are most important to reading comprehension. In this study, we tested two models of comprehension. One model, a bottom-up model of reading comprehension, suggests that phonological processes play a more important role in reading comprehension deficits than does the executive system. The rationale for this model is consistent with the work of Crain, Shankweiler, Macaruss, and Bar-Shalom (1990), which showed that poor readers are deficient in setting up phonological structures. Reading comprehension is compromised because inefficient phonological analysis creates a "bottleneck" that constricts information flow to higher levels of processing. In effect, lower-level deficits masquerade as deficits at higher levels. Thus, executive processing in the Crain et al. model has the task of relaying the results of lower-level linguistic analyses upward through the language system. The executive processor's regulatory duty is to begin at the lowest level by bringing phonetic processes into contact with "word-level" analysis. Phonologically analyzed information is then transferred to WM storage, which in turn is then transferred (thus freeing storage for the next chunk of phonological information) upward through the system to promote online extraction of meaning. The study also tested a second model (Baddeley, 1986), which suggested that executive processing may relay the results of lower-level linguistic analyses upward through the language system, but it also serves as a general storage and/or monitoring system independent of those skills. Thus, the model suggests that there is variance unique to particular components of WM (executive processing, phonological coding) that predict reading comprehension, but that also operate independently of reading comprehension ability. According to this view, skilled readers have relatively higher WM capacity than readers with RD, and therefore will have more resources related to the executive system to perform a task, regardless of the nature of the task.

In this study, Swanson (1999a) found significant differences between students with RD and counterparts matched for age and nonverbal IQ on measures of phonological-processing accuracy (phonemic deletion, digit recall, phonological choice, pseudoword repetition), phonological-processing speed (timed responses from phonemic deletion, digit recall, phonological choice, pseudoword repetition task), long-term memory (LTM) accuracy (orthographic choice, semantic choice, vocabulary), LTM time (timed response from orthographic choice, semantic choice, vocabulary), and executive processing (sentence span, counting span, visual-matrix). The results showed that the chronologically age (CA)-matched group outperformed the children with RD reading group whereas the readers with RD were comparable to reading-level (RL)-matched children. The important findings, however, were that the results brought together two alternative models of WM and their influence on reading comprehension. How so?

Swanson (1999a) examined each hypothesis through a series of hierarchical regression analyses to assess the independent contribution of phonological, LTM, and executive processes to reading comprehension. The general pattern was that the significant relationship between executive processing and reading comprehension was maintained when LTM and phonological-processing composite scores were partialed from the analysis. More importantly, Swanson found that the contribution of phonological processes, LTM, and executive processes to reading comprehension was statistically comparable. Thus, on the one hand, Swanson found support for the notion that the phonological system plays an important role in predicting reading ability group differences in reading comprehension. However, Swanson did not find support for the notion that the phonological system accounted for the influence of executive processing on reading comprehension. The attenuating effect of executive processing on reading comprehension also did not appear to be due to phonological-processing speed or to LTM. The implication of this finding was that no one process dominated another as underlying reading comprehension deficits.

Swanson was also interested in determining whether there were some fundamental processing differences between readers with RD and skilled readers that supersede their problems in reading comprehension. He analyzed the processing variables as a function of reading conditions by reframing the comparison groups in terms of the regression-based design outlined by Stanovich and Siegel (1994). When reading comprehension was statistically controlled (i.e., partialed out of the analysis), the results showed that significant differences exist in WM and the speed of processing phonological information between readers with RD and controls, independently of their reading comprehension level (this finding is discussed below).

In another study, Swanson and Ashbaker (2000) tested whether the operations related to STM and WM operated independently of one another. In this study, they compared readers with RD and skilled readers and younger reading level-matched children on a battery of WM and STM tests to assess executive and phonological processing, respectively. The Swanson and Ashbaker study yielded two important results. First, although the group with RD was inferior to skilled readers in WM, verbal STM, and articulation speed, the differences in verbal STM and WM revealed little relation with articulation speed. That is, reading-related differences on WM and STM measures remained when articulation speed was partialed from the analysis. These reading group differences were pervasive across verbal and visual–spatial WM tasks, even when the influence of verbal STM was statistically removed, suggesting that reading-group differences are domain-general. Second, WM tasks and verbal STM tasks contributed unique variance to word recognition and reading comprehension beyond articulation speed. These results are consistent with those of Daneman and Carpenter (1980) and others (e.g., Engle et al., 1999) who have argued that verbal STM tasks and WM tasks are tapping different processes. The findings from Swanson and Ashbaker's (2000) study were consistent with earlier work on RD samples (Swanson, 1994; Swanson & Berninger, 1995). In a 1994 study, Swanson tested whether STM and WM contributed unique variance to academic achievement in children and adults with RD. He found that STM and WM tasks loaded on different factors. Further, these two factors both contributed unique variance to reading comprehension performance.

In summary, our earlier studies on RD are consistent with studies on individual differences that suggest that general resources (e.g., executive processing) from a WM system play a critical role in integrating information during reading comprehension (e.g., Engle et al., 1992), as well as those that highlight the importance of a domain-specific language system (e.g., see Miyake, 2001, for a review). Our inference is that executive-processing deficits exist in children with RD independent of their deficits in phonological processing.

RECENT WORK

In the remainder of this chapter, we review our most recent work that attempts to dig deeper in identifying specific components of WM that may account for comprehension deficits in children with RD. We consider a model that suggests that both the phonological loop (i.e., STM) and the executive (WM) system play an important role in the reading comprehension deficits experienced by children with RD. We recognize that because STM and WM tasks are strongly correlated, it is difficult to determine whether reading deficits and poor WM performance are primarily due to a system related to storage (i.e., to STM) or to a system that taps both storage and executive processing (i.e., WM). We assume, however, that one means to untangle these possible sources of difficulties in reading is to compare different subgroups of less-skilled readers. Evidence for the contribution of different memory systems to reading deficits is suggested when different types of reading problems exhibit different cognitive profiles.

Thus, a hypothesis we have recently tested (Swanson, Howard, & Sáez, 2006) is whether children with RD in both word recognition and comprehension perform poorly on WM tasks primarily because of deficits in both the executive system and the phonological loop. We have also attempted to test whether children fluent in word recognition but deficient in comprehension exhibit specific deficits in the executive system. The rationale behind these hypotheses follows.

WM is seen as reflecting the contents of STM plus limited-capacity controlled-attention processes (e.g., Conway, Cowan, Bunting, Therriault, & Minkoff, 2002; Engle et al., 1999; Kane & Engle, 2003). This limited capacity of attention refers to what Baddely views as the central executive. STM is viewed as a simple storage component. This storage component includes, among other pieces of information, phonological codes. Controlled attention includes activities that maintain (e.g., update) information in the face of interference (see Engle et al., 1999, and Kane & Engle, 2003, for reviews).

As stated previously, there is strong consensus in the literature that poor phonological coding is related to poor word recognition (see, e.g., Shankweiler et al., 1995; also see Stanovich, 1990; see Stanovich & Siegel, 1994, for a review); thus a significant relationship between STM and word recognition would be expected in the present study. Further, the relationship between WM and reading comprehension is well established (Daneman & Merikle, 1996; Engle et al., 1992). What is unclear from the literature, however, is whether specific deficits in phonological storage and/or controlled attention underlie differences in reading comprehension. It seems to us that if WM plays a major role in reading comprehension, then poor comprehenders with average decoding skills (i.e., average word recognition) would experience memory problems only related to the executive system. In contrast, children with both word recognition and comprehension deficits (referred to as children with RD in our study) would be impaired on both STM (storage) and WM (storage + controlled attention or executive-processing) tasks. However, because it has been argued that deficits in phonological processes for children at risk for RD create a bottleneck in the processing of information within the executive system (e.g., Shankweiler & Crain, 1986), it is possible that performance differences between less-skilled readers (e.g., children with RD) and skilled readers on WM tasks would be eliminated once performance related to phonological processing was partialed out in the analysis.

Of course, an important question to be considered is whether problems in STM and WM can contribute to different types of reading problems. On this issue, we have found that children with RD (low word recognition, which in turn yields low comprehension) suffer defi-

cits in both the phonological and the executive system that are independent of each other. For example, Swanson and Berninger (1995)
examined potential differences between STM and WM by testing
whether STM and WM accounted for different cognitive profiles in
children with average intelligence. They used a double dissociation
design to compare children who varied on reading comprehension
and/or word recognition on WM and phonological STM measures.
Participants were divided into four ability groups: High Comprehen-
sion/High Word Recognition, Low Comprehension/High Word Recognition, High Comprehension/Low Word Recognition, and Low
Comprehension/Low Word Recognition. The results were straightforward: WM measures were related primarily to reading comprehension,
whereas phonological STM measures were related primarily to reading recognition. Most critically, because no significant interaction
emerged, the results further indicated that the comorbid group (i.e.,
children with RD low in both comprehension and word recognition)
had combined deficits in both WM and STM. These findings suggested
that performance on WM and STM tasks were independent of one
another.

What is unclear with the Swanson and Berninger study, as well as
other studies that have attributed STM and WM to reading deficits,
was whether "storage" and/or activities related to executive processing
(controlled attention) underlie the deficits in WM. That is, studies that
have attributed reading deficits to both STM and WM may have made
these attributions because both tasks draw on a common source (e.g.,
the phonological system). In addition, those studies that assume that
poor WM performance reflects problems in executive processing are
imprecise. This is because the executive component of WM includes a
variety of processes (e.g., inhibition, task switching, and updating; see
Miyake, Friedman, Emerson, Witzki, & Howerter, 2000) that may
underlie reading problems.

Activities of the Executive System

In the study we review (Swanson et al., 2006) we also explore some
activities related to the executive system as playing a possible role in
separating children with varying reading abilities. One activity relates
to inhibition. Recent studies suggest that deficits in poor monitoring,
such as an inability to suppress (i.e., inhibit) irrelevant information (e.g., De Beni & Palladino, 2000; Passolunghi & Siegel, 2001;
Passolunghi, Cornoldi, & De Liberto, 1999; Palladino et al., 2001) may
underlie executive-processing deficits in less-skilled readers (e.g., chil-

dren with RD). For example, a child with RD may be asked to identify a sequence of events in a story just read, but have a difficult time sorting out the relevant from the irrelevant information. When asked to retell the story to a teacher or a peer, the child may exhibit an inability to retell the main events in the story because he or she has difficulty ignoring incidental information. The ability to inhibit irrelevant information from entering WM is thought to be a component of executive functioning measured by a random generation task. Baddeley (1986) suggested that during random generation, the central executive acts as a filtering device, screening out automatically generated (and therefore nonrandom) responses. Several studies suggest that random generation can be used to load the central executive selectively within the WM system (Towse, 1998). In our study, we asked children to write letters and/or numbers (from 0 to 9) "out of order" as quickly as possible within a 30-second time period. Successful performance reflected the number of random digits produced. Our scoring included an index for randomness, information redundancy, and percentage of paired responses to assess the tendency of participants to suppress response repetitions.

A second executive activity considered was updating (e.g., Morris & Jones, 1990). Updating requires the monitoring and coding of incoming information for relevance to the task at hand and then appropriately revising the items held in WM by replacing old, no longer relevant information with newer, more relevant information (Miyake et al., 2000). It is assumed that the updating function goes beyond the simple maintenance of task-relevant information because it actively requires the manipulation of relevant information in WM. This task has relevance to reading comprehension. For example, when reading a mystery, one may have to go back and sort out the key players in the story, remembering who is related to whom, and the like, before continuing on further with the story. Thus, the reader engages in updating to fully understand text. In this study, we administered an updating task that required the monitoring of numerical information. Children were presented a list of numbers of varying lengths and asked to remember the last three digits. Children were not told the list length, and therefore had to keep the last few digits active in memory to successfully perform the task.

Another possible source of difficulties that may impair the efficient use of the central executive system is speed of processing. Several authors argue that processing speed accounts for the relationship between WM and cognitive performance on a multitude of tasks (e.g., Johnston & Anderson, 1998; Kail, 1993; Salthouse, 1996). The assumption is that processing speed determines capacity because processing (encoding, transforming, retrieving) is time-related. That is, faster rates of processing allow for more information to be processed, allowing for more functional WM capacity (e.g., Salthouse, 1996). A significant linear relationship between naming speed and verbal memory span has been found in many experimental situations (e.g., Hulme, Thomson, Muir, & Lawrence, 1984).

In summary, this next study examined the degree to which variations in WM performance among skilled and less-skilled readers were related to activities of the central executive and the phonological loop. An assessment of the phonological loop included the administration of STM measures. Our battery included traditional measures of digit and word span as well as the recall of nonwords. This was done because performance on traditional immediate memory tasks (serial recall of familiar items, e.g., digits) can reflect the contribution of LTM knowledge (Hulme, Maughan, & Brown, 1991). We expected to gain a more sensitive measure of phonological information in STM by using memory items for which there are few, if any, long-term lexical representations. Measures of the executive system were modeled after Daneman and Carpenter's (1980) WM tasks. These tasks demand the coordination of both processing and storage (e.g., Oberauer, 2002; Whitney, Arnett, Driver, & Budd, 2001).

To extend our earlier work (e.g., Swanson, 1999a; Swanson & Ashbaker, 2000; Swanson & Berninger, 1995), the presented study tested whether activities attributed to the executive system of WM underlie two types of reading deficits among children with average intelligence: children with both word recognition and comprehension deficits (children with RD) and children with comprehension-only deficits. We also determined whether WM differences between reading groups were tied to STM (storage), specific executive-processing activities (inhibition, updating), and/or a combination of storage (STM) and executive-processing activities.

Children with RD and children with comprehension-only deficits were also compared to children with comparable comprehension deficits but low in verbal intelligence. Because reading comprehension is associated with Verbal IQ, it was necessary to determine whether group differences found on WM measures were merely an artifact of verbal ability. Thus, also included in the comparison were poor readers with low Verbal IQ scores. Nation et al. (1999) have suggested that the relationship between WM and comprehension is mediated by verbal intelligence and not by executive-processing skills. They argued that poor comprehenders have a weakness in verbal skills that restricts their ability to store verbal information in STM. Likewise, Stothard and Hulme (1992) suggested that WM differences between good and poor comprehenders would be eliminated if differences in Verbal IQ were controlled. However, no evidence was provided to support this prediction.

Sampling and Classification

In this study, 66 children were selected from a school in southern California. The sample included 22 girls and 44 boys. The mean age of the sample was 12 years old. All children were from upper-middle- to upper-class homes. Ninety percent of the participants' fathers had a bachelor's degree and 70% of the mothers had a bachelor's degree. Thirty percent of the fathers and 10% of the mothers in the sample had graduate degrees (MA, PhD, or MD).

Classification was based upon standard scores from the word reading subtest of the Wide Range Achievement Test—Third Edition (WRAT3; Wilkinson, 1993), and from the subtests related to pseudoword and real word reading speed from the TOWRE (Test of Word Reading Efficiency; Wagner & Torgesen, 1999). Standard scores from the Gray Oral Reading Test, Third Edition (GORT-3; Wiederholt & Bryant, 1986) comprehension accuracy subtest and passage comprehension of the Woodcock Reading Mastery subtest (Woodcock, 1987) were used to define reading comprehension performance. The criterion for the skilled reading group was a score above the 50th percentile in reading comprehension and word recognition fluency, as well as a Verbal IQ score above 100. Operational criteria for children defined as RD were based upon (1) Verbal IQ > 100; (2) reading scores at or below the 25th percentile on a standardized measure of sight word reading accuracy (WRAT3) and fluency (TOWRE); and reading comprehension (GORT-3); and (3) lack of indication from school folders of brain injury. The cutoff score criteria for children with RD matched the operational definition of RD outlined by Siegel and Ryan (1989). Children who tested low in both comprehension and word recognition, but yielded Verbal IQs < 80, were defined as poor readers. Children with average IQs who tested above the 25th percentile in word recognition, but below the 25th percentile in comprehension, were classified as children with comprehension-only deficits.

In general, the groups were carefully matched on nonverbal intelligence, socioeconomic status (SES), gender, ethnicity, and chronological age, but varied significantly on reading and verbal intelligence measures.

Tasks and Materials

The battery of group and individually administered tasks is briefly described below (see Swanson & Beebe-Frankenberger, 2004, for a complete description). The majority of phonological measures are commonly used and derived from published standardized measures (i.e., WRAT3, WISC-III, Comprehensive Test of Phonological Processing [CTOPP; Wagner, Torgesen, & Rashotte, 2000]) that can be consulted for further detail.

Classification Measures
1. Real-word and pseudoword reading tasks. Two subtests were administered from the Test of Word Reading Efficiency (TOWRE; Wagner & Torgesen, 1999).
2. Word recognition (WRAT3).
3. Reading comprehension (GORT-3) and Passage Comprehension subtest from the Woodcock Reading Mastery Test—Revised (WRMT-R; Woodcock, 1988).
4. Fluid intelligence (Raven Colored Progressive Matrices [RCPM]; Raven, 1976).
5–7. Verbal intelligence (derived from two subtests of the WISC-III: general information and vocabulary).

Comparison Measures
Speed of processing
8–10. Rapid letter-, digit-, and object-naming speed (subtests from CTOPP).
11. Coding speed. Coding subtest from the Wechsler Intelligence Scale for Children–III.

Phonological processing
12. Phonological deletion (Elision subtest from the CTOPP).
13. Pseudowords (Word Attack subtest of the WRMT-R).

STM
14–16. Forward Digit Span, Word Span, and Pseudoword Span.

WM (see Swanson, 1996, for review of tasks).
17–20. Digit/sentence span, semantic association task, listening sentence span, backward digit span.

Inhibition and Updating Measures

21–22. Random generations of letters and numbers. These tasks measure inhibition because participants were required to actively monitor candidate responses and suppress responses that would lead to well-learned sequences, such as 1–2–3–4 or a–b–c–d (Baddeley, 1996).

23. Updating. The updating task was adapted from Morris and Jones (1990).

Math Achievement

24. Written computation (Mathematics subtest from the WRAT3).

Overview of Results

The general pattern across all these measures was that skilled readers outperformed the less-skilled readers (children with RD, children with comprehension-only deficits, poor readers). Skilled readers outperformed all the other ability groups on measures of WM, naming speed, and updating. Skilled readers were statistically comparable to poor comprehenders with average word recognition skills on measures of STM and phonological processing. This findings replicate other studies that show that comprehension and WM deficits emerge between children of comparable word recognition skills (e.g., Marshall & Nation, 2003; Swanson & Ashbaker, 2000; Swanson & Berninger, 1995). For example, Marshall and Nation (2003) found that children demonstrate difficulties in reading comprehension even when they possess normal levels of reading accuracy and speed and perform within age-appropriate levels in verbal STM.

What we did find that has not been extensively reported in the literature is that children with comprehension-only deficits were superior to children with RD on measures of WM, STM, phonological processing, and speed. Children with RD were superior to poor readers (children with low Verbal IQs and reading scores) on measures of WM and phonological processing. Also shown was that children with RD were inferior to skilled readers on the composite measures of inhibition. However, no significant differences emerged between children with RD, poor readers, and children with comprehension-only deficits on measures of inhibition and updating scores.

Although the above findings show that ability group differences emerged on WM measures, we have yet to identify the processes that mediate these differences. To address this issue we again used a regression design outlined in Stanovich and Siegel (1994). In this design, we partialed from the criterion variables the linear trend of the processes we assume underlie WM. This was done by comparing subgroup performance with or without partialing the influence of STM, processing speed, updating, and inhibition, or phonological skills. Scores related to STM, processing speed, and phonological skill were composite scores. Age served as a covariate in each model. The criterion measure was a composite WM performance score.

To analyze the source of ability group differences, three contrast variables were created for the subsequent regression analysis. The first contrast variable compared skilled readers (coded +1) and the comprehension deficit-only group (coded as –1, the remaining groups were coded as 0). The second contrast variable compared poor readers (children low in Verbal IQ, reading comprehension, and word recognition, coded as +1) to children with RD (coded –1; the remaining groups were coded as 0—see Cohen & Cohen, 1983, for discussion of contrast variables in regression models). The third contrast variable compared children who were fluent in sight word recognition, but low in comprehension (comprehension deficit-only children, coded at +1) to children with RD (word recognition + comprehension deficit, coded as –1; the remaining groups were coded as 0).

As shown in Table 6.1, we entered the three aforementioned contrast variables simultaneously into a regression analysis. The extent to which WM performance is associated with the contrast variables independent of age, STM, speed, phonological processing, inhibition, and updating will be reflected in the significant beta weights. A significant positive beta weight for the first contrast variable indicates that the WM performance of children skilled in reading exceeds the comprehension deficit-only group when the covariates (e.g., age, phonological processing) and other contrasts are partialed out. The second contrast reflects comparisons between children who are poor readers and children with RD. A significant positive beta weight indicates that the WM performance of poor readers exceeds that of children with RD. The final contrast reflects the comparison between children with comprehension deficits-only and children with RD. A significant positive beta weight indicates that children with comprehension deficits-only outperform children with RD when the effect of the covariates and other contrast variables are partialed out.

As shown in Table 6.1, for Model 1 we entered age and the contrast variables into the model. The results in Model 1 show that skilled readers outperform all less-skilled readers, children with RD outperform poor readers, and poor comprehenders outperform children with

TABLE 6.1. Hierarchical Regression Predicting Working Memory as a Function of Subgroups of Readers

	B	SE	β	*t*-ratio
Model 1				
Age	.53	.11	.53	5.19***
Contrast 1	.38	.09	.38	3.99**
Contrast 2	-.22	.11	-.22	-1.93*
Contrast 3	.27	.11	.27	2.25*
Model 2a				
Age	.42	.08	.42	4.67***
STM	.44	.09	.44	4.75**
Contrast 1	.25	.08	.25	2.90**
Contrast 2	-.17	.11	-.17	-1.71
Contrast 3	.10	.12	.10	.91
Model 2b				
Age	.50	.10	.50	4.71**
Update	.32	.09	.32	3.50**
Inhibition	-.01	.10	-.01	-.15
Contrast 1	.31	.09	.32	3.40**
Contrast 2	-.22	.10	-.22	-2.11*
Contrast 3	.29	.11	.29	2.63*
Model 2c				
Age	.43	.12	.43	3.64***
Speed	-.16	.12	-.16	-1.33
Contrast 1	.32	.10	.32	3.12**
Contrast 2	-.20	.11	-.19	-1.69
Contrast 3	.21	.12	.21	1.66
Model 3				
Age	.37	.08	.37	4.20***
Phon.	.18	.10	.18	1.77
Update	.17	.08	.17	1.90
STM	.34	.09	.34	3.59**
Contrast 1	.20	.08	.20	2.34*
Contrast 2	-.11	.10	-.11	-1.31
Contrast 3	.05	.11	.05	.50
Model 4				
Age	.40	.10	.39	3.74**
Verbal IQ	-.04	.11	-.04	-.39
Phon.	.17	.10	.17	1.63
Update	.19	.09	.19	2.02*
STM	.37	.09	.37	3.66**
Contrast 1	.20	.09	.20	2.16*
Contrast 2	-.12	.11	-.17	-1.14
Contrast 3	.05	.11	.05	.43

(continued)

TABLE 6.1. *(continued)*

Model 1	$R_2^2 = .42$, $F(4,61) = 11.35$***
Model 2a	$R_2^2 = .58$, $F(5,60) = 16.79$***
Model 2b	$R_2^2 = .52$, $F(6,59) = 10.93$***
Model 2c	$R_2^2 = .44$, $F(5,60) = 9.40$***
Model 3	$R_2^2 = .63$, $F(7,58) = 14.69$***
Model 4	$R^2 = .64$, $F(8,55) = 12.27$***

Note. The first contrast variable compared skilled readers and the comprehension deficit-only group. The second contrast variable compared poor readers (children low in Verbal IQ, reading comprehension, and word recognition) to children with RD. The third contrast variable compared children who were fluent in sight word recognition, but low in comprehension to children with RD (word recognition + comprehension deficits). Phon., phonological processing.
*$p < .05$, **$p < .01$, ***$p < .001$.

RD on measures of WM. We next engaged in subsequent testing by entering measures related to various processes assumed to underlie WM performance in ability groups. This subsequent model testing shown in Table 6.1 was based on the assumption that the processes that mediate WM differences between subgroups would eliminate significant subgroup differences (which occurred in Model 1) when entered into the regression analysis.

So what did we find? Three important findings emerged. First, the significant contrast variables related to children with RD versus children with comprehension deficit-only (contrast 3) and children with RD versus poor readers (contrast 2) found in Model 1 were completely eliminated in Models 2a and 2c. Model 2a entered STM and Model 2c entered naming speed. However, only in Model 2a was the assumed mediating variable (i.e., STM) found to contribute significant variance to WM. Speed of processing contributed no significant unique variance to WM performance. Second, none of the models eliminated the significant contribution of the skilled readers (skilled readers vs. comprehension deficit-only children) in predicting WM performance. Finally, Model 2b shows that partialing-out activities that relate to the executive system (i.e., updating and inhibition) does not eliminate the significant contribution of the contrast variables in predicting WM. Although Model 2b was a significant improvement over Model 1, all contrast variables contributed unique variance to WM performance. In addition, the results show that the updating measure, and not the inhibition measure, contributed unique variance to WM.

We also determined whether the variables that emerge as significant in Models 2a, 2b, and 2c contributed significant variance to WM once phonological processing was entered into the regression model. Thus, Model 3 entered into the regression model phonological processing and other measures that contributed unique variance in previous models (STM, updating). However, this model did not eliminate the significant differences between skilled readers and children with comprehension-only deficits. Further, none of the variables eliminated the significant contribution of STM to WM performance found in previous models. Thus, although we found that subgroup differences between less-skilled readers are due to differences in storage (Model 2a), it cannot be argued that these deficits were primarily isolated to phonological processes. Because some authors have argued that differences between skilled readers and those with comprehension deficits are related to Verbal IQ (e.g., Nation et al., 1999), we entered Verbal IQ into the next regression model. As shown in Model 4, performance differences between skilled children and children with comprehension-only deficits remain significant even when Verbal IQ was partialed from the analysis. The results also show that only updating and STM storage contributed unique variance to WM performance. Phonological processing contributed no significant variance to WM performance.

Summary

Taken together, our results to date show that children of normal intelligence who vary in word recognition and reading comprehension differ on measures related to WM. More importantly, we find that (1) the storage aspect of WM, not the executive system, underlies differences between comprehension deficit-only children and children with RD (combined word recognition and comprehension deficits); (2) the executive system, and not the phonological loop, accounts for the superior WM performance of skilled readers when compared to all comprehension deficit-only children; and (3) superior WM performance in children with RD when compared to poor readers is related to advantages in executive processing and not to the phonological loop.

Perhaps the most important finding to emerge in our recent work relates to the regression results in Model 4 shown in Table 6.1. This model shows that STM and updating contribute unique variance to WM beyond variables that relate to reading group classification. These findings are important for two reasons. First, the results are consistent with Engle et al.'s (1999) formulation that WM performance is made up of two components: STM and controlled attention. Our results support this contention in that both STM and updating (as a measure of controlled attention) contribute unique variance to WM performance. Our research also suggests, however, some independence between WM and STM as a function of reading comprehension ability. Children with comprehension-only deficits are inferior to skilled readers on WM measures, even when measures of STM, phonological processing, and Verbal IQ are partialed from the analysis. This is an important finding because WM differences between poor and good comprehenders have been primarily attributed to verbal skills (e.g., Nation et al., 1999) and Verbal IQ (Stothard & Hulme, 1992). These persistent problems in WM complement our previous work that has shown that problems in WM have been found to persist in children with RD even after partialing out the influence of verbal articulation speed (Swanson & Ashbaker, 2000), reading comprehension (Swanson, 1999a), STM (Swanson, Ashbaker, & Lee, 1996), or IQ scores (Swanson & Sachse-Lee, 2001).

Second, individual differences in storage and updating supersede any classifications attributed to reading proficiency. That is, even when significant differences between reading groups are partialed out, updating and STM storage contribute unique variance to WM. These results are consistent with the notion that WM performance is not a consequence of reading skill. This notion is consistent with the earlier work of Turner and Engle (1989; also see Engle et al., 1992; Kane & Engle, 2003), who suggest that people are less-skilled readers because they have a small "general" WM capacity and that this capacity is "independent" of reading. That is, less-skilled readers are viewed as having a weaker WM than skilled readers, not as a direct consequence of their poor reading skills, but because they have less WM capacity available for performing a reading task. As stated by Turner and Engle, "Working memory may be a unitary individual characteristic, independent of the nature of the task in which the individual makes use of it" (p. 150). Engle et al. (1992) also suggested that individual differences on various cognitive tasks are due to the "total level of activation" in a general WM (i.e., executive) capacity system. This amount of activation is a *constant* characteristic of an individual, and therefore changes little with increases or decreases in reading ability. Consistent with findings in adult samples, we find that children with comprehension difficulties are deficient in the executive-processing component of WM, not because of their reading level, but because executive-processing deficits (i.e., deficits in a general WM system) are a characteristic of this sample. Thus, the co-occurrence of poor reading and poor executive processing is not because the working memory tasks in our study require the subject to use the same specific processes as the reading comprehension measure, but because working memory is a general skill that underlies various domains.

In summary, we find that skilled readers outperform all less-skilled readers on measures related to WM, processing speed, and updating. Children with comprehension-only deficits, however, are superior on WM tasks to children with RD, and children with RD are superior in WM performance to poor readers. However, these differences among less-skilled readers are primarily due to variations in the *storage* aspect of WM and not to variations in phonological processing. Further, WM differences that emerge between skilled and less-skilled readers appear to be related to processes that are nonspecific to reading.

Implications for Remediation

Before leaving the discussion of our recent work on WM and compre-hension problems in children with LD in reading, some comments about remediation are necessary. Unfortunately, we have found no experimental intervention studies showing that direct intervention on WM functioning in children with RD leads to increased reading com-prehension performance. We have found, however, that studies using strategy intervention have improved comprehension performance in children with LD in reading. These findings may be related to some aspects of WM because instruction in strategy use would be expected to reduce demands on WM load. At present, we have done a fair amount of work summarizing the existing intervention literature that has attempted to directly improve reading comprehension and other skills in children with LD (Swanson, 1999b; Swanson & Hoskyn, 1998; Swanson et al., 1999); the reader is referred to these sources. Most of the studies included in our synthesis held to the view that students with LD underutilize access to knowledge unless they are explicitly prompted to use certain strategies. The most important contribution in our synthesis was the uncovering of the components of instruction that increased the positive outcomes (in this case, the magnitude of effect sizes). We found that effective instructional models follow a *sequence of events*:

1. State the learning objectives and orient the students to what they will be learning and what performance will be expected of them.
2. Review the skills necessary to understand the concept.
3. Present the information, give examples, and demonstrate the concepts/materials.

4. Pose questions (probes) to students and assess their level of understanding and correct misconceptions.
5. Provide group instruction and independent practice. Give students an opportunity to demonstrate new skills and learn the new information on their own.
6. Assess performance and provide feedback. Review the independent work and give a quiz. Give feedback for correct answers and reteach skills if answers are incorrect.
7. Provide distributed practice and review.

We also found that some instructional components are far more important than others. For reading comprehension, those key instructional components (as stated in the treatment conditions) that contributed in significantly improving the magnitude of effect sizes were:

1. *Directed response/questioning.* Treatment description related to dialectic or Socratic teaching, the teacher directing students to ask questions, the teacher and student or students engaging in reciprocal dialogue.
2. *Control difficulty or processing demands of task.* Treatment statements about short activities, level of difficulty controlled, teacher providing necessary assistance, teacher providing simplified demonstration, tasks sequenced from easy to difficult, and/or task analysis.
3. *Elaboration.* Statements in the treatment description about additional information or explanation provided about concepts, procedures, or steps, and/or redundant text or repetition within text.
4. *Modeling by the teacher of steps.* Statements or activities in the treatment descriptions that involve modeling by the teacher in terms of demonstration of processes and/or steps the students are to follow to solve the problem.
5. *Small-group instruction.* Statements in the treatment description about instruction in a small group, and/or verbal interaction occurring in a small group with students and/or teacher.
6. *Strategy cues.* Statements in the treatment description about reminders to use strategies or multisteps, use of "think-aloud models," and/or teacher presenting the benefits of strategy use or procedures.

In contrast, the important instructional components that increased the effect sizes for word recognition from our analysis were:

1. *Sequencing.* Statements in the treatment description about breaking down the task, fading of prompts or cues, sequencing short activities, and/or using step-by-step prompts.
2. *Segmentation.* Statements in the treatment description about breaking down the targeted skill into smaller units, breaking into component parts, segmenting and/or synthesizing components parts.
3. *Advanced Organizers.* Statements in the treatment description about directing children to look over material prior to instruction, children directed to focus on particular information, providing prior information about task, and/or the teacher stating objectives of instruction prior to commencing.

The importance of these findings is that only a few components from a broad array of activities enhance treatment outcomes.

Discussion

In general, we find, as do others, that children with high WM capacity (in this case, skilled readers) appear to have more attentional resources available to them than individuals with low WM capacity (in this case, less-skilled readers). Perhaps where we most differ from other authors is that we think that children with RD have difficulties related to the general WM (i.e., executive) system. We recognize that there is a problem in arguing that comprehension deficits are related to a domain-general system. This problem relates to the common assumption that specific lower order processing deficits (e.g., phonological deficits) are the core contributors to RD. One means of reconciling this issue is to suggest that problems in specific activities of the executive system can exist in children with RD independent of their problems in low-order processing (Swanson & Alexander, 1997). That is, higher order cognitive processing problems can exist in children with RD, *independently* of their specific problems in low-order processes, such as phonological processing. There may also be problems in coordinating these two levels of processing. For example, children with RD may be viewed as having difficulty accessing higher level information and/or lower order skills (phonological codes), or switching between the two levels of processing. Several studies have characterized children with RD as having difficulties in executive processing that relate to checking, planning, testing, and evaluating their performance. Various information-processing models and strategy intervention programs have attributed difficulties in coordinating multiple pieces of information to children with RD. Thus, one may speculate that the processing problems in children with RD reflect a deficit in the coordination of information in the executive system, which in turn fails to compensate for a deficient lower order specialized process. This lack of compensatory processing may be characterized by a WM system either not contributing enough information to a specialized system or failing to provide an adequate capacity of processing resources given that there are problems in a specialized system (see Swanson & Alexander, 1997, for a related discussion).

Another possibility is to suggest that a generic storage system may indirectly account for low-order processing deficits (especially on language-related tasks) because of excessive processing demands. For example, in Baddeley's (1986) earlier model the central executive system is an undifferentiated generic system that stores information that is used to support low-order systems. (Note: Baddeley and Logie, 1999, no longer suggest a storage system for executive processing.) However, if the executive system is overtaxed, it cannot contribute resources to low-order processing. That is, given that the phonological loop is controlled by the central executive, any deficits in phonological functioning may partially reflect deficiencies in the controlling functions of the central executive itself (see Gathercole & Baddeley, 1993). As stated by Gathercole and Baddeley (1993), related to reading deficiencies, "the limitation could be either in the operation of the phonological loop, or the central executive" (p. 228). They further suggest that one could create the argument that executive processing may play a more critical role in some stages of reading for poor readers than for skilled readers. That is, because poor readers do not have fully automatized procedures, they may need to rely heavily on the general resources furnished by the central executive component of working memory. This assumption is consistent with the notion that a limited-capacity WM system plays a role in the translation of phonemic and orthographic codes into a semantic representation while simultaneously storing the output from previous processing. Overall, we think our results are consistent with most information-processing models of individual differences that suggest that elementary processes are best understood in the context of their combination with other operations. Although it is important to identify elementary processes that underlie the performance of readers with LD, such an approach may not be sufficient in explaining how cognitive processes are organized and work in unison in accounting for general impairments in learning.

Another possibility is that the executive-processing problems experienced by children with RD is related to problems in inhibition. Several studies show that children with RD have difficulty suppressing irrelevant information under high-processing demand conditions (e.g., Chiappe, Hasher, & Siegel, 2000; Swanson & Cochran, 1991). Our earlier studies have established that children with RD vary from controls in their ability to selectively attend to word features (e.g., Swanson & Cochran, 1991). Several recent studies have also shown that children with RD have difficulties suppressing irrelevant information on WM tasks (Chiappe et al., 2000; Passolunghi et al., 1999). Consistent with these studies, we find that children poor in reading comprehension but average in word recognition suffer deficits in WM. In contrast to several studies that focus on comprehension (e.g., De Beni, Palladino, Pazzaglia, & Cornoldi, 1998; Passolunghi et al., 1999), however, we could not attribute these deficits in WM to problems in inhibition when several variables are entered into a regression model. We do find, however, that children with RD suffered deficits in inhibition on the random generation task relative to skilled readers. However, inhibition in children with RD was comparable to inhibition in children with higher WM scores but poor reading scores (children with comprehension deficit only), suggesting that processes other than inhibition may be moderating the results.

One executive-processing activity we did find that played an important role in WM was "updating" (Miyake et al., 2000). As stated earlier, updating requires monitoring and coding of information for relevance to the task at hand, and then appropriately revising items held in WM. We found that *both* STM and updating predicted individual differences in WM performance. Thus, our results suggest that there is residual variance in WM performance that has not been adequately captured in our analysis that can be attributed to the executive system. Although we argue that WM tasks require the active monitoring of events and these events are distinguishable between simple attention and stimuli held in STM, there are monitoring demands placed on STM tasks. It is possible that both STM and WM tasks may invoke controlled attentional processes, such as updating. Controlled processing emphasizes maintaining information in the face of interference. Several studies suggest that controlled processing on WM tasks emerges in the context of high demands on attention (e.g., maintaining a memory trace in the face of interference) and the drawing of resources from the executive system (see Engle et al., 1999, pp. 311–312, for discussion). In contrast, controlled processing on STM tasks attempts to maintain memory traces above some critical threshold. This maintenance does not directly draw resources from the central executive system (see Engle et al., 1999, for a review). Thus, there is some point on a continuum of monitoring where STM tasks can be distinguished from WM tasks.

CONCLUSION

In summary, future research must be directed toward developing intervention programs that compensate for WM demands on children with RD. These intervention programs would include, for example, the teaching of strategies to help compensate for or reduce WM demands. However, we also contend that concerted effort needs to be made in identifying the cognitive processes that underlie reading comprehension difficulties. Thus, future research must focus on the interaction between the executive and the phonological systems during the act of reading and across a broad age span to disentangle the alternative interpretations of the results. It appears from our most recent work, however, that WM factors that contribute to comprehension-only deficits relative to skilled readers emerge at the executive-processing level. Factors that contribute to poor WM performance in children with RD are related to both the executive and the phonological system.

ACKNOWLEDGMENTS

Preparation of this chapter was partially funded by Peloy Funds awarded to H. Lee Swanson from the University of California, Riverside.

REFERENCES

Baddeley, A. D. (1986). *Working memory*. London: Oxford University Press.

Baddeley, A. D. (1996). Exploring the central executive. *Quarterly Journal of Experimental Psychology, 49A,* 5–28.

Baddeley, A. D. (2000). The episodic buffer: A new component of working memory? *Trends in Cognitive Sciences, 4,* 417–422.

Baddeley, A. D., & Logie, R. H. (1999). The multiple-component model. In A. Miyake & P. Shah (Eds.), *Models of working memory: Mechanisms of active maintenance and executive control* (pp. 28–61). Cambridge, UK: Cambridge University Press.

Bishop, D. V. M., & Snowling, M. J. (2004). Developmental dyslexia and specific language impairment: Same or different? *Psychological Bulletin, 130,* 858–886.

Bull, R., Johnston, R. S., & Roy, J. A. (1999). Exploring the roles of the visual–spatial sketch pad and central executive in children's arithmetical skills: Views from cognition and developmental neuropsychology. *Developmental Neuropsychology, 15,* 421–442.

Cain, K., Oakhill, J., & Bryant, P. (2000). Phonological skills and comprehension failure: A test of the phonological deficit hypothesis. *Reading and Writing: An Interdisciplinary Journal, 13,* 31–56.

Cain, K., Oakhill, J., & Bryant, P. (2004). Children's reading comprehension ability: Concurrent prediction by working memory, verbal ability, and component skills. *Journal of Educational Psychology, 96,* 31–42.

Cain, K., Oakhill, J., & Lemmon, K. (2004). Individual differences in the inference of word meanings from context: The influence of reading comprehension, vocabulary knowledge, and memory capacity. *Journal of Educational Psychology, 96*(4), 671–681.

Chiappe, P., Hasher, L., & Siegel, L. S. (2000). Working memory, inhibitory control, and reading disability. *Memory and Cognition, 28,* 8–17.

Cohen, J., & Cohen, P. (1983). *Applied multiple regression/correlation analysis for the behavioral sciences* (2nd ed.). Hillsdale, NJ: Erlbaum.

Conway, A. R., Cowan, N., Bunting, M. F., Therriault, S., & Minkoff, S. R. (2002). A latent variable analysis of working memory capacity, short-term memory capacity, processing speed, and general fluid intelligence, *Intelligence, 30,* 163–183.

Crain, S., & Shankweiler, D. (1990). Explaining failures in spoken language comprehension by children with reading disabilities. In D. Balota, G. Flores d'Arcais, & K. Rayner (Eds.), *Comprehension processes in reading* (pp. 539–555). Hillsdale, NJ: Erlbaum.

Crain, S., Shankweiler, D., Macaruss, P., & Bar-Shalom, E. (1990). Working memory and sentence comprehension: Investigation of children and reading disorders. In G. Valler & T. Shallice (Eds.), *Impairments of short-term memory* (pp. 539–552). Cambridge, UK: Cambridge University Press.

Daneman, M., & Carpenter, P. A. (1980). Individual differences in working memory and reading. *Journal of Verbal Learning and Verbal Behavior, 19,* 450–466.

Daneman, M., & Merikle, P. M. (1996). Working memory and language comprehension: A meta-analysis. *Psychonomic Bulletin and Review, 3,* 442–433.

De Beni, R., & Palladino, P. (2000). Intrusion errors in working memory tasks: Are they related to reading comprehension ability? *Learning and Individual Differences, 12*(2), 131–143.

De Beni, R., Palladino, P., Pazzaglia, F., & Cornoldi, C. (1998). Increases in intrusion errors and working memory deficit of poor comprehenders. *Quarterly Journal of Experimental Psychology: Human Experimental Psychology, 51,* 305–320.

de Jong, P. (1998). Working memory deficits of reading disabled children. *Journal of Experimental Child Psychology, 70,* 75–95.

Engle, R. W., Cantor, J., & Carullo, J. J. (1992). Individual differences in working memory and comprehension: A test of four hypotheses. *Journal of Experimental Psychology: Learning, Memory and Cognition, 18,* 972–992.

Engle, R. W., Tuholski, S. W., Laughlin, J. E., & Conway, A. R. (1999). Working memory, short-term memory, and general fluid intelligence: A latent variable approach. *Journal of Experimental Psychology: General, 128,* 309–331.

Fletcher, J. M., Francis, D. J., Rourke, B. P., Shaywitz, S. E., & Shaywitz, B. A. (1992). The validity of discrepancy-based definitions of reading disabilities. *Journal of Learning Disabilities, 25,* 555–561.

Gathercole, S. E. (1998). The development of memory. *Journal of Child Psychology and Psychiatry, 39,* 3–27.

Gathercole, S. E., & Baddeley, A. D. (1993). *Working memory and language.* Hove, UK: Erlbaum.

Geary, D. (1993). Mathematical disabilities: Cognitive, neuropsychological, and genetic components. *Psychological Bulletin, 114,* 345–362.

Geary, D. (2003). Learning disabilities in arithmetic: Problem solving differences and cognitive deficits. In H. L. Swanson, K. M. Harris, & S. Graham (Eds.), *Handbook of learning disabilities* (pp. 199–212). New York: Guilford Press.

Haarmann, H. J., Davelaar, E. J., & Usher, M. (2003). Individual differences in semantic short-term memory capacity and reading comprehension. *Journal of Memory and Language, 48*(2), 320–345.

Hammill, D. (1990). On defining learning disabilities: An emerging consensus. *Journal of Learning Disabilities, 23,* 74–84.

Hulme, C., Maughan, S., & Brown, G. D. A. (1991). Memory for familiar and unfamiliar words: Evidence from a long-term memory contribution to short-term memory span. *Journal of Memory and Language, 30,* 685–701.

Hulme, C., Thomson, N., Muir, C., & Lawrence, A. (1984). Speech rate and the development of short-term memory span. *Journal of Experimental Child Psychology, 47,* 72–87.

Johnston, R. S., & Anderson, M. (1998). Memory span, naming speed, and memory strategies in poor and normal readers. *Memory, 6,* 143–163.

Just, M. A., Carpenter, P. A., & Keller, T. A. (1996). The capacity theory of comprehension: New frontiers of evidence and arguments. *Psychological Review, 103,* 773–780.

Kail, R. (1993). The role of global mechanisms in developmental change in speed of processing. In M. Howe & R. Pasnak (Eds.) *Emerging themes in cognitive development* (Vol. 1, pp. 97–116). New York: Springer-Verlag.

Kane, M. J., & Engle, R. W. (2003). Working-memory capacity and the control of attention: The contributions of goal neglect, response competition, and task set to Stroop interference. *Journal of Experimental Psychology: General, 132,* 47–70.

Marshall, C. M., & Nation, K. (2003). Individual differences in semantic and structural errors in children's memory for sentences. *Educational and Child Psychology, 20,* 7–18.

Miyake, A. (2001). Individual differences in working memory: Introduction to the special section. *Journal of Experimental Psychology, 130,* 163–168.

Miyake, A., Friedman, N. P., Emerson, M. J., Witzki, A. H., & Howerter, A. (2000). The unity and diversity of executive functions and their contributions to complex "frontal lobe" tasks: A latent variable analysis. *Cognitive Psychology, 41,* 49–100.

Morris, N., & Jones, D. M. (1990). Memory updating in working memory: The role of central executive. *British Journal of Psychology, 91,* 111–121.

Nation, K., Adams, J. W., Bowyer-Crane, C. A., & Snowling, M. J. (1999). Working memory deficits in poor comprehenders reflect underlying language impairments. *Journal of Experimental Child Psychology, 73,* 139–158.

Oberauer, K. (2002). Access to information in working memory: Exploring the focus of attention. *Journal of Experimental Psychology: Learning, Memory, and Cognition, 29*, 411–421.

Oberauer, K., Sub, H., Wilhelm, O., & Wittman, W. W. (2003). The multiple faces of working memory: Storage, processing, supervision, and coordination. *Intelligence, 31*, 167–193.

O'Shaughnessy, T., & Swanson, H. L. (1998). Do immediate memory deficits in students with learning disabilities in reading reflect a developmental lag or deficit?: A selective meta-analysis of the literature. *Learning Disability Quarterly, 21*, 123–148.

Palladino, P., Cornoldi, C., De Beni, R., & Pazzaglia, F. (2001). Working memory and updating processes in reading comprehension. *Memory and Cognition, 29*(2), 344–354.

Passolunghi, M. C., Cornoldi, C., & De Liberto, S. (1999). Working memory and intrusions of irrelevant information in a group of specific poor problem solvers. *Memory and Cognition, 27*, 779–790.

Passolunghi, M. C., & Siegel, L. S. (2001). Short-term memory, working memory, and inhibitory control in children with difficulties in arithmetic problem solving. *Journal of Experimental Child Psychology, 80*, 44–57.

Psychological Corporation. (1991). *Wechsler Intelligence Scale for Children–3rd edition.* San Antonio, TX: Harcourt Brace Jovanovich.

Ransby, M. J., & Swanson, H. L. (2003). Reading comprehension skills of young adults with childhood diagnoses of dyslexia. *Journal of Learning Disabilities, 36*(6), 538–555.

Raven, J. C. (1976). *Colored progressive matrices.* London, UK: H. K. Lewis & Co.

Salthouse, T. A. (1996). The processing-speed theory of adult age differences in cognition. *Psychological Review, 103*, 403–428.

Seigneuric, A., Ehrlich, M. F., Oakhill, J. V., & Yuill, N. M. (2000). Working memory resources and children's reading comprehension. *Reading and Writing, 13*, 81–103.

Shankweiler, D., & Crain, S. (1986). Language mechanisms and reading disorder. *Cognition, 24*, 139–168.

Shankweiler, D., Crain, S., Katz, L., Fowler, A. E., Liberman, A. M., Brady, S. A., et al. (1995). Cognitive profiles of reading disabled children: Comparison of language skills in phonology, morphology, and syntax. *Psychological Science, 6*, 149–156.

Shaywitz, S. E., Fletcher, J. M., Holahan, J. M., Schneider, A. E., Marchione, K. E., Stuebing, K. K., et al. (1999). Persistence of dyslexia: The Connecticut Longitudinal Study at Adolescence. *Pediatrics, 104*, 1351–1359.

Siegel, L. S. (1992). An evaluation of the discrepancy definition of dyslexia. *Journal of Learning Disabilities, 25*, 618–629.

Siegel, L. S. (1994). Working memory and reading: A life-span perspective. *International Journal of Behavioral Development, 17*, 109–124.

Siegel, L. S. (2003). Basic cognitive processes and reading disabilities. In H. L. Swanson, K. M. Harris, & S. Graham (Eds.), *Handbook of learning disabilities* (pp. 158–181). New York: Guilford Press.

Siegel, L. S., & Ryan, E. B. (1989). The development of working memory in normally achieving and subtypes of learning disabled. *Child Development, 60*, 973–980.

Stanovich, K. E. (1990). Concepts in developmental theories of reading skill: Cognitive resources, automaticity, and modularity. *Developmental Review, 10*, 72–100.

Stanovich, K. E., & Siegel, L. S. (1994). Phenotypic performance profile of children with reading disabilities: A regression-based test of the phonological–core variable–difference model. *Journal of Educational Psychology, 86*, 24–53.

Stothard, S., & Hulme, C. (1992). Reading comprehension difficulties in children. *Reading and Writing: An Interdisciplinary Journal, 4*, 245–256.

Swanson, H. L. (1989). Operational definitions of LD: An overview. *Learning Disability Quarterly, 14*, 242–254.

Swanson, H. L. (1994). Short-term memory and working memory: Do they contribute to our understanding of academic achievement in children and adults with learning disabilities? *Journal of Learning Disabilities, 27*, 34–50.

Swanson, H. L. (1995). *Swanson-Cognitive Processing Test*. Austin, TX: PRO-ED.

Swanson, H. L. (1996). Individual and age-related differences in children's working memory. *Memory and Cognition, 24*, 70–82.

Swanson, H. L. (1999a). Reading comprehension and working memory in skilled readers: Is the phonological loop more important than the executive system? *Journal of Experimental Child Psychology, 72*, 1–31.

Swanson, H. L. (1999b). Reading research for students with LD: A meta-analysis of intervention outcomes. *Journal of Learning Disabilities, 32*, 504–532.

Swanson, H. L. (2000). Searching for the best model for instructing students with LD: A component and composite analysis. *Educational and Child Psychology, 17*, 101–121.

Swanson, H. L. (2003). Age-related differences in learning disabled and skilled readers' working memory. *Journal of Experimental Child Psychology, 85*, 1–31.

Swanson, H. L., & Alexander, J. (1997). Cognitive processes as predictors of word recognition and reading comprehension in learning disabled and skilled readers: Revisiting the specificity hypothesis. *Journal of Educational Psychology, 89*, 128–158.

Swanson, H. L., & Ashbaker, M. H. (2000). Working memory, short-term memory, speech rate, word recognition and reading comprehension in learning disabled readers: Does the executive system have a role? *Intelligence, 28*, 1–30.

Swanson, H. L., Ashbaker, M. H., & Lee, C. (1996). Learning disabled reader's working memory as a function of processing demands. *Journal of Experimental Child Psychology, 61*, 242–275.

Swanson, H. L., & Beebe-Frankenberger, M. (2004). The relationship between working memory and problem solving in children at risk and not at risk for math disabilities. *Journal of Educational Psychology, 96*, 471–491.

Swanson, H. L., & Berninger, V. (1995). The role of working memory and STM in skilled and less skilled readers' word recognition and comprehension. *Intelligence, 21,* 83–108.

Swanson, H. L., & Cochran, K. (1991). Learning disabilities, distinctive encoding, and hemispheric resources. *Brain and Language, 40,* 202–230.

Swanson, H. L., & Hoskyn, M. (1998). Experimental intervention research on students with learning disabilities: A meta-analysis of treatment outcomes. *Review of Educational Research, 68,* 277–321.

Swanson, H. L., Hoskyn, M., & Lee, C. (1999). *Interventions for students with learning disabilities: A meta-analysis of treatment outcomes.* New York: Guilford Press.

Swanson, H. L., Howard, C., & Sáez, L. (2006). Components of working memory that are related to poor reading comprehension and word recognition performance in less skilled readers. *Journal of Learning Disabilities, 39,* 252–269.

Swanson, H. L., & Howell, M. (2001). Working memory, short-term memory, and speech rate as predictors of children's reading performance at different ages. *Journal of Educational Psychology, 93,* 720–734.

Swanson, H. L., & Sachse-Lee, C. (2001). Mathematical problem solving and working memory in children with learning disabilities: Both executive and phonological processes are important. *Journal of Experimental Child Psychology, 79,* 294–321.

Swanson, H. L., & Siegel, L. S. (2001). Learning disabilities as a working memory deficit. *Issues in Education: Contributions from Educational Psychology, 7,* 1–48.

Towse, J. (1998). On random generation and the central executive of working memory. *British Journal of Psychology, 89,* 77–101.

Turner, M. L., & Engle, R. W. (1989). Is working-memory capacity task dependent? *Journal of Memory and Language, 28,* 27–154.

Wagner, R., & Torgesen, J. (1999). *Test of Word Reading Efficiency.* Austin, TX: PRO-ED.

Wagner, R., Torgesen, J., & Rashotte, C. (2000). *Comprehensive Test of Phonological Processes.* Austin, TX: PRO-ED.

Weiderholt, L., & Bryant, B. (1986). *Gray Oral Reading Test–III.* Austin, TX: PRO-ED.

Whitney, P., Arnett, P., Driver, A., & Budd, D. (2001). Measuring central executive functioning: What's in a reading span? *Brain and Cognition, 45,* 1–14.

Wilkinson, G. S. (1993). *The Wide Range Achievement Test–3.* Wilmington, DE: Wide Range.

Woodcock, R. W. (1988). *Woodcock Reading Mastery Test–Revised.* Minneapolis, MN: American Guidance.

Yuill, N., Oakhill, J., & Parkin, A. (1989). Working memory, comprehension ability and the resolution of text anomaly. *British Journal of Psychology, 80,* 351–361.

PART III

Comprehension Impairments in Association with Neurological Damage and Sensory Impairment

This part includes three chapters. Two explore the language comprehension impairments of children who have suffered neurological damage, the other is a contrastive chapter on a population with language comprehension difficulties but no apparent cognitive deficit: children with hearing impairment. The findings that come out of these three research areas are shown to be relevant not only to the assessment and treatment of comprehension difficulties in these specific populations, they also inform models of typical function by identifying the cognitive functions that are crucial to success in language comprehension.

Chapter 7, by Barnes, Johnston, and Dennis concerns the language strengths and weaknesses of children with spina bifida myelomeningocele (SBM). SBM is a common birth defect that affects the development of spine and brain. Children with SBM often have preserved word-reading and single-word comprehension, but impaired comprehension of text. In a review of their recent work, Barnes and colleagues present evidence that children with SBM have accurate and fluent access to surface codes for word and text comprehension, but have specific difficulties with the construction of text-based meaning. This group's work strongly suggests that the problems experienced by children with SBM arise from deficits in a relatively constrained set of comprehension and memory processes. This work has clear parallels with the profile of poor comprehenders presented elsewhere in this volume (e.g., Cain & Oakhill, Chapter 2; Swanson, Howard, & Sáez, Chapter 6).

Chapter 8, by Cook, Chapman, and Gamino, reviews research into the cognitive-linguistic deficits associated with pediatric traumatic brain injury (TBI). Children often experience decreased academic achievement after a brain injury, yet many measures of everyday language function and ability do not capture the nature and extent of their language and cognitive deficits because they tend to focus on word- and sentence-level comprehension and automatic skills. Chapman and colleagues have used discourse production and comprehension measures to explore these children's difficulties and have identified specific problems with their ability to extract the *gist* of written and spoken language. Similar to the analysis of the difficulties experienced by children with SBM, these children's difficulties may be related to memory processes and key comprehension processes, such as the selection of crucial information. A detailed case study provides an insight into the specific difficulties in gist discourse experienced by a child who has experienced a TBI and possibilities for intervention.

In Chapter 9, Kelly and Barac-Cikoja begin with an overview of the extent of deaf readers' problems. They discuss four aspects of competence and how they may limit deaf children's reading development: word reading, syntactic knowledge, discourse comprehension, and reading strategies. The main focus of their chapter is on word reading and the ways in which deaf readers' comprehension is compromised by the quality of their phonological and orthographic representations. Kelly and Barac-Cikoja point out that the other problems evidenced by deaf readers are likely to be secondary to, and possibly even caused by, their problems at the word level. Thus, they advise that instructional efforts should be concentrated on improving word reading in this population.

CHAPTER 7

Comprehension in a Neurodevelopmental Disorder, Spina Bifida Myelomeningocele

MARCIA A. BARNES
AMBER M. JOHNSTON
MAUREEN DENNIS

What characterizes the difference between good and poor comprehension for oral and written texts? Studies of individual differences in text comprehension designed to answer this question have used a number of approaches (correlating comprehension with other cognitive skills or decomposing comprehension into component processes), methods (studying comprehension in isolation or on-line, in real time), and study populations (children or adults, skilled or less skilled at comprehension, neurologically intact or impaired).

Correlational approaches to comprehension involve studying how skills such as vocabulary or inferencing or resources such as memory and attention account for individual differences in comprehension (e.g., Yuill, Oakhill, & Parkin, 1989). Skilled and less-skilled comprehenders can differ in both skills such as inference making and in resources such as working memory. Likewise, cognitive resources such as working memory may be related to comprehension skills such as inferencing and learning new vocabulary (e.g., Cain, Oakhill, & Lemmon, 2004). On-line approaches to comprehension, designed to understand how comprehension unfolds in time, involve studying how representations of what is heard or read are constructed and revised over time in response to the current text and the knowledge and goals of the listener and reader (Kintsch, 1988; Schmalhofer, McDaniel, & Keefe, 2002). On-line approaches to comprehension typically use cognitive models of text comprehension to investigate the integrity of comprehension processes *during* listening or reading in children of different ages and skill levels (e.g., Nation, Marshall, & Altmann, 2003), or in individuals with brain injuries (e.g., Barnes, Faulkner, Wilkinson, & Dennis, 2004; Brownell, Simpson, Bihrle, Potter, & Gardner, 1990; Gagnon, Goulet, Giroux, & Joanette, 2003; Tompkins, Baumgaertner, Lehman, & Fassbinder, 2000).

Most studies of text comprehension after brain compromise have been conducted with adults, yet developmental injury to the brain is of considerable interest to comprehension models. In particular, the study of off-line and on-line text comprehension in a neurodevelopmental disorder that preserves word-reading and single-word comprehension may reveal how text comprehension skills are acquired. This chapter presents a review of our research group's studies of text comprehension in children with spina bifida myelomeningocele (SBM), a common birth defect that affects the development of spine and brain and that is associated with selective deficits in comprehension.

SBM AND ITS COGNITIVE PHENOTYPE

SBM, a common severely disabling birth defect, arises from a failure of neural tube closure early in gestation. Even though folic acid fortification of grain-based foods in the late 1990s has reduced the prevalence of all types of neural tube defects (Persad,Van den Hof, Dube, & Zimmer, 2002), SBM still occurs in 0.3–0.5 per 1,000 live births (Williams, Rasmussen, Flores, Kirby, & Edmonds, 2005). SBM arises from a complex pattern of gene–environment interactions (Kirkpatrick & Northrup, 2003) that produce a neural tube defect that is associated at birth with distinctive physical, neural, and cognitive phenotypes. The physical phenotype of SBM, with its spinal cord defect and orthopedic sequelae such as significant paraplegia and limited ambulation, is what is most commonly associated with this developmental disorder. Less well known and less well studied is the neural phenotype of SBM that involves significant disruption of brain development. Disruptions in neuroembryogenesis produce anomalies in the regional development of the brain, especially the corpus callosum, midbrain and tectum, and cerebellum. Additional injury to the brain is produced because of hydrocephalus, which arises from a blockage of cerebral spinal fluid flow due to a malformed cerebellum and hindbrain. Hydrocephalus necessitates shunt treatment in 80–90% of cases of SBM (Reigel & Rotenstein, 1994), and it affects both corpus callosum and cortical neuronal development through thinning of the posterior brain regions (Del Bigio, 1993).

Mental retardation is not common in SBM. Verbal IQ is generally in the average range, though upper spinal lesions and social and economic disadvantage are associated with lower IQs, particularly in the verbal domain (Fletcher et al., 2004). SBM is associated with specific cognitive and academic deficits. As a group, children with SBM are stronger in language and weaker in perceptual and motor skills (Dennis et al., 1981; Fletcher et al., 1992). However, within the language domain, there is uneven skill development such that basic language skills including vocabulary and syntax are intact, but inferential and text-level skills are deficient (Barnes, 2002; Barnes & Dennis, 1998; Barnes et al., 2004). In terms of academic competencies, math and reading comprehension are impaired relative to word recognition skills, and writing problems are common (Fletcher, Brookshire, Bohan, Brandt, & Davidson, 1995; Barnes, Dennis, & Hetherington, 2004).

A neurodevelopmental disorder such as SBM affords several windows into the study of comprehension. First, it produces skill dissociations that are useful for testing cognitive models. SBM is associated with the adequate development of word-decoding, vocabulary, and grammatical skills, but less well developed oral and written text comprehension. Although these dissociations can also be found in individuals with no neurological impairment (Muter, Hulme, Snowling, & Stevenson, 2004; Oakhill, Cain, & Bryant, 2003), they are common in children with SBM, which makes this disorder valuable for the investigation of comprehension difficulties. Second, SBM is a lifelong condition, so individuals with SBM can be followed from birth to adulthood to ask questions about comprehension such as developmental precursors, developmental trajectories, the effects of aging, and the consequences of comprehension problems for everyday functioning and quality of life.

In children with no neurological disorder, comprehension disabilities tend to be identified later in schooling than are disabilities in word reading (Leach, Scarborough, & Rescorla, 2003) and have been estimated to affect between 5 and 10% of the school-age population (Cornoldi, De Beni, & Pazzaglia, 1996). In North American samples, children diagnosed with reading disabilities after third grade include equal numbers with word-reading problems only, with both word-reading and comprehension problems, and with comprehension problems only (Leach et al., 2003). Regardless of word-reading ability, children with comprehension difficulties experience problems in understanding what they hear and read (Shankweiler et al., 1999).

In SBM, the dissociation between preserved word decoding and poor text comprehension is common (Barnes, 2002; Barnes & Dennis, 1992; Barnes, Faulkner, & Dennis, 2001). Decoding and phonological skills may even be enhanced in individuals with SBM (Barnes et al., 2006; see Nation, Clarke, & Snowling, 2002, for a similar finding in neurologically normal good decoders/poor comprehenders). More than four-fifths of adults with SBM have stronger word-decoding skills than reading comprehension skills (Barnes et al., 2004). In a recent large-scale study in Ontario and Texas, we looked at reading and listening comprehension in a large sample of children with SBM and no mental retardation. Using a low achievement definition of learning disabilities (Francis et al., 2005), one-third of the sample had a disability in reading comprehension; this was higher than the rate of word-reading disability (Fletcher et al., 2004). The average achievement level for word reading in the group with SBM was age-appropriate, whereas the average achievement level for reading comprehension was below average when the reading comprehension measure tapped literal, inferential, and thematic aspects of comprehension. Oral as well as reading comprehension is impaired. On an oral-inferencing task, nearly half of the children with SBM scored below the low achievement cutoff, and inferencing skills predicted unique variance in reading comprehension even after controlling for word decoding and vocabulary (Fletcher et al., 2004). In sum, children and adults with SBM are typically accurate at reading words, but they have difficulties with both oral and written text comprehension.

In SBM, development across a number of domains (including motor function, perception, language, reading, and mathematics) can be explained by a model that includes a small number of core deficits that are closely tied to the primary brain dysmorphologies of SBM, present from birth and persist throughout the lifespan, and result in a combination of spared and deficient processing within domains such as language and reading (Dennis, Landry, Barnes, & Fletcher, 2006). Some of the processing assumptions of this model are useful for the study of comprehension and its relation to other cognitive domains, specifically, the idea that core deficits limit the ability to integrate information during cognitive processing, although not to activate stored information. The specific entailment of the SBM model for oral and written comprehension is that directly activated representations are stipulated as a result of learning, whereas assembled representations that guide on-line performance in novel contexts require revision as the situation unfolds in time.

STUDIES OF TEXT COMPREHENSION IN SBM

Our studies of text comprehension in SBM have used two approaches. Reasoning that the manner in which skills cohere or fall apart in SBM should be informative for cognitive models of comprehension development, we have investigated the integrity of comprehension processes identified in cognitive models of discourse and text comprehension (e.g., Barnes, Faulkner, et al., 2004). Because we are interested in exploring the ways in which neurobiology constrains cognitive models (e.g., Dennis et al., 2006), we have also situated investigation of comprehension processes in a broader neurobiological context that considers how intact and deficient language development in SBM is related to intact and deficient development of skills outside the language domain.

Sophisticated models of text-level comprehension processes, developed from cognitive studies of fluent adult readers, are sometimes applied to study developmental and individual differences. Discourse comprehension builds on vocabulary and on syntactic constraints (Clifton & Duffy, 2001), sometimes referred to as the "surface code," but comprehension also requires construction of meaning as the text unfolds in time and interacts with the knowledge and goals of the reader (Kintsch, 1988; Schmalhofer et al., 2002; Snow & the RAND Reading Study Group, 2001). Active construction processes are important in building representations of the "text base" (a representation of the explicit meaning of the text in which context is used to specify meaning, and various sources of information within the text are integrated through pronominal reference and bridging inferences) and the "situation model" (integration of the text with a reader's knowledge and goals in order to situate text in a real-world context) (Clifton & Duffy, 2001; Kintsch, 1988; Schmalhofer et al., 2002; Zwaan & Radvansky, 1998).

Memory has multiple functions in comprehension. It may facilitate vocabulary development (Jarrold, Baddeley, Hewes, Leeke, & Phillips, 2004), and it supports a number of cognitive and academic tasks. During comprehension, short-term memory holds or maintains current text-based information for short periods of time. Long-term memory stores knowledge about the world as well as previously encountered propositions from the text. In contrast to these two relatively static memory systems, working memory is a dynamic system, or "mental workspace," in which information from long-term memory and current text can be integrated or where information in short-term verbal memory can be integrated, manipulated, or revised to enable comprehension of current text. Working memory, in particular, is often poorly developed in individuals with academic and developmental disorders (Gathercole & Pickering, 2000; Geary & Hoard, 2005; Swanson & Sachse-Lee, 2001). Memory is integral to the operation of particular comprehension mechanisms. As comprehension proceeds in time, the products of one processing cycle, which includes the integration of surface code, text base, and situation model, feed forward into the next processing cycle; that is to say, representation of what is heard or read involves frequent integration and revision (van den Broek, Young, Tzeng, & Linderholm, 1999; Graesser, Millis, & Zwaan, 1997). Integration and revision require memory processes. For example, working memory facilitates revision within a current processing cycle, and sustains activation of information from previous processing cycles so that it can be integrated with information from the current cycle (Graesser et al., 1997). A proposition in a current processing cycle may resonate with information in long-term memory from a previous processing cycle or may serve to activate general knowledge from long-term memory, thereby facilitating retrieval of that information to make inferences across text or inferences between general knowledge and text (Albrecht & Myers, 1998; van den Broek et al., 1999).

In theory, individual differences in comprehension could arise from failures in comprehension processes at the level of the surface code, the text base, or the situation model, or with the memorial processes that are necessary for integration and revision. The studies presented below investigate the integrity of comprehension processes that relate to the surface code, the text base, and the situation model in children with SBM as well as the role of memorial processes through manipulations of information-processing load.

Accessing Meaning from the Surface Code

Children with SBM have ready access to the literal meanings provided by surface codes. Despite significant disruptions to their brain development, most children with SBM master phonology and learn to read words (Barnes & Dennis, 1992), and develop vocabulary knowledge and syntax, whether measured through comprehension of oral language (Dennis, Hendrick, Hoffman, & Humphreys, 1987; Horn, Lorch, Lorch, & Culatta, 1985; Parsons, 1986), comprehension of written language (Barnes & Dennis, 1992), or through language production (Barnes & Dennis, 1998; Dennis, Jacennik, & Barnes, 1994). For example, in a story narrative task, children with hydrocephalus, most with SBM, produced as many clauses and propositions of comparable syntactic complexity as normal same-age peers (Barnes & Dennis, 1998). In a longitudinal study of outcomes at 36 and 60 months in children with SBM and no mental retardation, vocabulary skills were developed to age-appropriate levels (Barnes, Smith-Chant, & Landry, 2005). If the environment of children with SBM is socially and economically disadvantaged, however, then basic vocabulary skills may be deficient (Fletcher et al., 2004). Young and middle-age adults with SBM also show age-appropriate vocabulary (Barnes et al., 2004).

Some figurative language comprehension involving surface codes also develops well in individuals with SBM. Common idioms are formulaic expressions (e.g., "Let me give you a hand") whose meaning may be stored like the meanings of words and accessed as units during text comprehension. Children of average intelligence with hydrocephalus, most with SBM, do not differ from age peers in their comprehension of common idioms (Barnes & Dennis, 1998).

Because text comprehension requires processing in real time, it is important to distinguish knowledge from fluent knowledge access during comprehension (Cain et al., 2004). In SBM, which is associated with slowed performance on a number of cognitive and motor tasks (Dennis et al., 1987; Fletcher et al., 1996), fluency in accessing the surface code appears to be intact.

Several comprehension models propose that a passive semantic process initially activates word meanings regardless of context such that more semantic information is activated than will actually be fed forward to the next processing cycle (Gernsbacher, 1990; Schmalhofer et al., 2002). Normal adult readers are slower to say that *ace* does *not* fit the meaning of the sentence "He dug with the spade" than they are to say that *ace* does *not* fit the meaning of the sentence "He dug with the shovel" when tested immediately (i.e., within 250 milliseconds) after having read the last word of each sentence (Seidenberg, Tanenhaus, Leimen, & Bienkowski, 1982). Context is irrelevant to activation, by which a broad range of semantic information is activated immediately upon reading a word, but, as comprehension proceeds in time, context suppresses context-irrelevant semantic information. Difficulty in rejecting the context-irrelevant meaning of the word right after reading it is called an interference effect.

Children with hydrocephalus, most with SBM, and normal controls (matched on word-reading levels, but differing in reading comprehension) read sentences containing an ambiguous word (e.g., *spade*) in a context that biased the meaning of the ambiguous word (e.g., "He dug with the spade") and control sentences that did not contain an ambiguous word (e.g., "He dug with the shovel"). The task was to say whether a test word fitted the meaning of the previously read sentence. In some cases the test word was related to the contextually irrelevant meaning of the ambiguous word (e.g., *ace*). Both children with SBM and their age peers showed similar interference effects, demonstrating that children with SBM activate word meanings during comprehension and access the same range of meanings as age peers (Barnes et al., 2004). Of note, children with SBM also show intact semantic priming in implicit memory tasks (Yeates & Enrile, 2005) and they read words fluently (Barnes et al., 2001).

A number of comprehension studies in children with SBM reveal intact skills in understanding of literal meanings for single words, understanding of idioms, and activation of word-level meaning during sentence comprehension. The data suggest that these children have accurate and fluent access to surface codes for word and text comprehension.

Construction of Text-Based Representations

Two operations support the construction of text-based meaning: context–dependent suppression and bridging. An important component of comprehension is successful suppression of context-irrelevant activated meanings (Gernsbacher, 1990). Failure to suppress extraneous propositional information creates an incoherent text representation. Meaning is constructed through bridging inferences that link two propositions in a text (Albrecht & O'Brien, 1993). We studied how children with SBM use context to *suppress irrelevant semantic information* and how they *bridge propositions within a text* to infer meaning.

Suppression was investigated in the meaning activation task described above, but in which the judgment about whether the test word *ace* fitted the meaning of the sentence "He dug with the spade," or "He dug with the shovel" was delayed for 1,000 milliseconds after the presentation of the last word of the sentence. If contextually irrelevant information is efficiently suppressed as processing proceeds in time, there should be no interference effect, that is, it should take the same amount to time to decide that the word *ace* does not fit the meaning of the sentence containing the ambiguous word ("He dug with the spade") and the meaning of the control sentence ("He dug with the shovel"). Unlike the control group, children with SBM continued to show a substantial interference effect (Barnes et al., 2004).

Similar findings are reported for adult readers with weak reading comprehension skills (Gernsbacher & Faust, 1991) who showed intact initial activation of word meanings, but deficient contextual suppression. Consistency in findings such as these across different groups of individuals with poor comprehension, some children, some adults, some with frank brain injury, and others without, provides constraints on models of comprehension disability and converging evidence for core deficits in individuals with comprehension problems.

Bridging inferences in children with SBM were studied in relation to manipulations of the textual distance between sentences that had to be integrated to make the inference. Children read six-sentence paragraphs and had to decide whether a seventh test sentence was a coherent continuation of the previous paragraph. The critical sentence was ambiguous with respect to its meaning (e.g., "John laughed as he picked up a spade") and relied on context to specify whether the *spade* was a card or a digging implement. In one condition (the near integration condition), the bridging was between information in adjacent sentences; in the other condition (the far integration condition), bridging was between information separated by three filler sentences. In the example below, the critical sentence in parentheses appeared as either the second sentence (far integration) or fifth sentence (near integration) of the paragraph. This critical sentence needed to be integrated with the sixth sentence in order to judge whether the test sentence was a coherent continuation.

> *John and Eddie always get together on Saturdays.*
> *(This Saturday John and Eddie were planting some bushes for John's*
> *mother.)*
> *John especially likes Eddie for his sense of humor.*
> *Eddie wants to be a stand-up comedian so he is always practicing jokes on*
> *John.*
> *The two have a great time together.*
> *(This Saturday John and Eddie were planting some bushes for John's*
> *mother.)*
> *John laughed as he picked up a spade.*
> Test Sentence: *He began to dig.*

All children were highly accurate in both the near and the far integration conditions, and all required more time to make decisions in the far distance versus the near distance condition, but the children with SBM were significantly more disadvantaged by textual distance (Barnes et al., 2004). The data suggest accurate but slow bridging inferences in children with SBM, who would thereby be less efficient than typically developing children in constructing a coherent and integrated representation of the text base.

What role might memorial processes play in the construction of text representations? Children with SBM have intact immediate verbal memory spans or verbal short-term memory (Backman, Beattie, & Bawden, 1999), but difficulties with delayed recall and recognition or long-term memory (Ewing-Cobbs, Barnes, & Fletcher, 2003; Scott et al., 1998; Yeates, Enrile, Loss, Blumenstein, & Delis, 1995) and with working memory (Dennis & Barnes, 2002; Purzner, Wilkinson, Boudousquie, Fletcher, & Barnes, 2004). Memory problems contribute to slow integration of information during reading. This lack of fluency in integration processes could lead to processing bottlenecks at the text level (Long, Oppy, & Seely, 1997), similar to those of slow readers at the word and the sentence level (Perfetti, 1985). In normal reading situations in which the performance demands differ from those encountered in psychological testing, effortful processing may or may not serve comprehension. Children may be strongly motivated to perform comprehension tasks with accuracy in experimental testing situations, and less motivated to perform in more typical reading situations, whether for pleasure or for learning. To the extent that the motivations or goals of the reader contribute to comprehension, children with comprehension problems, like those with SBM, may fail to make some of these bridging inferences if they are too time-consuming. Deficits in fluent access to previous propositions may be particularly detrimental for comprehension in situations where the pace of information delivery is not always under the control of the listener or the discourse partner.

The role of working memory in comprehension seems similar in children with SBM and young, neurologically intact children with poorly developed comprehension skills. Cain, Oakhill, and Elbro (2003) showed that the learning of new vocabulary from context was impaired in less-skilled comprehenders when the context was not adjacent to the new word, and that working memory capacity, but not immediate memory span, was related to the ability to infer meanings of novel words from context (Cain et al., 2004). Again, the consistency of findings in children with poor comprehension, regardless of the presence of early brain injury, provides converging evidence for the idea that comprehension problems arise from deficits in a relatively constrained set of comprehension and memorial processes.

Construction of a Situation Model

A "situation model" is the representation of text that situates it in the real world and includes inferences about space, time, causality, and the goals of the characters that are made when meaning cannot be established solely through information provided in the text (Zwaan & Radvansky, 1998). At the sentence level, situation models require *construction*; at the text level, they typically require *construction and revision*. We have investigated the construction of situation models during comprehension both at the sentence level and at the text level. In the former case, the child had to construct a situation model, but there was no requirement to revise the model. In the latter case, the child had to retrieve information from a knowledge base and use that knowledge to make inferences as events in a story unfolded.

In investigating the construction process for situation models, we have studied the ability to form a mental model of the spatial layout described by a sentence (Johnston & Barnes, 2006). Because inferences in situation models are commonly tested by spatial layouts, which are an area of relative weakness for individuals with SBM, we tested situation models inferred from spatial layouts (following Bransford & Franks, 1972) as well as models from which characters' goals and feelings could be inferred. In a two-sentence study phase followed by a two-sentence recognition test, the child's task is to decide whether each test sentence is *exactly* the same in wording as one of the sentences from the study phase. For example, if a study sentence was "Three turtles rested on a floating log and a fish swam beneath them," a test sentence could be "Three turtles rested on a floating log and a fish swam beneath them" (identical wording), or "Three turtles rested on a floating log and a fish swam beneath it" (changed wording, but identical spatial mental model), or "Three turtles rested on a floating log and a fish swam beside them" (changed wording and changed spatial model). Typical adult performance involves accurately accepting test sentences that preserve both wording and meaning, accurately rejecting test sentences that change both wording and situation model, but difficulty rejecting test sentences that change the wording while preserving the spatial model (this is called the "false recognition" effect). Whether the model contained spatial or social-emotional information, children with SBM and age peers performed similarly, with both groups correctly accepting identical sentences, correctly rejecting sentences with wording and meaning changes, and showing a false recognition effect on sentences that changed wording, but preserved the situation model. For all children, recognition decisions were made from a situation model invoked by what is read, with exact wording being rapidly forgotten. Even when they had to infer spatial information, children with SBM could construct situation models as well as typically developing children during sentence comprehension, suggesting that children with SBM do not have difficulty constructing situation models at the sentence level.

Knowledge is a powerful determinant of performance on many cognitive tasks. Indeed, knowledge has been shown to reduce or eliminate some developmental and individual differences in memory, problem solving, and comprehension (Chi, 1978; Bjorklund & Bernholtz, 1986; Schneider, Korkel, & Weinert, 1989). This means that studies of individual differences in situation model construction must control for knowledge in order to determine the source of any observed deficits in model construction during comprehension of oral or written texts. Constructing situation models requires the integration of knowledge with text, which we will refer to as "knowledge-based inference." One of the issues in investigating individual differences in the construction of situation models during comprehension is that individual differences in knowledge might account for differences in situation model construction.

To investigate the construction of a situation model in text comprehension, we have investigated knowledge-based inferencing in typical development (Barnes, Dennis, & Haefele-Kalvaitis, 1996), in poor readers with both word-decoding and comprehension problems (Barnes & Dennis, 1996), in neurologically normal good decoders with poor comprehension (Cain, Oakhill, Barnes, & Bryant, 2001), in children with hydrocephalus—most with SBM—who were good decoders and less-skilled comprehenders (Barnes & Dennis, 1998), and in children with poor comprehension as a result of acquired brain injuries (Barnes & Dennis, 2001). Our paradigm controls for knowledge by teaching children a new knowledge base about a make-believe world, and having them hear or read a story consisting of several episodes in which they have opportunities to integrate their newly learned knowledge with events in the text. Two types of inferences are tested: those that are necessary for comprehension and serve to maintain story coherence (coherence inferences), and those that, while not necessary for comprehension, elaborate on objects and people in the text (elaborative inferences). We analyzed only those inferences for which children were able to remember the requisite knowledge all the way through the task (i.e., they could recall the requisite knowledge at the end of the task). Further details on this paradigm can be found in the papers cited above.

The main findings across the studies cited above on knowledge-based inferencing are remarkably similar. When knowledge is equated between children with different comprehension abilities, older but less-skilled comprehenders look, in many ways, like younger, skilled comprehenders: like younger children, less-skilled older comprehenders make fewer inferences than older skilled comprehenders, and the sources of their inferencing failures are similar (Barnes & Dennis, 1998; Cain et al., 2001). Differences between skilled and less-skilled comprehenders are magnified when the processing load is high (i.e., when inferences have to be made by retrieving knowledge from memory as stories unfold in time), and the differences are attenuated when the processing load is low (i.e., when knowledge and text needed to make an inference are cued; see Barnes & Dennis, 2001; Cain et al., 2001). Despite the fact that elaborative inferences are easier to make than coherence inferences (Barnes et al., 1996), regardless of comprehension skill, more coherence than elaborative inferences are made during story comprehension, showing that even less-skilled comprehenders attempt to maintain semantic coherence. Less-skilled comprehenders, regardless of their word-reading abilities or brain injury status, take longer to learn the knowledge base (Barnes & Dennis, 2001).

These results from the studies on the construction of situation models are of interest for two reasons. First, they replicate the processing load findings obtained for constructing text-based representations. Whether children with SBM are constructing text-based representations or situation models, manipulations that increase the processing load (greater textual distance or retrieval of knowledge from long-term memory during on-line processing) result in particularly deficient construction of meaning. Similarly, conditions in which the processing load is relatively light result in more accurate and more fluent construction of both text-based representations and situation models. This could be seen when a bridging inference required integration of adjacent sentences in the text, when knowledge and text needed to make an inference were cued, and when situation models that inferred spatial or social-emotional information did not need to be revised or used in on-line processing. Second, because the pattern of findings for knowledge-based inferencing is very similar across different groups of less-skilled comprehenders, the integration of knowledge and discourse or text may be a fundamental deficit in less-skilled comprehenders, and there would appear to be constraints on how deficits in knowledge-based inferencing come about. Although deficits related to memorial processes and processing load may play a role in these individual differences, it would be of interest to further explore the causes and consequences of slower knowledge base learning in less-skilled comprehenders. This is particularly relevant in light of a finding by Cain et al. (2001) that skilled and less-skilled comprehenders were similar in their recall of the knowledge base at the end of the task, but that less-skilled comprehenders recalled less of the knowledge base than more-skilled comprehenders 1 week later.

RELEVANCE OF COMPREHENSION DEFICITS IN SBM
TO MODELS OF TEXT COMPREHENSION

The comprehension processes that are intact in SBM correspond in broad strokes to those that are related to accessing meaning of the surface code, while those that are deficient tend to be the processes needed to construct representations of the text base and the situation model. To the extent that the construction of the text base and the situation model draw on memorial processes, greater processing loads result in less coherent semantic representations, particularly for less-skilled comprehenders. Although the representational distinctions provided by cognitive models are quite good at capturing the comprehension data in both SBM and in other groups with comprehension problems, we propose a somewhat different view of individual differences in comprehension based, in part, on our model of neurocognitive function in SBM (Dennis et al., 2006) discussed earlier. Broadly, we suggest that two types of information processing can account for the uneven comprehension profile in SBM. Meaning that can be activated through reference to stipulated memory representations is intact in SBM, while meaning that requires construction either through information integration or through revision of previous representations is deficient in SBM (also see Van Lancker Sidtis, 2004).

This generalization finds support from studies of cognitive domains other than language, and for processes other than comprehension. The distinction between stipulated and constructed processing captures intact and deficient performance of individuals with SBM across a number of motor, cognitive, and social/behavioral domains. Performance that is guided by information that has been learned through repetition and that is based on the formation of associations or for which there is early preferential or specialized processing (e.g., faces; Johnson & de Haan, 2001) is relatively intact in SBM. Thus, children with SBM show strengths in activation of stipulated representations, including the ability to recognize faces, perceive objects from degraded visual cues (Dennis, Fletcher, Rogers, Hetherington, & Francis, 2002), and retrieve small math facts (e.g., $2 + 3 = 5$) from memory (Barnes et al., 2006), and adaptive motor learning (Colvin, Yeates, Enrile, & Coury, 2003; Edelstein et al., 2004). In contrast, cognitive and motor functions that rely on the integration of information from various sources and on-line adjustments to performance are uniformly deficient in individuals with SBM. Deficits in on-line revision occur in cognitive domains seemingly far removed from language comprehension, and include on-line control of movement (Salman et al., 2005), perception that requires the ability to shift between visual representations (Dennis et al., 2002), and performance on larger sum problems (e.g., 8 + 7) that more often must be computed rather than be retrieved (Barnes et al., 2006). An evaluation of comprehension that combines cognitive models of comprehension and neurocognitive models of cognitive functions provides an integrated view of comprehension disabilities that may be useful for investigating how deficits in comprehension are related to dysfunction in other cognitive domains, perhaps not just in SBM. In the process, such investigations may also be relevant for constructing hypotheses about the neurobiology of comprehension disorders in childhood.

A number of entailments follow from our interpretations of the data on text comprehension in SBM. One is that comprehension of phrases may be achieved either by stipulated or by constructed meanings. Another is that processing load interacts with comprehension processing. A third is that the broad dissociations in text comprehension appear more similar than different in children and adults with and without brain compromise.

While it is generally the case that access to meaning through the surface code is more likely to involve stipulated meanings, and that representations of the text base and the situation model are more likely to be constructed through integration and revision processes, this is not always the case. Comprehension of formulaic expressions such as idioms might be intact or deficient depending on the comprehension processing required. For example, presentation of formulaic expressions that are rated as being highly literal (e.g., "a piece of cake") may result in the simultaneous activation of their literal meaning and their figurative meaning, requiring that the literal meaning be suppressed over time in relation to context. Given the need to use context to suppress literal meaning, comprehension of such idioms in on-line processing tasks is deficient for children with SBM even if they are familiar with the figurative meaning (see Huber-Okrainec, Blaser, & Dennis, 2005). Children with SBM with more extensive damage to corpus callosum structures that link the cerebral hemispheres also had the greatest difficulty when comprehension of figurative expression required integration of context or the suppression of literal meaning (Huber-Okrainec et al., 2005).

Processing load intersects with these two comprehension processes. Which predictions follow from this assumption? Although construction of representations of the text base and the situation model typically draws on memorial processes to a greater extent than accessing meaning through the surface code, there are situations in which accessing the meaning of the surface code will draw more heavily on these memorial resources (Just & Carpenter, 1992). For example, comprehension of more complex syntactic constructions should be deficient in SBM. Conversely, intact construction of spatial and social-emotional situation models in SBM occurs with no requirement for resource-heavy processes involved in model revision or use of the model in on-line comprehension.

Studies of adult neurological patients have shown that comprehension breaks down along some of the fault lines that correspond to distinctions within our analysis of comprehension, described above. In different neurologically compromised groups, Caplan and Waters (2006) have distinguished between comprehension failures that arise because of structural processes and those stemming from limitation in resources such as working memory. The neurobiology of comprehension failure in children with developmental brain disorders has been much less studied, although recent work suggests that the integrity of cross-hemispheric communication may be important for language comprehension in both adults (Funnell, Corballis, & Gazzaniga, 2000) and children (Huber-Okrainec et al., 2005).

CONCLUSIONS AND IMPLICATIONS

A recent review led by the RAND Reading Study Group, a panel of experts in reading research (Snow & the RAND Reading Study Group, 2001), described the current knowledge base on reading comprehension as "sketchy, unfocused, and inadequate as a basis for reform in reading comprehension instruction" (p. xii). Understanding how children learn to read words and why some children have difficulty with word decoding has benefited from multidisciplinary research in cognitive development, learning disabilities, and neurobiological factors. This integrated knowledge base has led to substantial changes in public policy that have affected both the assessment of reading and teaching practices (Fletcher et al., 2002). Understanding how children acquire comprehension skills and why some find listening and reading comprehension difficult may require a similar sustained research effort that builds knowledge across several domains of inquiry including studies of comprehension in children with neurological disorders (Lyon, Fletcher, & Barnes, 2003).

Studies of individual differences in comprehension, whether of children or of adults, or of individuals with or without neurological impairment, need to include hypotheses derived from models of comprehension that specify how discourse and texts are understood as they unfold across time and that allow one to address questions about mechanisms that underlie skill differences in comprehension (e.g., Cain et al., 2004). We have used cognitive models of comprehension to decompose the components of comprehension in SBM for determining potential sources of disability, and for highlighting the consistency in findings across groups of less-skilled comprehenders. These models have also proved useful in identifying commonalities between processes related to comprehension and those required for other cognitive skills.

In summary, four important generalizations may be extracted from our studies of comprehension in SBM that are of interest to understanding individual differences in comprehension. First, activation of stipulated meanings and surface codes is more robust than construction of text representations and situation models. Developmental brain compromise need not prevent learning of and access to stipulated meanings, which are important for accessing the meaning of the surface code that serves as initial inputs into comprehension. At the same time, developmental brain compromise disrupts those aspects of comprehension that require the construction of text-based representations and situation models. Second, memory is important for the construction of meaning, especially for representations of the text base and the situation model, which require integration of textual and extratextual material and revisions of representations over time.

Third, the similarity in findings in comprehension and memorial processes between groups of less-skilled comprehenders (both those with and those without explicit brain compromise) is substantial, which has implications for theories of comprehension disability. Deficient components of comprehension that are shared by different groups of less-skilled comprehenders are those that likely represent key comprehension operations, so that a relatively constrained set of comprehension and memorial processes may account for most individual differences in comprehension. Fourth, the evaluation of comprehension that combines cognitive models of comprehension and neurocognitive models of a broad range of cognitive functions provides an integrated view of comprehension disabilities that may be useful for investigating how deficits in comprehension are related to dysfunction in other cognitive domains, thereby revealing features of the neurobiology of comprehension disorders in childhood.

Our research also has implications for the clinical conceptualization of comprehension difficulties in children with neurodevelopmental disorders, which has consequences for both assessment and treatment. Better comprehension of more concrete or literal aspects of language and poorer comprehension of more abstract aspects of language is sometimes said to characterize children with both congenital and acquired neurodevelopmental disorders such as SBM and traumatic brain injury. This distinction does not accurately characterize the typical development and operation of the comprehension system. Moreover, it fails to capture the ways in which that system breaks down under conditions of brain injury. Although children with neuro-developmental disorders may have relatively more difficulty in dimensions of language such as inference and figurative language compared to literal language comprehension, the reason for this pattern has less to do with a literal/abstract dimension of language than it has to do with the specific comprehension and memorial processes that are often, but not always, implicated in understanding inferential and figurative language. In our studies of children with traumatic brain injuries, for example, inferential skills are deficient in the context of story comprehension, but not under conditions in which the memory load is reduced (Barnes & Dennis, 2001). In all, our findings suggest that it is important to accurately characterize the nature of comprehension problems in children with neurodevelopmental disorders as well as the conditions under which they are most likely to succeed or fail in understanding what they hear or read. Such information is critical for accurate assessment of comprehension abilities and disabilities in children with neurodevelopmental disorders as well as for informing the choice of evidence-based interventions that are appropriate for treating those disabilities as discussed below.

Comprehension difficulties can be missed if assessment tools do not explicitly measure those aspects of comprehension that are particularly deficient in children with neurodevelopmental disorders. For example, there are some children with congenital and acquired brain injuries whose difficulties in comprehension are not related to problems in word-level reading or comprehension, yet they experience significant problems in understanding and learning from text. Language and reading comprehension tests that require little text integration and revision and few memorial resources may significantly underestimate the difficulties that these children face in typical comprehension contexts such as classroom learning. In our studies, children with SBM are more likely to be identified as having comprehension disabilities when the reading comprehension test involves questions that draw on inferential comprehension than when it taps more local aspects of text integration such as pronominal reference (Fletcher et al., 2004). So, although tests of vocabulary and sentence structure are important aspects of assessment, evaluations of listening and reading comprehension should also include tasks that measure inference and text integration.

Because there are more similarities than differences in the comprehension processes that are deficient across groups of less-skilled comprehenders, comprehension interventions that are effective for neurologically intact children may also prove useful for children with neurodevelopmental disorders. Intervention programs that explicitly teach both comprehension skills and comprehension strategies are most effective regardless of whether the comprehension disability is accompanied by problems in word decoding (National Reading Panel, 2000; Swanson, 1999). Although we do not think deficits in metacognitive aspects of comprehension are the cause of comprehension difficulties in many less-skilled comprehenders, we do not deny that strategy instruction has proven to be an effective intervention for comprehension problems. Strategy instruction may help to compensate for deficits in text integration and revision processes and for weaknesses in the memorial resources that support these comprehension processes. As is the case for other learning disabilities, interventions that address the academic manifestations of the disability are more effective than interventions that treat cognitive processes such as memory. This is likely to be the case regardless of whether or not the comprehension disability is related to neurodevelopmental disorder (Lyon, Fletcher, Fuchs, & Chhabra, 2006).

In conclusion, model-driven investigations of comprehension in children with neurodevelopmental disorders provide information that has implications for both theory and practice. The findings reviewed above are relevant to models of comprehension, to neurocognitive models that integrate across a broad range of cognitive functions, and to the assessment and treatment of comprehension difficulties in children with neurodevelopmental disorders.

REFERENCES

Albrecht, J. E., & Myers, J. L. (1998). Accessing distant text information during reading: Effects of contextual cues. *Discourse Processes, 26,* 87–107.

Albrecht, J. E., & O'Brien, E. J. (1993). Updating a mental model: Maintaining both local and global coherence. *Journal of Experimental Psychology: Learning, Memory and Cognition, 19,* 1061–1070.

Backman, J., Beattie, T., & Bawden, H. (1999). Learning and memory abilities in children with spina bifida and hydrocephalus. *Journal of the International Neuropsychological Society, 5,* 148.

Barnes, M. A. (2002). The decoding–comprehension dissociation in the reading of children with hydrocephalus: A reply to Yamada. *Brain and Language, 80,* 260–263.

Barnes, M. A., & Dennis, M. (1992). Reading in children and adolescents after early-onset hydrocephalus and in normally developing peers: Phonological analysis, word recognition, word comprehension, and passage comprehension skill. *Journal of Pediatric Psychology, 17,* 445–465.

Barnes, M. A., & Dennis, M. (1996). Reading comprehension deficits arise from diverse sources: Evidence from readers with and without developmental brain pathology. In C. Cornoldi & J. Oakhill (Eds.), *Reading comprehension difficulties* (pp. 251–278). Hillsdale, NJ: Erlbaum.

Barnes, M. A., & Dennis, M. (1998). Discourse after early-onset hydrocephalus: Core deficits in children of average intelligence. *Brain and Language, 61,* 309–334.

Barnes, M. A., & Dennis, M. (2001). Knowledge-based inferencing after childhood head injury. *Brain and Language, 76,* 253–265.

Barnes, M. A., Dennis, M., & Haefele-Kalvaitis, J. (1996). The effects of knowledge availability and knowledge accessibility on coherence and elaborative inferencing in children from six to fifteen years of age. *Journal of Experimental Child Psychology, 61,* 216–241.

Barnes, M. A., Dennis, M., & Hetherington, R. (2004). Reading and writing skills in young adults with spina bifida and hydrocephalus. *Journal of the International Neuropsychological Society, 10,* 655–663.

Barnes, M. A., Faulkner, H., & Dennis, M. (2001). Poor reading comprehension despite fast word decoding in children with hydrocephalus. *Brain and Language, 76,* 35–44.

Barnes, M. A., Faulkner, H., Wilkinson, M., & Dennis, M. (2004). Meaning construction and integration in children with hydrocephalus. *Brain and Language, 89,* 47–56.

Barnes, M. A., Smith-Chant, B., & Landry, S. (2005). Number processing in neurodevelopmental disorders: Spina bifida myelomenigocele. In J. I. D. Campbell (Ed.), *The handbook of mathematical cognition* (pp. 299–313). New York: Psychology Press.

Barnes, M. A., Wilkinson, M., Boudousquie, A., Khemani, E., Dennis, M., & Fletcher, J. M. (2006). Arithmetic processing in children with spina bifida: Calculation accuracy, strategy use, and fact retrieval fluency. *Journal of Learning Disabilities, 39,* 174–187.

Bjorkland, D. F., & Bernholtz, J. F. (1986). The role of knowledge base in the memory performance of good and poor readers. *Journal of Experimental Child Psychology, 41,* 367–373.

Bransford, J. D., & Franks, J. J. (1972). The abstraction of linguistic ideas: A review. *Cognition, 1,* 211–249.

Brownell, H. H., Simpson, T. L., Bihrle, A. M., Potter, H. H., & Gardner, H. (1990). Appreciation of metaphoric alternative word meanings by left and right brain-damaged patients. *Neuropsychologia, 28,* 375–383.

Cain, K., Oakhill, J. V., Barnes, M. A., & Bryant, P. E. (2001). Comprehension skill, inference making ability and their relation to knowledge. *Memory and Cognition, 29,* 850–859.

Cain, K., Oakhill, J. V., & Elbro, C. (2003). The ability to learn new word meanings from context by school-age children with and without language comprehension difficulties. *Journal of Child Language, 30,* 681–694.

Cain, K., Oakhill, J. V., & Lemmon, K. (2004). Individual differences in the inference of word meanings from context: The influence of reading comprehension, vocabulary knowledge, and memory capacity. *Journal of Educational Psychology, 96,* 671–681.

Caplan, D., & Waters, G. (2006). Language disorders in aging. In E. Bialystok & F. I. M. Craik (Eds.), *Life span cognition: Mechanisms of change* (pp. 253–273). Oxford, UK: Oxford University Press.

Chi, M. T. H. (1978). Knowledge structures and memory development. In R. S. Siegler (Ed.), *Children's thinking: What develops?* (pp. 73–96). Hillsdale, NJ: Erlbaum.

Clifton, C., Jr., & Duffy, S. A. (2001). Sentence and text comprehension: Roles of linguistic structure. *Annual Review of Psychology, 52,* 167–196.

Colvin, A. N., Yeates, O. K., Enrile, B. G., & Coury, D. L. (2003). Motor adaptation in children with myelomeningocel: Comparison to children with ADHD and healthy siblings. *Journal of the International Neuropsychological Society, 9,* 642–652.

Cornoldi, C., De Beni, R., & Pazzaglia, F. (1996). Profiles of reading comprehension difficulties: An analysis of single cases. In C. Cornoldi & J. Oakhill (Eds.), *Reading comprehension difficulties: Processes and intervention* (pp. 113–136). Mahwah, NJ: Erlbaum.

Del Bigio, M. R. (1993). Neuropathological changes caused by hydrocephalus. *Acta Neuropathologica, 18,* 573–585.

Dennis, M., & Barnes, M. A. (2002). Math and numeracy skills in young adults with spina bifida and hydrocephalus. *Developmental Neuropsychology, 21,* 141–155.

Dennis, M., Fitz, C. R., Netley, C. T., Sugar, J., Harwood-Nash, D. C. F., Hendrick, E. B., et al. (1981). The intelligence of hydrocephalic children. *Archives of Neurology, 38,* 607–615.

Dennis, M., Fletcher, J. M., Rogers, S., Hetherington, R., & Francis, D. (2002). Object-based and action-based visual perception in children with spina bifida and hydrocephalus. *Journal of the International Neuropsychological Society, 8,* 95–106.

Dennis, M., Hendrick, E. B., Hoffman, H. J., & Humphreys, R. P. (1987). The language of hydrocephalic children and adolescents. *Journal of Clinical and Experimental Neuropsychology, 9,* 593–621.

Dennis, M., Jaccenik, B., & Barnes, M. A. (1994). The content of narrative discourse in children and adolescents after early-onset hydrocephalus and in normally-developing age peers. *Brain and Language, 46,* 129–165.

Dennis, M., Landry, S. H., Barnes, M. A., & Fletcher, J. M. (2006). A model of neurocognitive function in spina bifida over the lifespan. *Journal of the International Neuropsychological Society, 12,* 285–296.

Edelstein, K., Dennis, M., Copeland, K., Francis, D., Frederick, J., Brandt, M., et al. (2004). Motor learning in children with spina bifida: Dissociation between performance level and acquisition rate. *Journal of the International Neuropsychological Society, 10,* 877–887.

Ewing-Cobbs, L., Barnes, M. A., & Fletcher, J. M. (2003). Early brain injury in children: Development and reorganization of cognitive function. *Developmental Neuropsychology, 24,* 671–706.

Fletcher, J. M., Bohan, T. P., Brandt, M. E., Brookshire, B. L., Beaver, S. R., Francis, D. J., et al. (1992). Cerebral white matter and cognition in hydrocephalic children. *Archives of Neurology, 49,* 818–824.

Fletcher, J. M., Brookshire, B. L., Bohan, T. P., Brandt, M. E., & Davidson, K. C. (1995). Early hydrocephalus. In B. P. Rourke (Ed.), *Syndrome of nonverbal learning disabilities: Neurodevelopmental manifestations* (pp. 206–238). New York: Guilford Press.

Fletcher, J. M., Dennis, M., Northrup, H., Barnes, M. A., Hannay, H. J., Landry, S. H., et al. (2004). Spina bifida: Genes, brain, and development. *International Review of Research in Mental Retardation, 29,* 63–117.

Fletcher, J. M., Lyon, G. R., Barnes, M. A., Stuebing, K. K., Francis, D. J., Olson, R. K., et al. (2002). Classification of learning disabilities: An evidence-based evaluation. In R. Bradley, L. Danielson, & D. Hallahan (Eds.), *Identification of learning disabilities: Research in practice* (pp. 185–250). Mahwah, NJ: Erlbaum.

Fletcher, J. M., McCauley, S. R., Brandt, M. E., Bohan, T. P., Kramer, L. A., Francis, D. J., et al. (1996). Regional brain tissue composition in children with hydrocephalus. *Archives of Neurology, 53,* 549–557.

Francis, D. J., Fletcher, J. M., Stuebing, K. K., Lyon, G. R., Shaywitz, S. E., & Shaywitz, B. A. (2005). Psychometric approaches to the identification of learning disabilities. Test scores are not sufficient. *Journal of Learning Disabilities, 38,* 545–552.

Funnell, M. G., Corballis, P. M., & Gazzaniga, M. S. (2000). Insights into the functional specificity of the human corpus callosum. *Brain, 123,* 920–926.

Gagnon, L., Goulet, P., Giroux, F., & Joanette, Y. (2003). Processing of metaphoric and non-metaphoric alternative meanings of words after right- and left-hemisphere lesions. *Brain and Language, 87,* 217–226.

Gathercole, S. E., & Pickering, S. J. (2000). Working memory deficits in children with low achievement in national curriculum at 7 years of age. *British Journal of Educational Psychology, 70,* 177–194.

Geary, D. C., & Hoard, M. K. (2005). Learning disabilities in arithmetic and mathematics: Theoretical and empirical perspectives. In J. I. D. Campbell (Ed.), *Handbook of mathematical cognition* (pp. 253–267). New York: Psychology Press.

Gernsbacher, M. A. (1990). *Language comprehension as structure building.* Hillsdale, NJ: Erlbaum.

Gernsbacher, M. A., & Faust, M. E. (1991). The mechanism of suppression: A component of general comprehension skill. *Journal of Experimental Psychology: Learning, Memory, and Cognition, 17,* 245–262.

Graesser, A. C., Millis, K., & Zwaan, R. A. (1997). Discourse comprehension. *Annual Review of Psychology, 48,* 163–189.

Horn, D. G., Lorch, E. P., Lorch, R. F., & Culatta, B. (1985). Distractibility and vocabulary deficits in children with spina bifida and hydrocephalus. *Developmental Medicine and Child Neurology, 27,* 713–720.

Huber-Okrainec, J., Blaser, S. E., & Dennis, M. (2005). Idiom comprehension deficits in relation to corpus callosum agenesis and hypoplasia in children with spina bifida meningomyelocele. *Brain and Language, 93,* 349–368.

Jarrold, C., Baddeley, A. D., Hewes, A. K., Leeke, T. C., & Phillips, C. E. (2004). What links verbal short-term memory performance and vocabulary level? Evidence of changing relationships among individuals with learning disability. *Journal of Memory and Language, 50,* 134–148.

Johnson, M. H., & de Haan, M. (2001). Developing cortical specialization for visual–cognitive function: The case of face recognition. In J. L. McClellan & R. S. Siegler (Eds.), *Mechanisms of cognitive development: Behavioral and neural perspectives* (pp. 253–270). Mahwah, NJ: Erlbaum.

Johnston, A. M., & Barnes, M. A. (2006). Comparing situational model building in children with spina bifida and typically developing children. *Canadian Psychology, 47,* 185.

Just, M. A., & Carpenter, P. A. (1992). A capacity theory of comprehension: Individual differences in working memory. *Psychological Review, 99,* 122–149.

Kintsch, W. (1988). The role of knowledge in discourse comprehension: A construction integration model. *Psychological Review, 95,* 163–182.

Kirkpatrick, T. L., & Northrup, H. (2003). Neural tube defects: Genetics. In D. N. Cooper (Ed.), *Nature encyclopedia of the human gemone* (Vol. 4, pp. 302–307). New York: Macmillan.

Leach, J. M., Scarborough, H. S., & Rescorla, L. (2003). Late-emerging reading disabilities. *Journal of Educational Psychology, 95,* 211–224.

Long, D. L., Oppy, B. J., & Seely, M. R. (1997). Individual differences in readers' sentence- and text-level representations. *Journal of Memory and Language, 36,* 129–145.

Lyon, G. R., Fletcher, J. M., & Barnes, M. A. (2003). Learning disabilities. In E. J. Mash & R. Barkley (Eds.), *Child psychopathology* (2nd ed., pp. 520–588). New York: Guilford Press.

Lyon, G. R., Fletcher, J. M., Fuchs, L. S., & Chhabra, V. (2006). Learning disabilities. In E. Mash & R. Barkley (Eds.), *Treatment of childhood disorders* (3rd ed., pp. 512–591). New York: Guilford Press.

Muter, V., Hulme, C., Snowling, M. J., & Stevenson, J. (2004). Phonemes, rimes, vocabulary, and grammatical skills as foundations of early reading development: Evidence from a longitudinal study. *Developmental Psychology, 40,* 665–681.

Nation, K., Clarke, P., & Snowling, M. J. (2002). General cognitive ability in children with poor reading comprehension. *British Journal of Educational Psychology, 72,* 549–560.

Nation, K., Marshall, C. M., & Altmann, T. M. (2003). Investigating individual differences in children's real-time sentences comprehension using language-mediated eye movements. *Journal of Experimental Child Psychology, 86,* 314–329.

National Reading Panel. (2000). *Teaching children to read: An evidence-based assessment of the scientific research literature on reading and its implications for reading instruction.* Washington, DC: National Institute of Child Health and Human Development.

Oakhill, J., Cain, K., & Bryant, P. E. (2003). The dissociation of word reading and text comprehension: Evidence from component skills. *Language and Cognitive Processes, 18,* 443–468.

Parsons, J. G. (1986). An investigation into the verbal facility of hydrocephalic children with special reference to vocabulary, morphology, and fluency. *Developmental Medicine and Childhood Neurology, 10,* 109–110.

Perfetti, C. A. (1985). Reading ability. New York: Oxford University Press.

Persad, V. L., Van den Hof, M. C., Dube, J. M., & Zimmer, P. (2002). Incidence of open neural tube defects in Nova Scotia after folic acid fortification. *Canadian Medical Association Journal, 167,* 241–245.

Purzner, J., Wilkinson, M., Boudousquie, A., Fletcher, J., & Barnes, M. A. (2004). Verbal and visual working memory in children with spina bifida. *Final Program Thirty-Second Annual International Neuropsychological Society Conference Abstracts,* 60.

Reigel, D. H., & Rotenstein, D. (1994). Spina bifida. In W. R. Cheek (Ed.), *Pediatric neurosurgery* (3rd., pp. 51–76). Philadelphia: Saunders.

Salman, M. S., Sharpe, J. A., Eizenman, M., Lillakas, L., To, T., Westall, C., et al. (2005). Saccades in children with spina bifida and Arnold–Chiari Type II malformation. *Neurology, 64,* 2098–2101.

Schmalhofer, F., McDaniel, M. A., & Keefe, D. (2002). A unified model for predictive and bridging inferences. *Discourse Processes, 33,* 105–132.

Schneider, W., Korkel, J., & Weinert, F. E. (1989). Domain specific knowledge and memory performance: A comparison of high and low aptitude children. *Journal of Educational Psychology, 81,* 306–312.

Scott, M. A., Fletcher, J. M., Brookshire, B. L., Davidson, K. C., Landry, S. H., Bohan, T. C., et al. (1998). Memory functions in children with early hydrocephalus. *Neuropsychology, 4,* 578–589.

Seidenberg, M. S., Tanenhaus, M. K., Leiman, J. M., & Bienkowski, M. (1982). Automatic access of the meaning of ambiguous words in context: Some limitations of knowledge-based processing. *Cognitive Psychology, 14,* 489–537.

Shankweiler, D., Lundquist, E., Katz, L., Stuebing, K., Fletcher, J., Brady, S., et al. (1999). Comprehension and decoding: Patterns of association in children with reading difficulties. *Scientific Studies of Reading, 3,* 69–94.

Snow, C., & the RAND Reading Study Group. (2001). Reading for understanding: Toward an R & D program in reading comprehension. Santa Monica, CA: RAND Education.

Swanson, H. L. (1999). *Interventions for students with learning disabilities: A meta-analysis of treatment outcomes.* New York : Guilford Press.

Swanson, H. L., & Sachse-Lee, C. (2001). A subgroup analysis of working memory in children with reading disabilities: Domain-general or domain-specific deficiency? *Journal of Learning Disabilities, 34,* 249–263.

Tompkins, C. A., Baumgaertner, A., Lehman, M. T., & Fassbinder, W. (2000). Mechanisms of discourse comprehension impairment after right hemisphere brain damage: Suppression in lexical ambiguity resolution. *Journal of Speech, Language, and Hearing Research, 43,* 62–78.

van den Broek, P., Young, M., Tzeng, Y., & Linderholm, T. (1999). The landscape model of reading: Inferences and the online construction of a memory representation. In H. van Oostendorp & S. R. Goldman (Eds.), *The construction of mental representations during reading* (pp. 71–98). Mahwah, NJ: Erlbaum.

Van Lancker Sidtis, D. (2004). When novel sentences spoken or heard for the first time in the history of the universe are not enough: Toward a dual-process model of language. *International Journal of Language and Communication Disorders, 39*, 1–44.

Yeates, K. O., & Enrile, B. G. (2005). Implicit and explicit memory in children with congenital and acquired brain disorder. *Neuropsychology, 19*, 618–628.

Yeates, K. O., Enrile, B. G., Loss, N., Blumenstein, E., & Delis, D. (1995). Verbal learning and memory in children with myelomeningocele. *Journal of Pediatric Psychology, 20*, 801–815.

Yuill, N. M., Oakhill, J. V., & Parkin, A. J. (1989). Working memory, comprehension skill and the resolution of text anomaly. *British Journal of Psychology, 80*, 351–361.

Williams, L. J., Rasmussen, S. A., Flores, A., Kirby, R. S., & Edmonds, L. D. (2005). Decline in the prevalence of spina bifida and anencephaly by race/ethnicity: 1995–2002. *Pediatrics, 116*, 580–586.

Zwaan, R. A., & Radvansky, G. A. (1998). Situation models in language comprehension and memory. *Psychological Bulletin, 123*, 162–185.

CHAPTER 8

Impaired Discourse Gist in Pediatric Brain Injury
Missing the Forest for the Trees

LORI G. COOK
SANDRA B. CHAPMAN
JACQUELYN F. GAMINO

A "traumatic brain injury" (TBI) is defined as an injury to the brain that is typically associated with motor vehicle, motor–pedestrian, or motorcycle accidents; sports-related injuries; or falls. Approximately 475,000 TBIs occur among children ages 0 to 14 years each year in the United States, with nearly 2,700 of the injuries resulting in death (Langlois, Rutland-Brown, & Thomas, 2004).

Sustaining a TBI in childhood can result in many long-term effects, including deficits in language, cognition, behavior, motor skills, and psychosocial function, particularly in severe injury (e.g., Chapman, Levin, Matejka, Harward, & Kufera, 1995; Chapman et al., 2001; Dennis & Barnes, 2001; Fletcher, Miner, & Ewing-Cobbs, 1987). Although children commonly exhibit decreased academic performance after a brain injury (Ewing-Cobbs et al., 2004; Ewing-Cobbs, Fletcher, Levin, Iovino, & Miner, 1998), the nature of their difficulties

218

is often difficult to identify. Consequently, they rarely receive the specialized help they need.

The purpose of this chapter is threefold: (1) to discuss comprehension and production of discourse and associated cognitive processes, (2) to elucidate the potential of discourse gist to assess higher level cognitive-linguistic deficits in children with TBI, and (3) to illustrate the clinical utility of evaluating discourse gist with a case study. With regard to discourse, the focus in this chapter is on verbal summarization skills, selective learning abilities, and written discourse competence.

INJURY VARIABLES

Several variables related to pediatric brain injury can play a role in the recovery of higher level cognitive processes, including age at injury, severity of injury, lesion site, and premorbid factors. The full scope of these processes is often masked by what appears to be complete recovery of simple cognitive function.

Age at Injury

A child's age at the time of his or her brain injury is a key factor in the recovery of cognitive-linguistic skills. It has been well documented that an individual's stage of development greatly influences neurobehavioral recovery in children (Chapman, 1995; Chapman, Levin, Matejka, et al., 1995; Fletcher et al., 1987). In fact, language-related abilities that are undergoing rapid development have been shown to be more vulnerable to brain injury than well-established abilities, meaning that a younger age at injury is associated with a poorer outcome of higher-level linguistic abilities (Chapman, Levin, & Lawyer, 1999; Chapman et al., 2004; Ewing-Cobbs, Levin, Eisenberg, & Fletcher, 1987).

When a brain injury occurs during any of the critical developmental stages, subsequent development of higher-level skills can be hindered, which has a direct influence on the abilities necessary for success in the classroom (e.g., Ewing-Cobbs et al., 1987; Fletcher et al., 1987). Moreover, as a child with TBI progresses through school, the gap between his or her abilities and those of a typically developing peer is likely to increase over time. The expanding gap is not so much a result of losses in already acquired skills as it is due to failure to develop later emerging skills (Brookshire, Chapman, Song, & Levin, 2000; Chapman, Levin, Wanek, Weyrauch, & Kufera, 1998; Chapman et al., 2001; Yorkston, Jaffe, Polissar, Liao, & Fay, 1997).

Severity and Site of Lesion

The severity of a brain injury is commonly determined by three factors: the child's initial score on the Glasgow Coma Scale (GCS), structural brain-imaging findings, and duration of posttraumatic amnesia. The GCS, a score reflecting level of consciousness, is usually determined upon admittance to the hospital (Teasdale & Jennett, 1974). A GCS score ≤ 8 indicates a severe injury, a score falling between 9 and 12 is usually classified as moderate, and a score of 13–15 represents a mild injury. Taking into consideration positive CT (computed tomography, or CT scan) findings and/or magnetic resonance imaging (MRI) helps elucidate the extent of structural damage. For example, a child with an injury classified as mild (GCS ≥ 13) who has positive CT findings would be expected to have a more substantial injury than a child with mild TBI who has no remarkable CT findings. The duration of post-traumatic amnesia sheds light on brain function after the initial injury and has also been shown to be of great importance when classifying injury severity (e.g., Levin et al., 1993; Mendelsohn et al., 1992).

The more severe the brain injury, the worse the prognosis for long-term language outcome. At least 50% of children who present with a severe TBI incur a residual neuropsychological deficit (Ewing-Cobbs, Barnes, & Fletcher, 2003). Emerging evidence suggests that even children with mild brain injury may exhibit subtle neurocognitive deficits, particularly of higher level cognitive skills, including discourse impairments (Chapman, Gamino, et al., 2006; Dennis, Purvis, Barnes, Wilkinson, & Winner, 2001).

However, the severity of the injury does not always clarify specific endogenous factors, such as the site, size, and extent of the brain lesions. Most severe TBI cases entail a combination of diffuse and focal injury, indicating more widespread damage than concentrated, less severe injuries (Ewing-Cobbs et al., 2003). MRI studies have revealed that the most common lesions that occur in children with moderate or severe TBI are frontal and anterior temporal contusions (e.g., Levin et al., 1993; Mendelsohn et al., 1992). In fact, the size of frontal lobe lesions enhances the relationship between injury severity and cognitive performance (Levin et al., 1993). Additional evidence indicates that children with severe TBI regularly present with prefrontal tissue loss, even if there are no focal brain lesions in the area (Berryhill et al., 1995).

For example, Chapman and colleagues (1992) found that children with relatively large severe frontal lobe injuries (as determined from MRI findings) exhibited greater deficits than other children with severe injuries when asked to retell a story. In particular, children with frontal lesions struggled with organizing information, tending to omit more essential story components (setting, action, resolution, and evaluation), in addition to demonstrating decreased ability to retain the gist of a story.

Premorbid Factors

Although studies of children with TBI have established that age and severity/locus of injury are central to understanding long-term effects, multiple premorbid factors play an important role in an individual child's recovery. For example, effective research designs may require use of comparison groups consisting of children with orthopedic (i.e., broken bone) injuries rather than just typically developing children in order to control for risk factors that may predispose a child to injury. Additionally, preinjury environmental factors such as lower socioeconomic status, poor child and family functioning, and high levels of family stress have been shown to have a detrimental effect on later outcome from brain injury (Ewing-Cobbs et al., 2004).

INADEQUACY OF EXISTING
STANDARDIZED MEASURES IN TBI

The cognitive-linguistic sequelae typically associated with pediatric TBI include problems of a communicative nature (e.g., disorganized discourse, slow and inefficient word retrieval, impulsive communication style), academic difficulties (e.g., problems with new learning and strategic learning, concrete thinking, inefficient note-taking and study skills, disorganized writing), and social/behavioral problems (e.g., impulsive and context-insensitive social interaction, anger and aggression, withdrawal from social situations; see Ylvisaker et al., 2005, for a review).

The cognitive-linguistic deficits in children with TBI can be difficult to detect through commonly used standardized measures. For example, achievement tests often assess verbal and math abilities that are either overlearned or automatic, skills that are often found to be relatively spared following TBI (Ewing-Cobbs et al., 1998, 2004). In fact, Ewing-Cobbs and colleagues (1998) found that children who received average achievement test scores 2 years after their TBI often had failed a grade and/or required special education assistance. This evidence indicates that achievement tests do not fully reflect postinjury deficits.

Standardized language measures, such as those used to identify whether a child qualifies for special education services, also fall short in evaluating deficits after TBI. This is largely due to the focus on word- and sentence-level measures rather than text- or discourse-based competence. One principle that has become increasingly more apparent in recent years is the lack of correspondence between performances on isolated measures of language function and everyday functionality (e.g., Chapman, Levin, & Culhane, 1995; Chapman et al., 2001; Ulatowska & Chapman, 1994). Specifically, many children with TBI have marked difficulty conveying their ideas in discourse, as discussed later in this chapter, although their scores on traditional language measures, as well as their use of complex syntax, are typically within normal limits (Chapman, 1997; Chapman, Levin, & Culhane, 1995; Chapman, Levin, Matejka, et al., 1995).

DISCOURSE MEASURES

Definition of Discourse

Emerging evidence points to discourse measures as a promising paradigm by which to address complex language comprehension in children with TBI. "Discourse" is defined as connected language, or the "linguistic expression of ideas, wishes, and opinions in everyday life, typically conveyed as a sequence of sentences that has coherent organization and meaning" (Chapman & Sparks, 2003, p. 754). Discourse is both spoken and written, and in written form is manifested in both informal and formal texts. In regard to the development of discourse-specific abilities concerning the narrative genre, several essential stages have been identified and are exemplified in studies including typically developing children (Applebee, 1978; Brookshire et al., 2000; Chapman, Levin, Matejka, et al., 1995; Chapman et al., 1997, 1998; Johnson, 1983; Stein & Glenn, 1979; Westby, 1984). See Table 8.1 for a summary of these developmental stages.

Discourse production relies upon complex cognitive processes that primarily involve the interplay of comprehending information, manipulating the content in working memory, and organizing the ideas in a coherent manner. In particular, discourse processing necessitates comprehension of the text presented, as well as the ability to update meaning as the text unfolds. In addition, discourse processing requires the ability to combine world knowledge with the textual information in order to generate inferences and comprehend the gist of the text (Barnes & Dennis, 2001; Dennis & Barnes, 2001).

TABLE 8.1. Development of Narrative Discourse Abilities

Age	Narrative discourse ability development
2 years	Begin to refer to past events in discourse.
3 years	Able to combine two events in discourse.
4–5 years	Able to produce well-formed stories, incorporating the basic narrative structure of setting, action, and resolution.
6 years	Able to transform verbal information, as is necessary for producing summaries.
7 years	Able to synthesize and interpret information from a simple narrative.
8–10 years	Continue to show development in deriving a central theme and building elaborated narratives.

Discourse production is of particular interest because it is sensitive to the higher level cognitive deficits typically seen in TBI (Biddle, McCabe, & Bliss, 1996; Brookshire et al., 2000; Reilly, Bates, & Marchman, 1998). In a clinical setting, narrative discourse production is assessed by means of eliciting a straightforward retell or a complex summarization of a story or text, either orally or in written form. A good story retell incorporates conveyance of explicit story content within a narrative structure, including an initiating event, goal-directed actions, and a conclusion. A summary is characterized as a shortened version of an original text that retains the main idea (Chapman, Nasits, Challas, & Billinger, 1999). A summary differs from a retell in that it entails condensing and synthesizing information, with less focus on specific details. Table 8.2 further highlights the similarities and differences between retells and summaries.

Gist-Based Discourse Processing

Definition of Discourse Gist

As the familiar adage states, "Do not miss the forest for the trees," that is, it is possible to become so focused on the details that one fails to see the bigger picture. One of the most fundamental and fascinating aspects of information processing is the brain's ability to encode and reduce massive amounts of incoming stimuli to an abstracted or generalized meaning that we refer to as "gist" (van Dijk, 1995). Children are able to achieve this amazing feat of abstracting a gist, with the ability emerging at a relatively early age (approximately age 7), at least for

TABLE 8.2. Comparison of Retells and Summaries

Both retells and summaries tap:
- Comprehension
- Memory
- Decontextualized language
- Language and information
- Coherence and cohesion

How are they different?

Retell
- Retells provide a story schemata, including an initiating event, goal-directed actions, and a conclusion.
- Explicit story content is required.
- Emerges in the early preschool years.

Summary
- Summaries provide a shortened version of the original text while retaining the main idea (Chapman, Nasits, Challas, & Billinger, 1999).
- More inferencing and paraphrasing of information, with less focus on details and content than retells.
- Requires more condensing and synthesizing of information.
- Heavier demands are placed on abilities to provide coherence and cohesion.
- Emerges in the early elementary years with refinement through high school.

Note. Adapted from Chapman, Levin, and Hart (2006).

familiar information. Gist abilities become increasingly more sophisticated into young adulthood (e.g., Johnson, 1983). The ability to derive gist is achieved through the application of "macrostrategies," which allow individuals to conceptualize rules and generalize meaning across different informational sources. Specifically, macrostrategies facilitate comprehension, organization, and reduction of complex discourse information (Ulatowska & Chapman, 1994). As a result of macrostrategies, we typically remember the *gist* of what we see in a movie, hear from a lecture, or read in a book far better than we recall the specific *details*, especially after a delay.

In discourse, gist is manifested by the ability to encode, comprehend, and convey the central meaning from connected language (van Dijk, 1995). Gist responses are realized in the form of minitexts such as titles, synopses, summaries, main ideas, and interpretative statements (Ulatowska & Chapman, 1994). Each minitext, in its optimal form, is constructed to express the gist meaning at a more global level than the component details that comprise the lengthier original information.

This is to say that a gist-based text conveys the same central meaning as the original text but does so in a reduced and generalized version that omits the details. Moreover, a gist-based text should demonstrate both cohesion and coherence. "Cohesion" refers to the syntactic and thematic links between the words and sentences comprising a text (Lehman & Schraw, 2002). "Coherence" entails the global interpretation of the original discourse text by means of bridging information across ideas (Singer & Ritchot, 1996).

Discourse gist is of interest in pediatric TBI because it is a newly developed construct that more fully characterizes communicative competence than word- and sentence-level measures (Chapman et al., 2004; Chapman, Gamino, et al., 2006; Ulatowska & Chapman, 1994). In addition, evidence suggests that discourse gist is closely related to learning capacity, at least for children with learning problems (Johnson, 1983; Stein & Kirby, 1992). In order to attain learning at a deeper level, one must progress beyond the common pitfalls of recalling verbatim information, learning everything regardless of importance, sticking only with stated facts, and providing single-word answers.

The few existing studies of discourse gist in pediatric populations with TBI focus predominantly on production tasks (e.g., Chapman et al., 2004; Chapman, Gamino, et al., 2006). Nonetheless, discourse models indicate that production has an intimate relation with comprehension and associated cognitive abilities (e.g., Bracewell, Frederickson, & Frederickson, 1982). Moreover, evidence from other pediatric populations such as low-comprehending readers reveals that discourse production provides a window to view the adequacy of comprehension skills (Cain, 2003; Cain & Oakhill, 1996; Yuill & Joscelyne, 1988). Gist-based production deficits are associated with poor inferential comprehension and impaired cognitive control in that extracting meaning from text involves the careful selection, manipulation, and integration of information to derive the central meaning. Previous approaches to gist production have centered largely on the surface-level main points (Chapman et al., 1992, 1998; Yuill & Joscelyne, 1988). Whereas such key points may involve some inferential processing, they are readily accessible to normal language processors as part of the explicit text. Discourse gist paradigms discussed in the current chapter expand upon previous work by involving the abstraction of the deeper level meaning.

Gist Problems after Severe TBI

Children with severe TBI exhibit difficulties in producing gist-based responses when compared to typically developing children (Chapman et al., 1997, 2004; Chapman, Gamino, et al., 2006; Reilly et al., 1998). Deficits in gist-based processing are manifested in at least four major ways. First, children with severe TBI show marked difficulties in combining information into more generalized statements when producing a summary; instead, they tend to remember specific details from the original discourse text (Chapman et al., 2004). In contrast, typically developing children are able to spontaneously combine two or three ideas into a more global meaning that is paraphrased in their own words (Chapman et al., 2004). Second, children with TBI produce decreased thematic complexity in narrative productions (Reilly et al., 1998). Third, children with severe TBI show a significant impairment in producing an interpretive statement after hearing a narrative (Chapman et al., 1997). Instead, they tend to repeat or minimally paraphrase one of the explicit statements from the original text. In contrast, typically developing children produce generalized statements built around the entire content. Fourth, children with mild to severe TBI do not fare well in constructing cohesive and coherent summaries. Despite the fact that they reportedly reduce the information appropriately (Chapman, Gamino, et al., 2006), their summaries fail to convey the central meaning or build the main message in a cohesive manner (Chapman, Gamino, et al., 2006). Examples of these four aspects of gist-based processing are illustrated in the case study later in the chapter.

What Accounts for the Breakdown in Gist Processing after Severe TBI in Childhood?

One major question that arises is, What accounts for the breakdowns in gist processing after severe TBI in childhood? Do children with severe TBI fail to develop macrostrategies, or are they inefficient in their application of macrostrategies to achieve gist-based processing of information? Whereas the answers to these two questions are unknown, insight from recent studies sheds light on the relation of macrostrategies to individual cognitive processes, as discussed below.

WORKING MEMORY

Macrostrategies require the integration of cognitive processes with specific, goal-directed language behaviors. The prerequisite macrostrategies to comprehend and produce discourse gist include processes of information reduction, organization, and transformation, as well as the ability to abstract the central meaning (Chapman, Gamino, et al., 2006; Hanten et al., 2004; Hanten, Zhang, & Levin, 2002).

Although the specific cognitive mechanisms that contribute to discourse processing are still under investigation, working memory has been shown to be the umbrella under which the processes that facilitate comprehension and production operate (e.g., Dennis & Barnes, 2001; Levin et al., 2002; Roncadin, Guger, Archibald, Barnes, & Dennis, 2004). More specifically, the working memory aspects of memory storage and executive function work in tandem to accommodate discourse processing and production (Chapman, Gamino, et al., 2006). In pediatric TBI, evidence suggests that deficits in discourse production are related to deficits in working memory executive functions (Chapman, Gamino, et al., 2006). Similarly, in typically developing children, there is evidence of a relation between working memory executive functions and reading comprehension ability (Swanson & Berninger, 1995; Yuill, Oakhill, & Parkin, 1989).

Working memory storage systems facilitate the maintenance of information for short-term recall and manipulation. On the other hand, long-term memory serves to retain information for future needs. Both memory systems in conjunction with executive functions are important for comprehension and production.

Working memory executive function subsystems, referred to by Baddley and Hitch (1974) as the "central executive," are similar to pieces of a puzzle that fit together to create the basis of discourse comprehension and production. These subsystems work in serial and parallel sequence to facilitate efficient strategies for the achievement of desired goals. The executive subsystems consist of various functions such as attention, inhibition, association, elaboration, and goal maintenance (Baddeley, 1992). Executive functions are regulated and coordinated by cognitive control. "Cognitive control" is the ability to willfully control thought processes in order to facilitate manipulation of information and goal maintenance.

During discourse processing, cognitive control allows for manipulation of information in memory storage. "Manipulation" refers to the ability to update information in short-term memory stores with new incoming information. In addition, manipulation is used as a means to retrieve information from long-term memory storage to interpret and synthesize with new information.

During discourse production, cognitive control facilitates organization and manipulation of the information necessary for cohesion and coherence. Thus, cognitive control allocates resources to achieve both logical semantic organization and global interpretation across the text (Singer & Ritchot, 1996). New evidence suggests that cognitive control may have a greater influence on discourse production abilities than immediate memory (Chapman, Gamino, et al., 2006). Specifically, executive functions of working memory have been shown to be significantly correlated with the ability to produce a cohesive and coherent summary (Chapman, Gamino, et al., 2006). Thus, higher level cognitive functioning, of the kind required for discourse processing and production, is postulated to be related to cognitive control.

In addition to manipulation and organization, cognitive control is proposed to play an important role in the ability to differentiate the important from the less important details during discourse processing (Chapman, Gamino, et al., 2006). The macrostrategies involved in discerning and selecting important information from a text are exemplified through selective learning.

SELECTIVE LEARNING

The ability to select key information from among many facts is important for inferencing and recognizing the gist of a text, two major components of discourse comprehension and production. The term "selective learning" refers to the ability to strategically select the most important information for learning while disregarding or suppressing less important information.

The ability to selectively learn is exemplified in summary production, whereby choosing the key information is a prerequisite to infer the gist of the discourse. In addition, the ability to prioritize information provides an organizational structure by which to recall important facts and facilitate production of a cohesive and coherent summary. More specifically, as Chapman and colleagues (2004, p. 51) noted, summarizing requires "comprehension of the isolated facts that make up the whole discourse text, sorting them according to importance, and appreciating the relation of the isolated facts to the central meaning of the whole discourse text."

Hence, assessment of selective learning of key information is a novel way to measure complex language comprehension skills. Selective learning ability is assessed by assigning differential values to information to be learned. Selective learning efficiency is demonstrated by the ability to determine and learn high-value information over low-value information. Consequently, information is prioritized for learning in relation to its value. In selective learning assessments, instructions provide the values of the information to be learned and an explanation of the objective to earn a substantial number of points by recalling information. Thus, in order to achieve the goal, high-value information must be strategically selected or prioritized over low-value information for learning and subsequent recall. However, a specific strategy for successfully achieving the goal must be inferred.

Selective learning has been assessed in children with TBI using word lists and expository discourse texts (Hanten et al., 2002, 2004). Hanten and colleagues (2002, 2004) found that children with TBI manifested deficits in selective learning abilities when compared to age-matched typically developing peers. However, no significant differences in memory capacity were found between children with TBI and the control groups. These findings suggest that cognitive processes other than basic memory capacity have greater impact on the ability to selectively learn information. In particular, Hanten and colleagues postulated that selective learning requires cognitive control. Cognitive control, as discussed previously, would allow one to strategically select information for learning while suppressing or ignoring irrelevant information.

Written Discourse Production in TBI

Although most studies examining discourse-related abilities after pediatric TBI have focused on oral production, a few studies have described the nature of written discourse production in children with TBI (Alajouanine & Lhermitte, 1965; Hecaén, 1976, 1983; Wilson & Proctor, 2000, 2002; Wilson, Smith, & Proctor, 2001; Yorkston, Jaffe, Liao, & Pollisar, 1999; Yorkston et al., 1997). Written discourse, like spoken discourse, relies upon cognitive processes such as encoding, organizing, storing, retrieving, manipulating, and reconstructing information. However, written discourse requires even more cognitive control, or online processing, than verbal discourse, because errors such as false starts, incomplete utterances, and revisions are better tolerated in oral than in written discourse production (Yorkston et al., 1997, 1999). As such, evidence has indicated that written discourse production may be more vulnerable to the effects of severe brain injury than oral expression of discourse (Ewing-Cobbs et al., 1987; Yorkston et al., 1997, 1999).

Written language abilities derive from spoken language abilities. Thus, because both spoken and written discourse production call upon many of the same component cognitive processes, typical development reveals similar patterns of performance for both modalities (Bracewell et al., 1982). For example, written discourse shares a similar but later emerging sequence in vocabulary and sentence construction to spoken discourse (deHirsch & Jansky, 1968; Scott, 1991). However, due to differences in the stylistic aspects of spoken versus written discourse, the mode of discourse production is likely to be differentially affected by TBI in children (Wilson & Proctor, 2002).

In fact, written language has been reported to be the most common and persistent area of academic difficulty following brain lesions in children (Aram, 1991). Ewing-Cobbs and colleagues (1987) identified a positive relationship between severity of TBI and errors in writing (omission, spelling, and capitalization) during a written dictation task in which sentences were presented as many times as the child requested. Additionally, Yorkston and colleagues (1997, 1999) identified patterns of impairment in written discourse 1 month following TBI that persisted at 1 year postinjury in children with severe TBI. Specifically, the children with severe TBI exhibited reduced efficiency in written expression (words per minute), lower discourse completeness (a composite score consisting of thematic maturity, number of words, and sentential units), decreased general readability (length of sentences and estimated grade level of vocabulary), and grammatical and spelling errors. Overall, the stories produced by children with TBI were shorter than those of typically developing children: they contained fewer words, fewer grammatical units, and fewer story elements. Moreover, Yorkston and colleagues (1997, 1999) found that written discourse abilities after TBI in children are dependent on injury severity and neuropsychological functioning, including aspects such as intelligence, memory, adaptive problem-solving skills, motor performance, and academic performance.

The ability to produce gist-based texts in written form has not yet been investigated in children with TBI, though some aspects of gist have been evaluated in written narratives (Chapman, Sparks, et al., 2006). In a study by Chapman, Sparks, and colleagues (2006), children with either mild or severe TBI were instructed to generate written narratives that corresponded with a picture stimulus. The narratives were analyzed at multiple levels, including language structure, information content and organization, and technical aspects of writing (e.g., spelling, punctuation, capitalization). Children with severe TBI exhibited reductions in both the amount of language and key (gist) information compared to children with mild TBI. Children with severe TBI also demonstrated marked impairment in organization of information (episodic structure) and technical aspects of writing. Although all written discourse variables were correlated with motor speed/dexterity, the reduced written expression exhibited by the children with severe TBI could not be entirely accounted for by slowed motor speed. Accordingly, the impairment in written discourse seen in children with severe TBI may be present at all levels of representation, including the gist-level content, amount and organization of information, and technical aspects of written language.

CLINICAL APPLICATION OF DISCOURSE GIST

Further understanding of higher level language deficits will guide teachers, special education service providers, and speech–language clinicians in how to provide meaningful, functional remediation for children with TBI that can apply throughout various stages of cognitive development and academic progression. The following case study illustrates how discourse-based assessment can benefit a child with severe TBI.

Case Example

While riding her bicycle, 11-year-old Emma was hit by a large truck. Emma lost consciousness at the scene and presented with a GCS score of 3, placing her in the severe range for a TBI. Medical evaluation identified a basilar skull fracture, a left temporal fracture with subarachnoid hemorrhage, a sacral fracture, a small splenic laceration, and multiple abrasions. MRI scans revealed abnormalities in the right frontal, right temporal, left temporal, and left occipital regions of her brain.

Prior to her injury, Emma was an "A" student. All of her developmental milestones were reportedly normal, with no concern or evidence of any learning disabilities. Emma continued to participate in a standard education classroom setting beginning 2 months following her injury, although a few modifications were implemented, including providing her with extra time for completion of exams and reading assignments. Emma's parents reported that, after her injury, she seemed to focus on the small details of her homework, causing her to spend excessive hours doing schoolwork each night. The parents also noted that in casual conversation Emma often included too much information, causing the "point" of her conversation to be unclear.

Emma participated in cognitive-linguistic assessments as a part of a longitudinal study of pediatric TBI at the Center for BrainHealth. These assessments included evaluation of discourse gist at 3 months, 12 months, and 3 years postinjury. The following are examples of summaries produced orally by Emma in reference to a long (578-word) didactic narrative about a man's life from the *Test of Strategic Learning* (Chapman, Levin, & Hart, 2006). The narrative was presented at a third-grade vocabulary level and included many details about the man and the eight jobs he attempted throughout his life. Whereas the details delineated a series of career failures, the gist-level meaning reflected the man's success in making life better for others (see also Chapman et al., 2002).

3-Month Evaluation

EMMA'S SUMMARY

"John was a failure at everything mostly that he did because he would always, like, in math, give, treat the students like easily and make their homework really easy and like make them get good grades when they really shouldn't have gotten that, and the stuff was too easy. And like when he was, um, selling things, he'd sell the things way too low. But the things that he could, he did get in, he quit. And he just quit because he didn't like the things that he got into. And when, when he was older, he um, wrote some poetry and some songs that we still use today."

ANALYSIS

Strengths. In this summary, Emma was able to remember several specific pieces of information from the story. Her summary is shortened from the original text (i.e., reduced information).

Weaknesses. Emma failed to combine information into more generalized statements. Her summary lacks cohesiveness (see definition on p. 225) in that the interconnections between propositions are poor. It is not clear how one statement leads to another, making the ideas seem isolated rather than related in a causal way. The summary also lacks coherence (see definition on p. 225), as demonstrated by the use of vague language (e.g., "But the things that he could, he did get in, he quit."). Emma demonstrated minimal paraphrasing, choosing to condense the information by using a "copy-delete" strategy. She failed to convey the overall meaning or gist of the story, instead misinterpreting the character's actions.

12-Month Evaluation

EMMA'S SUMMARY

"John Pierpont, well, he tried all these jobs and everything. And he tried everything from, um, school to law and everything, but he failed everything that he would do, but he kept on trying and trying, trying, but he would not do good in any of the things that he tried to do good at. And then, um, then when he was very old, he worked as a file clerk or whatever for, I think 5 years, but he wasn't good at that either. Um, and then, even though he failed, he wasn't good at everything, he was, because he, like, abolished slavery and made life different and easier for other people and everything."

ANALYSIS

Strengths. In terms of improvement, Emma exhibited more gist-level thought in her 12-month summary as compared to her 3-month summary, showing some ability to make inferences or "read between the lines," as seen in the statement, " . . . [he] made life different and easier for other people. . . . " She is also beginning to move away from the "copy-delete" approach by combining and transforming thoughts and ideas to make more generalized statements. Additionally, she did not provide any incorrect information (as she had done in her 3-month summary). Although Emma still focused largely on the unimportant details, they were less prominent than in her previous summary, and she was able to produce a global interpretive statement.

Weaknesses. Emma still demonstrated reduced cohesion and coherence, as her propositions were not logically connected and she was still somewhat vague in her descriptions (e.g., " . . . he tried all these jobs and everything."). Though the details became less specific, she did not convey the central meaning in her summary.

3-Year Evaluation

At 3 years postinjury, Emma, now in the ninth grade, underwent additional testing due to concern over her worsening school performance. Specifically, Emma reported that she often had trouble remembering and understanding information that she read, requiring her to read passages many times before comprehending them. The following is an example of the summary produced by Emma at 3 years postinjury:

EMMA'S SUMMARY

"It's about John Pierpont, and through his life he tried a lot of different jobs. But he'd have disappointments and he'd have to get out of them because he wouldn't earn enough money or he'd just be doing the wrong work or be doing it wrong. And his whole life even when he was really old he had really sad jobs. And he still didn't do well in those, but in the end he actually helped a lot of people and changed the world and made it a lot better, and he had a song made out, um, jingle bells, for how hard he's been working and how determined he was to get a job. And he actually changed lives forever."

ANALYSIS

Strengths. At the 3-year evaluation, Emma's summary reflected continued improvement in two areas. First, she was better able to use higher level macrostrategies to appropriately condense the information. Instead of a "copy-delete" approach, she made use of paraphrasing, transforming, and combining ideas into more generalized statements. Second, she was able to demonstrate use of global inferencing to abstract the central meaning of the story.

Weaknesses. Emma continued to exhibit difficulty, producing a cohesive summary, however, as the flow of information was poorly organized. Although a few details were mentioned, coherence also continued to be impeded by the impression that Emma did not fully comprehend the story scenarios, including a few vague interpretations (e.g., "sad jobs"). It appears that her improved ability to make use of global inferencing came at the cost of clarity. In order to effectively summarize, one needs to be able to combine and condense information while maintaining good organization and a degree of specificity. Emma was not able to achieve the delicate balance between gist-level thought and clarity of expression. As such, the specificity of content was overly reduced when she expressed gist-level ideas.

POSSIBLE REASONS FOR IMPAIRED DISCOURSE GIST

One reason for Emma's summary deficits may be an impaired ability to use selective learning. As mentioned previously, selective learning entails the prioritization of information based upon its importance. Emma performed two selective learning assessments, an auditory word list and an expository text (see Hanten et al., 2004, for further task information) to evaluate her selective learning ability. Information in each selective learning task was assigned a high or low value of "points." Emma was told the value of points associated with the various facts and was instructed to earn a high number of points by remembering the information.

In a selective learning word list task, Emma failed to prioritize the words she learned from each of 10 lists, demonstrating poor selective learning ability. In other words, she did not select words for recall based upon the highest value. Emma also included many words in her recall that were not on the list. Interestingly, selective learning for an expository discourse task was less problematic for Emma. The clinician read the text aloud while Emma read along silently. Emma was given 2 minutes to study the text prior to a cued recall of information from the text. Emma successfully recalled primarily high-value information, without intrusions of extraneous information not found in the text.

The disparity in Emma's performance on the two selective learning tasks is somewhat surprising. During the auditory word list task, Emma may have had difficulty using cognitive control to attend to both the speaker's voice (as the gender determined the value) and the individual words. Hence, she may have attempted to compensate by recalling any word that came to mind regardless of value or inclusion on the list. Rather than use a strategy, Emma appeared to guess words to recall.

The expository discourse task, on the other hand, had an inherent structure that may have contributed to her success with this measure. The text was broken down into categorical paragraphs and value was attributed to the category of information, rain forests, rivers, or food. In addition, the cued recall evoked a structure that may have facilitated Emma's ability to strategically recall high-value information. Thus, the expository discourse measure may have enhanced Emma's ability to successfully use cognitive control to improve her performance. Emma's selective learning ability was improved when the task provided a structure through directed probes for recalling information. In contrast, Emma may have found during free recall of the word list that the need to strategically select words without a direct probe to provide structure overwhelmed her cognitive resources.

In conclusion, even at 3 years postinjury, Emma struggled with the ability to strategically select and summarize information. One remediation approach for children with TBI who exhibit higher-level language deficits, as exemplified by Emma, is to use a gist-based intervention, as outlined below.

IMPLICATIONS FOR INTERVENTION

Gist-based intervention may facilitate academic performance and further skills such as reading comprehension and written expression. Two key questions arise as to what form gist-based remediation should take and why it might benefit children with TBI. Specifically, we propose a multilevel approach to improve gist-level comprehension and production after TBI in childhood. The focus involves top-down processing of information in conjunction with detail-based learning. The gist-based remediation process incorporates three major skills sequenced within a single session. The clinician first provides a topical lead-in to a particular text and subsequently elicits from the child: (1) a detailed recall, (2) a transformed summary, and (3) a synthesized interpretation of the text.

The first step is to provide the child with a title and main idea of a story or text prior to its presentation in order to enhance subsequent comprehension. Titles that explain the main point of a story have been shown to improve the story comprehension of children with reading comprehension difficulties (Yuill & Joscelyne, 1988). Moreover, presenting a topical lead-in can serve to enhance the child's interest level and activate the child's prior knowledge of the general subject matter by providing a frame of reference for the incoming information (Swanson, Fey, Mills, & Hood, 2005).

After the text is presented, in the second step, the child immediately retells the text in as much detail as possible. Detailed recalls provide insight into what pieces of information from the text he or she comprehends. In fact, recent evidence indicates that children with good comprehension skills may be better at recalling stories because they encode the story more fully in the first place (e.g., Norbury & Bishop, 2002).

For the third step, the child reduces the information by combining ideas and constructing a transformed summary. Pushing the child to move from a retell to a more challenging summarization task encourages the encoding of meaning at a more abstract level. The practice of storing information at higher levels of semantic representation can enhance encoding (e.g., Chapman, Nasits, et al., 1999; Frederikson, Bracewell, Breuleux, & Renuas, 1990; Ulatowska & Chapman, 1994; van Dijk, 1995). Specifically, summarization strategies have been found to be an effective tool in facilitating gains in comprehension skills (e.g., Kinnunen & Vauras, 1995; Palincsar & Brown, 1984). In order to produce a cohesive and coherent summary, one must process information at a more generalized level, transforming information rather than being bound solely to the explicit story details (Stein & Kirby, 1992). In effect, formulating a condensed version of the text can facilitate more efficient encoding and information retrieval by mandating prioritization of important content (Chapman, Nasits, et al., 1999; Kintsch, 1990). Component skills necessary for learning to strategically select and summarize information are outlined in greater detail in Table 8.3.

In the final step, the child conveys a synthesized interpretation of the text in a single statement or "take-home message." This step

TABLE 8.3. Components of Strategically Selecting and Summarizing Information

Component	Description
Select	Discard unimportant details. Focus on and learn most important information.
Paraphrase	Convey content in child's own words.
Combine	Reduce two statements into one.
Infer	Read "between the lines."
Connect	State relationship between two ideas.
Integrate	Combine new information with world knowledge. Interpret in light of own experience.
Organize	Convey thoughts in a logical sequence. Express beginning, middle, and end.
Generalize	Look at the "big" picture. Interpret in one sentence or "take-home message."
Self-monitor	Read the work critically. Have child answer questions: • Did I use my own words? • Did I give one main idea that was not stated? • What would my title be?
Self-correct	Make changes, reduce, and revise. Be concise.

benefits encoding by integrating the entire content of the text with world knowledge. New textual information is ultimately better comprehended, encoded, and retrieved when integrated with the child's personal knowledge base (Ulatowska & Chapman, 1995; Zwaan & Radvansky, 1998).

The type of multilevel approach to remediation described above is based upon recent findings in cognitive neuroscience. For example, evidence reveals that training directed at strengthening immediate memory, which relies heavily on hippocampal networks, may deter the development of frontally mediated cognitive systems such as working memory and discourse gist production by delaying or disrupting full maturation of these complex skills (e.g., Ramos et al., 2003). As such, we speculate that children with severe TBI strive to overcome immediate memory deficits by overfocusing on remembering the details, which has a detrimental impact on gist-based processing. That is, concentrating largely on the details may strengthen immediate memory at the cost of lowered working memory and poorer controlled retrieval of information, such as is required for summarization (Chapman, Gamino, et al., 2006). Moreover, evidence indicates that brain efficiency is achieved by decreasing the amount of resources required to implement a given task (e.g., Laughlin & Sejnowski, 2003). By teaching children with TBI to encode at a more generalized, abstract level, they are able to progress beyond working solely at inefficient, lower levels of information processing. Accordingly, the provision of a scaffold or support for gist-based learning can ultimately ease the processing load of a child with TBI by facilitating more efficient and economical use of cognitive resources.

Overall, evidence suggests that children with TBI can be trained to see both the forest (gist) and the trees (supporting details) by using a multilevel approach to gist-based intervention. In particular, discourse gist can likely be facilitated by explaining and coaching the steps required to produce macrolevel summaries.

CONCLUSION

We proposed in this chapter new approaches in discourse methodologies that advance clinical practice. Evidence from both theoretical and clinical perspectives supports the view that discourse gist and selective learning may serve to improve assessment of the long-term sequelae in pediatric TBI due to their close relation to learning capacity. Investigating macrostrategies, as reflected in discourse gist, bears theoretical importance in its potential to elucidate how children comprehend, remember, and use information for later learning.

The clinical utility of evaluating discourse gist appears promising as an informative index of comprehension as viewed through production. Measures of discourse gist are functionally relevant, as children are required to engage in learning activities that call upon higher level language skills on a daily basis. In particular, discourse comprehension and production are integral to learning in mainstream school practices. In order to achieve academic success, children are expected to progress beyond recalling verbatim information, learning everything regardless of importance, sticking only with stated facts, and providing single-word answers. Hence, future work should address whether remediation of discourse gist could enhance performance in children with TBI. Prodigious effort should be undertaken to examine the effects of gist-based interventions and whether such an approach promotes optimal learning in children who suffer a TBI, particularly at later stages of development postinjury.

REFERENCES

Alajouanine, T., & Lhermitte, F. (1965). Acquired aphasia in children. *Brain, 88*, 553–562.

Applebee, A. N. (1978). *The child's concept of story: Ages two to seventeen.* Chicago: University of Chicago Press.

Aram, D. M. (1991). Scholastic achievement after early brain lesions. In I. P. Martins et al. (Eds.), *Acquired aphasia in children* (pp. 203–212). Dordrecht, The Netherlands: Kluwer Academic.

Baddeley, A. D. (1992). Working memory. *Science, 255*, 556–559.

Baddeley, A. D., & Hitch, G. (1974). Working memory. In G. A. Bower (Ed.), *The psychology of learning and motivation* (Vol. 8, pp. 47–89). New York: Academic Press.

Barnes, M. A., & Dennis, M. (2001). Knowledge-based inferencing after childhood head injury. *Brain and Language, 76*, 253–265.

Berryhill, P., Lilly, M. A., Levin, H. S., Hillman, G. R., Mendelsohn, D., Brunder, D. G., et al. (1995). Frontal lobe changes after severe diffuse closed head injury in children: A volumetric study of magnetic resonance imaging. *Neurosurgery, 37*, 392–400.

Biddle, K. R., McCabe, A., & Bliss, L. S. (1996). Narrative skills following traumatic brain injury in children and adults. *Journal of Communication Disorders, 29*, 447–468.

Bracewell, R., Frederickson, C., & Frederickson, J. D. (1982). Cognitive processes in composing and comprehending discourse. *Educational Psychologist, 17*, 146–164.

Brookshire, B., Chapman, S. B., Song, J., & Levin, H. S. (2000). Cognitive and linguistic correlates of children's discourse after closed head injury: A three year follow-up. *Journal of the International Neuropsychological Society, 6*, 741–751.

Cain, K. (2003). Text comprehension and its relation to coherence and cohesion in children's fictional narratives. *British Journal of Developmental Psychology, 21*, 335–351.

Cain, K., & Oakhill, J. (1996). The nature of the relationship between comprehension skill and the ability to tell a story. *British Journal of Developmental Psychology, 14*, 187–201.

Chapman, S. B. (1995). Discourse as an outcome measure in pediatric head-injured populations. In S. H. Broman & M. E. Michel (Eds.), *Traumatic head injury in children* (pp. 95–116). New York: Oxford University Press.

Chapman, S. B. (1997). Cognitive-communication abilities in children with closed head injury. *American Journal of Speech–Language Pathology, 6*, 50–58.

Chapman, S. B., Culhane, K. A., Levin, H. S., Harward, H., Mendelsohn, D., Ewing-Cobbs, L., et al. (1992). Narrative discourse after closed head injury in children and adolescents. *Brain and Language, 43*, 42–65.

Chapman, S. B., Gamino, J. F., Cook, L. G., Hanten, G., Li, X., & Levin, H. S. (2006). Impaired discourse gist and working memory in children after brain injury. *Brain and Language, 97*, 178–188.

Chapman, S. B., Levin, H. S., & Culhane, K. (1995). Language impairment in closed head injury. In H. Kirschner (Ed.), *Handbook of neurological speech and language disorders* (pp. 387–414). New York: Marcel-Dekker.

Chapman, S. B., Levin, H. S., & Hart, J. (2006). *The Test of Strategic Learning.* Unpublished manuscript.

Chapman, S. B., Levin, H. S., & Lawyer, S. L. (1999). Communication problems resulting from brain injury in children: Special issues of assessment and management. In S. McDonald, L. Togher, & C. Code (Eds.), *Communication disorders following traumatic brain injury* (pp. 235–270). East Sussex, UK: Psychology Press.

Chapman, S. B., Levin, H. S., Matejka, J., Harward, H., & Kufera, J. A. (1995). Discourse ability in children with brain injury: Correlations with psychosocial, linguistic, and cognitive factors. *Journal of Head Trauma Rehabilitation, 10*, 36–54.

Chapman, S. B., Levin, H. S., Wanek, A., Weyrauch, J., & Kufera, J. (1998). Discourse after closed head injury in young children. *Brain and Language, 61*, 420–449.

Chapman, S. B., McKinnon, L., Levin, H. S., Song, J., Meier, M. C., & Chiu, S. (2001). Longitudinal outcome of verbal discourse in children with traumatic brain injury: Three-year follow-up. *Journal of Head Trauma Rehabilitation, 16*, 441–455.

Chapman, S. B., Nasits, J., Challas, J. D., & Billinger, A. P. (1999). Long-term recovery in paediatric head injury: Overcoming the hurdles. *Advances in Speech–Language Pathology, 1*, 19–30.

Chapman, S. B., & Sparks, G. (2003). Language and discourse. In M. Aminoff & R. Daroff (Eds.), *Encyclopedia of the neurological sciences* (pp. 753–755). San Diego: Academic Press.

Chapman, S. B., Sparks, G., Cook, L. G., Gamino, J. F., Levin, H. S., & Song, J. (2006). *Recovery of written discourse after pediatric closed head injury.* Unpublished manuscript.

Chapman, S. B., Sparks, G., Levin, H. S., Dennis, M., Roncadin, C., Zhang, L., et al. (2004). Discourse macrolevel processing after severe pediatric traumatic brain injury. *Developmental Neuropsychology, 25*, 37–61.

Chapman, S. B., Watkins, R., Gustafson, C., Moore, S., Levin, H. S., & Kufera, J. A. (1997). Narrative discourse in children with closed head injury, children with language impairment and typically developing children. *American Journal of Speech–Language Pathology, 6*, 66–76.

Chapman, S. B., Zientz, J., Weiner, M., Rosenberg, R., Frawley, W., & Burns, M. H. (2002). Discourse changes in early Alzheimer disease, mild cognitive impairment, and normal aging. *Alzheimer Disease and Associated Disorders, 16*, 177–186.

deHirsch, K., & Jansky, J. (1968). *Predicting reading failure.* New York: Harper & Row.

Dennis, M., & Barnes, M. A. (2001). Comparison of literal, inferential, and intentional text comprehension in children with mild or severe closed head injury. *Journal of Head Trauma Rehabilitation, 16*, 456–468.

Dennis, M., Purvis, K., Barnes, M. A., Wilkinson, M., & Winner, E. (2001).

Understanding of literal truth, ironic criticism and deceptive praise following childhood head injury. *Brain and Language 78*, 1–16.

Ewing-Cobbs, L., Barnes, M. A., & Fletcher, J. M. (2003). Early brain injury in children: Development and reorganization of cognitive function. *Developmental Neuropsychology, 24*, 669–704.

Ewing-Cobbs, L., Barnes, M. A., Fletcher, J. M., Levin, H. S., Swank, P. R., & Song, J. (2004). Modeling of longitudinal academic achievement scores after pediatric traumatic brain injury. *Developmental Neuropsychology, 25*, 107–133.

Ewing-Cobbs, L., Fletcher, J. M., Levin, H. S., Iovino, I., & Miner, M. E. (1998). Academic achievement and academic placement following traumatic brain injury in children and adolescents: A two-year longitudinal study. *Journal of Clinical and Experimental Neuropsychology, 20*, 769–781.

Ewing-Cobbs, L., Levin, H. S., Eisenberg, H. M., & Fletcher, J. M. (1987). Language functions following closed-head injury in children and adolescents. *Journal of Clinical and Experimental Neuropsychology, 9*, 575–592.

Fletcher, J. M., Miner, M., & Ewing-Cobbs, L. (1987). Age and recovery from head injury in children: Developmental issues. In H. S. Levin, J. Graufman, & H. M. Eisenberg (Eds.), *Neurobehavioral recovery from head injury* (pp. 279–292). New York: Oxford University Press.

Frederikson, C. H., Bracewell, F. J., Breleux, A., & Renuas, A. (1990). The cognitive representation and processing of discourse: Function and dysfunction. In Y. Joanette & H. H. Brownell (Eds.), *Discourse ability and brain damage: Theoretical and empirical perspectives* (pp. 69–112). New York: Springer-Verlag.

Hanten, G., Chapman, S. B., Gamino, J. F., Zhang, L., Benton, S. B., Stallings-Roberson, G., et al. (2004). Verbal selective learning after traumatic brain injury in children. *Annals of Neurology, 56*, 847–853.

Hanten, G., Zhang, L., & Levin, H. S. (2002). Selective learning in children after traumatic brain injury: A preliminary study. *Child Neuropsychology, 8*, 107–120.

Hecaén, H. (1976). Acquired aphasia in children and the ontogenesis of hemispheric functional specialization. *Brain and Language, 3*, 114–134.

Hecaén, H. (1983). Acquired aphasia in children: Revisited. *Neuropsychologia, 21*, 581–587.

Johnson, N. S. (1983). What do you do if you can tell the whole story?: The development of summarization skills. In K. E. Nelson (Ed.), *Children's language* (pp. 314–383). New York: Gardner Press.

Kinnunen, R., & Vauras, M. (1995). Comprehension monitoring and the level of comprehension in high- and low-achieving primary school children's reading. *Learning and Instruction, 5*, 143–165.

Kintsch, E. (1990). Macroprocesses and microprocesses in the development of summarization skill. *Cognition and Instruction, 7*, 161–195.

Langlois, J. A., Rutland-Brown, W., & Thomas, K. E. (2004). *Traumatic brain injury in the United States: Emergency department visits, hospitalizations, and deaths.* Atlanta: Centers for Disease Control and Prevention, National Center for Injury Prevention and Control.

Laughlin, S. B., & Sejnowski, T. J. (2003). Communication in neuronal networks. *Science, 301,* 1870–1874.

Lehman, S., & Schraw, G. (2002). Effects of coherence and relevance on shallow and deep text processing. *Journal of Educational Psychology, 94,* 738–750.

Levin, H. S., Culhane, K. A., Mendelsohn, D., Lilly, M. A., Bruce, D., Fletcher, J. M., et al. (1993). Cognition in relation to magnetic resonance imaging in head-injured children and adolescents. *Archives of Neurology, 50,* 897–905.

Levin, H. S., Hanten, G., Chang, C., Zhang, L., Schachar, R., Ewing-Cobbs, L., et al. (2002). Working memory after traumatic brain injury in children. *Annals of Neurology, 52,* 82–88.

Mendelsohn, D., Levin, H. S., Bruce, D., Lilly, M., Harward, H., Culhane, K. A., et al. (1992). Late MRI after head injury in children: Relationship to clinical features and outcome. *Child's Nervous System, 8,* 445–452.

Norbury, C. F., & Bishop, D. V. M. (2002). Inferential processing and story recall in children with communication problems: A comparison of specific language impairment, pragmatic language impairment, and high-functioning autism. *International Journal of Language and Communication Disorders, 37,* 227–251.

Palincsar, A. S., & Brown, A. L. (1984). Reciprocal teaching of comprehension-fostering and comprehension-monitoring activities. *Cognition and Instruction, 1,* 117–175.

Ramos, B. P., Birnbaum, S. G., Lindenmayer, I., Newton, S. S., Duman, R. S., & Arnsten, A. F. T. (2003). Dysregulation of protein kinase A signaling in the aged prefrontal cortex: New strategy for treating age-related cognitive decline. *Neuron, 40,* 835–845.

Reilly, J. S., Bates, E. A., & Marchman, V. A. (1998). Narrative discourse in children with early focal brain injury. *Brain and Language, 51,* 335–375.

Roncadin, C., Guger, S., Archibald, J., Barnes, M., & Dennis, M. (2004). Working memory after mild, moderate, or severe childhood closed head injury. *Developmental Neuropsychology, 25,* 21–36.

Scott, C. M. (1991). Learning to write: Context, form and process. In A. G. Kamhi & H. W. Catts (Eds.), *Reading disabilities: A developmental language perspective* (pp. 261–302). Boston: Allyn & Bacon.

Singer, M., & Ritchot, K. F. M. (1996). The role of working memory capacity and knowledge access in text inference processing. *Memory and Cognition, 24,* 733–743.

Stein, B. L., & Kirby, J. R. (1992). The effects of text absent and text present conditions on summarization and recall of text. *Journal of Reading Behavior, 24,* 217–232.

Stein, N. L., & Glenn, C. G. (1979). An analysis of story comprehension in elementary school children. In R. O. Freedle (Ed.), *New direction in discourse processing* (pp. 53–120). Norwood, NJ: Ablex.

Swanson, H. L., & Berninger, V. (1995). The role of working memory in skilled and less-skilled readers' comprehension. *Intelligence, 21,* 83–108.

Swanson, L. A., Fey, M. E., Mills, C. E., & Hood, L. S. (2005). Use of narrative-based language intervention with children who have specific language impairment. *American Journal of Speech–Language Pathology, 14,* 131–143.

Teasdale, G., & Jennett, B. (1974). Assessment of coma and impaired consciousness: A practical scale. *Lancet, 2,* 81–84.

Ulatowska, H. K., & Chapman, S. B. (1994). Discourse macrostructure in aphasia. In R. L. Bloom, L. K. Obler, S. DeSanti, & J. S. Ehrlich (Eds.), *Discourse analysis and applications* (pp. 29–46). Hillsdale, NJ: Erlbaum.

Ulatowska, H. K., & Chapman, S. B. (1995). Discourse changes in dementia. In R. Lubinski (Ed.), *Dementia and communication: Research and clinical implications* (pp. 115–130). Philadelphia: Decker.

van Dijk, T. A. (1995). On macrostructure mental models and other inventions: A brief personal history of the Kintsch–van Dijk theory. In C. A. Weaver, S. Mannes, & C. R. Flecher (Eds.), *Discourse comprehension* (pp. 383–410). Hillsdale, NJ: Erlbaum.

Westby, C. (1984). Development of narrative abilities. In G. Wallach & K. G. Butler (Eds.), *Language learning disabilities in school-age children* (pp. 103–127). Baltimore: Williams & Wilkins.

Wilson, B. M., & Proctor, A. (2000). Oral and written discourse in adolescents with closed head injury. *Brain and Cognition, 43,* 425–429.

Wilson, B. M., & Proctor, A. (2002). Written discourse of adolescents with closed head injury. *Brain Injury, 16,* 1011–1025.

Wilson, B. M., Smith, R., & Proctor, A. (2001). The validity of cognitive distance in oral and written discourse. *Brain and Cognition, 46,* 304–307.

Ylvisaker, M., Adetson, P. D., Braga, L. W., Burnett, S. M., Glang, A., Feeney, T., et al. (2005). Rehabilitation and ongoing support after pediatric TBI: Twenty years of progress. *Journal of Head Trauma Rehabilitation, 20,* 95–109.

Yorkston, K. M., Jaffe, K. M., Liao, S., & Polissar, N. L. (1999). Recovery of written language production in children with traumatic brain injury: Outcomes at one year. *Aphasiology, 13,* 691–700.

Yorkston, K. M., Jaffe, K. M., Polissar, N. L., Liao, S., & Fay, G. C. (1997). Written language production and neuropsychological function in children with traumatic brain injury. *Archives of Physical Medicine and Rehabilitation, 78,* 1096–1102.

Yuill, N. M., & Joscelyne, T. (1988). Effect of organisational cues and strategies on good and poor comprehenders' story understanding. *Journal of Educational Psychology, 80,* 152–158.

Yuill, N. M., Oakhill, J. V., & Parkin, A. J. (1989). Working memory, comprehension ability and the resolution of text anomaly. *British Journal of Psychology, 80,* 351–361.

Zwaan, R. A., & Radvansky, G. A. (1998). Situation models in language comprehension and memory. *Psychological Bulletin, 123,* 162–185.

CHAPTER 9

The Comprehension
of Skilled Deaf Readers

The Roles of Word Recognition and Other
Potentially Critical Aspects of Competence

LEONARD P. KELLY
DRAGANA BARAC-CIKOJA

If success in helping deaf children to read skillfully is an indicator of our knowledge about reading processes that are critical to their comprehension, then our knowledge of deaf readers must be assessed as very scant indeed. A recent study of deaf readers by the Gallaudet Research Institute (GRI; 2004) determined that the median reading comprehension performance of those deaf students nearing completion of their secondary education was comparable to the comprehension of hearing children in the third grade. Kuntz's (1998) description of deaf readers' achievement as "dismal" is as warranted as ever.

The GRI (2004) study also revealed, however, that 5% of the school-leaving sample comprehended text at a level equal to or superior to an average hearing reader in the 12th grade. If we could better understand the nature of the competence attainable by this minority of deaf readers, we might identify the targets of instruction that educators and students need to address with greater energy, creativity, and resources, in order to help the majority of deaf readers to better understand printed English.

Given its limited success in reading instruction, the field of deaf education has every reason to seek guidance from the theory and methods of the many studies conducted on the reading comprehension of readers with normal hearing. At the same time, the unique effect of deafness on language processing, particularly processing that is visual, suggests that new knowledge about the comprehension of skilled deaf readers could inform the larger field of reading research. That potential for reciprocal illumination is a key impetus for this chapter.

Four aspects of competence are considered in this chapter: word recognition, syntactic knowledge, discourse comprehension, and reading strategies. Theoretical and empirical reasons combine to indicate that the first of these, word recognition, is particularly instrumental to the comprehension of skilled deaf readers. Word recognition is also a topic about which the larger literature on the comprehension of hearing readers has much to offer both theoretically and methodologically. Finally, it is an area where a better understanding of skilled deaf readers might add authentic new knowledge about the comprehension of *all* readers, not just those who are deaf. For these reasons, the role of word recognition in comprehension is a major focus of this chapter. Limitations related to syntax, discourse comprehension, and reading strategies are also considered in light of their effects on reading comprehension.

DEAF READERS' COMPREHENSION PROBLEMS

Large recent studies in North America and Europe reveal that text-level comprehension poses an enormous challenge to many readers who are deaf. These same studies also reveal severe and widespread reading difficulties at the level of single words. The GRI periodically conducts studies to establish norms for the Stanford Achievement Tests (Harcourt Assessment, 2003), the measurement used most often to estimate the reading competence of deaf readers. These studies measure deaf readers' comprehension of a variety of extended passages including expository texts, narratives, and poems. According to the most recent investigation, GRI (2004), which included a sample of approximately 3,800 readers, the median score for a deaf 10-year-old was equivalent to the score of an average hearing child in the 7th month of the first grade, which is a grade-level deficit approaching 4 years. The median comprehension score for deaf readers age 17, roughly the age at which students are entering the 12th grade, was equivalent to the average score for a hearing child in the 5th month of the third grade, or 8 years below grade level. In other words, the grade-level deficit had virtually doubled between the ages of 10 and 17.

In addition to measuring comprehension of extended text, the same investigation also included measurement of reading competence at the word level, that is, reading vocabulary. Again, 10-year-old deaf readers scored on average at a level equivalent to an average hearing child in the 7th month of the first grade, a deficit approaching four grade levels. The 17-year-old readers generated reading vocabulary results that resembled their passage-level comprehension results. Their median score was equivalent to an average hearing child in the 5th month of the third grade, a deficit between eight and nine grade levels. As with the passage-level performance, the grade-level deficit in reading vocabulary almost doubled between ages 10 and 17.

Although these results are from just the most recent GRI investigation, similar patterns also are evident in the data from the previous norming studies, GRI (1996; N = 4,810), GRI (1991; N = 6,932), and Allen (1986, N = 7,557). The decline in the number of readers in these studies over the years reflects the proliferation of statewide testing programs, which is a harbinger of the consequences of this reading problem soon will extend beyond a severe deficit in comprehension. That is because statewide reading standards require performance well above the third–fourth-grade levels that are the average for deaf readers. As a result, an increasingly large number of deaf students face the specter of being denied a high school diploma because they cannot pass the reading portion of their state's minimum competency test.

Beyond these assessments of deaf readers' comprehension in North America, a recent study by Wauters, van Bon, and Tellings (2006) measured the reading comprehension and word recognition of 464 deaf readers in the Netherlands. The average text comprehension score for the Dutch deaf readers was equivalent to the score for a hearing child six levels lower in school. Comparison of deaf and hearing children at each instructional age showed significantly lower scores for the deaf readers. Of the entire sample, only 20 of the deaf children, approximately 4%, demonstrated reading comprehension at the same level as hearing children of the same instructional age.

The Wauters et al. (2006) study also measured automaticity and accuracy of word recognition. The results paralleled those found for text-level comprehension: Deaf students scored at a level significantly lower than hearing students. The correlation between text-level reading comprehension and word recognition was a significant and moderately strong .50. These results obtained even though the word stimuli used in the study comprised short, high-frequency words, which may have limited the measurements' sensitivity to higher levels of word recognition ability. In combination, these findings indicate that reading comprehension presents serious difficulties for many deaf readers across different languages and educational settings, and that deficits related to the reading of individual words contribute significantly to the problem.

THE WORD RECOGNITION AND COMPREHENSION OF DEAF READERS

In addition to the empirical findings presented previously, there are also theoretical reasons to suspect that a limitation in the fluent recognition of known words is central to the text comprehension problems of deaf readers. Olson, Forsberg, Wise, and Rack (1994) observed that the most severe reading comprehension problems in the hearing population stem from deficient word recognition. Related to this finding, an abundance of research indicates that severe deficiencies in word recognition stem from what Stanovich and Siegel (1994) describe as a "phonological core"deficit, and, as the following section will show, deaf readers face severe obstacles in using English phonology. It follows that this will limit their word recognition performance. In addition, Gough (1996) observes that it is extremely rare for a reader who comprehends well to suffer from deficient word recognition ability. Thus, it is likely that the minority of deaf readers who do comprehend well also enjoy effective word recognition.

A focus on word recognition also is warranted by interactive theories of reading processes (Carpenter & Just, 1981; Rumelhart, 1977; Stanovich, 1980), which stipulate that reading comprehension suffers when the cognitive resources needed to complete higher level comprehension tasks are usurped by effortful word recognition. An appreciable body of research (Kelly, 1993, 1995, 1996, 1998, 2003b) addresses differences between deaf readers who demonstrated skilled comprehension compared to those less skilled, and this work suggests that word recognition fluency distinguishes the two groups. For example, the word-reading rate of exceptional deaf readers comprehending text at the college level was measured in the Kelly (2003b) study to be 333 milliseconds for syntactically simple sentences and 367 milliseconds for complex sentences. The less-skilled deaf readers, comprehending at the fifth-grade level, demonstrated significantly slower rates of 462 and 503 milliseconds for words in the two types of sentences, respectively. By way of comparison, Just, Carpenter, and Masson (1982) measured hearing college readers as having an average word reading rate of 330 milliseconds, which is similar to that of the deaf college-level readers. In other words, for deaf readers comprehending at the college level, fluency when reading words appears to be a strength.

Word recognition will be examined by focusing on two aspects of word form, one that seems to be a particular weakness of deaf readers—phonology—and one that may tap into one of their potential strengths, namely, orthography. A guiding assumption of this discussion of word recognition is that readers must convert the letter strings of words into some form that is well known to them. One instance of this conversion process occurs when hearing children who have gained control of the initial stages of phonological awareness and learned letter–phoneme correspondences are able to systematically convert the complicated visual displays of printed words into a form that is already well known to them, namely, speech. By achieving some level of control over the alphabetic system, they take possession of a tool that is virtually indispensable to their skilled reading. Novel words can be deciphered, and the need to visually memorize exact sequences of letter combinations is eliminated. The mechanism used by skilled deaf readers to convert letter sequences into a form that is highly familiar to them has not yet been identified, but there is every reason to believe that, to them, such a system is equally indispensable.

Phonological Knowledge

Research principally with hearing readers shows that phonological knowledge participates in the analytical reading of developing readers, in the process that represents a novel word so that it can be recognized swiftly, and in the rapid word recognition of mature readers. First, it enables a reader to decipher new words as they are encountered in print, resulting in far greater independence as a reader and, according to Allington (1980), vastly increasing word recognition practice. Second, and critically, phonological analysis is precisely the manner of processing that represents a new word so that it can be recognized automatically or read, as Ehri (1997) says, as a "sight word." This is the conclusion from research with prealphabetic readers (Ehri & Wilce, 1985; Gough, 1996), with dyslexic readers (Ehri & Saltmarsh, 1995; Reitsma, 1989), and with normally developing alphabetic readers (Cunningham, Perry, Stanovich, & Share, 2002; Share, 1999). The phonological nature of this representation pays dividends during future encounters with a word, because, even when the reader is highly skilled and no intentional analysis occurs, the word's phonology is activated automatically, along with the meaning that is bonded to it. This automatic activation of a word's phonological representation has been found in research with mature skilled readers by, for example, Berent and Perfetti (1995), Van Orden (1987), and Van Orden, Johnston, and Hale (1988). This functioning of phonology as a sort of mnemonic device eliminates the monumental burden of remembering thousands of letter sequences in their exact order as if they were numbers in a phone book (see Gough, 1996; Share, 1995).

It follows from this research that, if the phonological knowledge of deaf readers is deficient, then they will have trouble decoding novel words into a form that is understandable. They will also be unable to represent words in a manner that capitalizes on the mnemonic benefit stemming from the bond between a word's phonology and its meaning. As a consequence, typical deaf readers may need to resort to a laborious, paired-associate approach to memorizing exact letter sequences and meanings, a tactic that produces diminishing benefit as the size of the lexicon increases.

Effects of Hearing Loss on Acquisition of English Phonology

It is important to understand the obstacles that deaf readers face stemming from the inescapable fact that printed English represents the spoken phonemes of the language. It is a surrogate for English speech. Unique individual abilities related to hearing, speechreading (i.e., lipreading), and pronunciation combined with differences in the phonetic distinctiveness among phonemes—both acoustic and optic—can shape the nature of the representation of English phonology that deaf people acquire and the fund of English words that are represented in their lexicons. These potential sources of variation are magnified by differences in the use of amplification, the speech and hearing training received, the amounts of time invested in practice outside of formal instruction, and the conduciveness of the environment to incidental language learning.

It may seem self-evident that a deaf person's most obvious obstacle to acquiring phonology is difficulty hearing voices. To clarify this somewhat, the loudness of average conversational speech from a speaker facing a listener at a distance of 1 meter is about 60 decibels (dB) (Cox, Matesich, & Moore, 1988). Thus, a person with a hearing loss measured at 60 dB will have difficulty hearing much of the speech signal. Hearing losses at this level are considered moderate, and amplification with a hearing aid permits virtually complete access to voices, and thus to phonological information. People with hearing losses above this level, however, are likely to face obstacles to hearing voices even with amplification.[1]

Hearing losses greater than 70 dB are considered severe and they constitute a serious impediment to understanding speech. More than differing in terms of sensitivity to soft sounds, severe and profound (greater than 90 dB) hearing losses commonly include deficiencies related to other aspects of auditory processing, which can complicate and often limit the benefit of amplification (see Moore, 1996, and Van Tasell, 1993, for more detailed reviews of the perceptual consequences of various degrees of hearing loss). For instance, natural fluctuations in the intensity of the speech signal may lead to the perception of speech peaks as excessively loud, sometimes to the point of discomfort, and usually to the point of distorting what is perceived. Another common deficiency is the listener's reduced frequency selectivity; the consequent smearing of the acoustic input results in loss of phonetic information that is normally carried in the fine spectral structure of the speech signal. In addition, poor temporal resolution and integration may further interfere with segmentation of the speech stream.

These audiological deficiencies can severely limit the formation of a lexicon of English words and the development of effective representations of English phonemes. Specifically, provided that there is appropriate amplification, individuals with a severe hearing loss may be able to differentiate some vowels, and show awareness of consonant voicing (e.g., /p/ vs. /b/) and manner (e.g., /n/ vs. /d/ vs. /l/) contrasts, but the differences in terms of the place of articulation (/p/ vs. /t/ vs. /k/) will not be audible. Individuals with a profound hearing loss may be able to distinguish only the speaker's gender, detect voicing for the presence of vowels and some consonants, and perceive the syllabic structure of the speech stream. They cannot, however, differentiate among the vowels and the consonants (see Boothroyd, 1984, for more information). Hearing loss in excess of 115 dB leaves no auditory capacity, and perceptual responses are mediated solely by the sense of vibration in the ear, conveying some information about the speech rhythm (Erber, 1979).

An additional obstacle to processing fluent speech is posed by the individual's reduced ability to differentiate simultaneous sounds. Individuals with severe and profound hearing loss have great difficulty understanding speech in the presence of any noise and, in particular,

---

[1]Use of amplification cannot be taken for granted. A study by GRI (2005) showed that of 38,744 students with a hearing loss surveyed for the 2003–2004 school year, 60% reported that they used a hearing aid during instruction, and 40% reported that they did not.

when the competition is from a rival source of speech. The lack of fine binaural cues to sound localization and spatial separation of sound sources (due to typically asymmetrical hearing loss across the ears) further aggravates this difficulty. Importantly, this deficiency also results in ineffective auditory attention capture and switching, limiting attention to incidental speech, which is so important to language acquisition.

In summary, for a person with mild or moderate hearing loss, appropriate sound amplification is likely to make speech intelligible most of the time from listening only, and therefore his or her oral language development can be expected to resemble that of hearing individuals. However, the obstacles that severe and profound hearing losses pose to the auditory reception of speech cannot be completely eliminated by aural enhancements. The auditory consequences of hearing loss to acquiring phonological representations of English are somewhat mitigated by the visual reception of spoken language input.

Speechreading, also called lipreading, can be a significant source of spoken information, and thus a potential resource for developing a phonologically represented lexicon. However, the articulatory gestures that are visually observable during speechreading, commonly referred to as "visemes," allow only limited speech comprehension (Fisher, 1968; Massaro, 1998). The limited effectiveness of visemes for conveying speech is a consequence of their lack of phonemic specificity. Several phonemes often correspond to a single viseme (e.g., /p/, /b/, /m/), while for other phonemes, the associated articulatory gestures are at best partially visible (e.g., the occluded place of articulation for /s/, /z/, /j/, /h/, /k/, /g/). An additional source of limited phonemic specificity stems from difficult visual segmentation due to coarticulation (e.g., as in the word *needles*).

It is estimated that the 40 phonemes of English map to only 9–14 visemes (Jeffers & Barley, 1971). It is therefore not surprising that the accuracy for speech-reading sentences is in the range of 5–45% words correct (Ronnberg, Samuelsson, & Lyxell, 1998). Accuracy can, however, reach 80% for some expert speech readers (e.g., college-educated deaf individuals who rely on auditorily augmented visual information for their daily communication) under favorable listening conditions (i.e., listening to single carefully produced sentences as opposed to conversational, fluent speech; Bernstein, Demorest, & Tucker, 2000). Notably, the accuracy and ease of visual recognition of a given spoken word depends not only on the visual intelligibility of its *segments* (i.e., the degree to which a word's different phonemes are confusable), but also on the word's visual similarity to other *words* in the lexicon (its visual uniqueness). Visually unique words have fewer competitors for recognition (Auer & Bernstein, 1997; Matys, Bernstein, & Auer, 2002), and hence are more understandable through speechreading.

For many individuals with hearing loss, combining speechreading with amplified auditory input allows speech recognition that is superior to either visual-only or auditory-only reception. Adding visual speech information may improve auditory word recognition accuracy by more than 40% (Grant, Walden, & Seitz, 1998). However, large individual differences exist in the ability to integrate audio and visual speech information in order to derive benefit from bimodal reception. One of the factors that affects the effectiveness of cross-modal integration is the degree of redundancy between the auditory and the visual speech information that an individual is capable of perceiving.

For individuals who have auditory access to speech information that is *complementary* to visually accessible information, the advantage of bimodal over unimodal speech reception is substantial. For instance, a person with severe hearing loss who can hear the contrasts in voicing and manner for consonants will be able to combine that information with the visible information about the place of articulation and achieve speech recognition that greatly exceeds the level of speechreading alone. An individual with a profound hearing loss, on the other hand, usually has access to information that is redundant across modalities, and therefore will experience much smaller benefits from audiovisual speech reception (Grant et al., 1998). It should be emphasized that an individual's ability to use phonological, syntactic, and semantic context to disambiguate auditory and/or visual phonetic information plays a prominent role in cross-modal integration. Use of linguistic and contextual constraints is important in speech recognition. For deaf individuals, it is not likely to develop without systematic training and practice.

Experience related to speech production can also affect the acquisition of a phonological representation of English. Development of speech, which occurs naturally through imitation of heard and seen speech, is constrained by the nature of the speech input that is available to a child with a severe or profound hearing loss. Limits on spontaneous imitation of ambient speech are imposed by reduced or no access to the spectral details of the speech signal that can specify articulatory gestures, along with insufficient articulatory information in the optical signal.

Importantly, self-hearing during speech articulation is affected as well. As a consequence, gradual tuning to the relevant acoustic and articulatory aspects of speech, which occurs naturally in the process of self-correction during speech imitation, is also less likely to take place. Because of insufficient self-hearing, speech self-monitoring may rely on somatosensory information (i.e., the feel of the entire articulatory apparatus when in use). Although the phonological specificity of the somatosensory feedback is poorly understood, it is evident that the resulting speech is usually hard to understand and maintains a distinct quality even after years of training. The benefits of oral and aural instruction obviously cannot exceed what is allowed by the child's capacity to utilize the available perceptual information.

Phonetic deviations observed in the speech of deaf people suggest possible concomitant changes in the representations of phonology that they form: some of the phonological distinctions may be collapsed (e.g., voiced vs. voiceless stops), may be based on rearranged and altered acoustic and optic cues (Monsen, 1983), or may be based primarily on articulatory feedback and production memory as acquired through oral/aural instruction and training. Consequently, we can expect that the phonological organization of the lexicon of a deaf individual is not likely to equal that of a hearing person.

It is useful to contrast the foregoing obstacles with those faced by a somewhat more familiar group of challenged readers, namely, hearing readers who are dyslexic. Although deaf and dyslexic readers share a serious problem related to word recognition and phonological processing, the sources and severity of their difficulty are not the same, nor is its resistance to instruction. According to Shaywitz (2003), dyslexic readers have formed representations of spoken phonemes that are relatively imprecise, and they experience difficulty developing phonemic awareness. As a consequence, it is more difficult for them to intentionally identify the phonemes in spoken words, divide words into phonemes, and combine phonemes into words.

Shaywitz (2003) maintains that, in spite of facing an extremely serious condition, dyslexic readers can be helped to catch up to their nondyslexic peers through the right kind of concentrated and prolonged instruction. This treatment requires a significant commitment of time and resources, as it can entail an extra 90 minutes daily for as long as 3 years. Among Shaywitz's highest priority instructional objectives are noticing, identifying, and manipulating the sounds of spoken language. In contrast to deaf readers, dyslexic readers enjoy at least one major ally in their efforts to achieve those objectives, namely, they are effective users of spoken communication. They thus have at their disposal their representations of the English phonemes and their lexicons of English words. The thousands of different words that dyslexic learners use in face-to-face communication constitute an abundance of examples, allowing teachers to orchestrate practice separating words into phonemes and combining phonemes into words. Shaywitz's description of the prospects for dyslexic readers is a hopeful one. Although the challenges faced by dyslexic readers are rarely considered trivial, the obstacles confronting deaf people as they learn to read can be far more daunting. This is largely because they do not share the disabled hearing reader's ability to use the spoken form of the language that the alphabet represents.

The Timing of Deaf Readers' Phonological Development

To the extent that phonological knowledge does develop in deaf readers, it appears to do so later than it does with hearing children. Studies of relatively young deaf readers either do not show evidence of phonological competence, or they show moderate evidence of phonological competence. By the same token, appreciable phonological knowledge has been shown in deaf readers who are somewhat older and who also are usually relatively skilled readers.

Evidence of phonological knowledge did not result from studies of relatively young deaf readers by Merrills, Underwood, and Wood (1994) (subject ages 11–15 years); by Sutcliffe, Dowker, and Campbell (1999) (ages 9 years, 1 month–12 years, 4 months); by Waters and Doehring (1990) (ages 7–20 years); and by Izzo (2002) (ages 4 years, 3 months–13 years, 4 months). Several other studies did find some evidence indicating phonological knowledge among younger deaf readers. Hanson, Liberman, and Shankweiler (1984) studied phonological processing among developing deaf readers (mean age approximately 9 years), and found that those in the sample classified as good readers (grade equivalent 2.2), were affected by the phonetic similarity of letter names used in a recall task. Sterne and Goswami (2000) tested deaf children's (average age 11 years, 2 months) phonological abilities at three levels: syllables, rhymes, and phonemes. On the syllable awareness task, the deaf subjects performed at a level equal to chronological-age hearing controls. Recall from earlier discussion of the auditory effects of hearing loss that even a profound hearing loss allows perception of the syllabic structure of the speech stream, provided there is appropriate amplification. Dyer, MacSweeney, Szczerbinski, Green, and Campbell (2003) conducted another study that found some evidence of phonological knowledge in the processing of deaf children (average age 13 years). Results revealed above-chance performance on phonological tasks, and there was a moderate correlation between reading ability and phonological performance.

It is important to note, however, that even when moderate phonological competence was evident, the children in these studies demonstrated uniformly deficient reading comprehension performance, which suggests that phonological knowledge was not enabling effective reading. Phonological knowledge does not appear to be an asset to the reading performance of deaf children. Note that the subjects in the studies cited were not exceptionally young. They were tested well beyond the ages when hearing children are already routinely demonstrating considerable phonological competence. Limited phonological knowledge in relatively young readers is not surprising in light of the obstacles to acquiring it that they face.

Again, studies that found evidence of appreciable phonological knowledge were those that included subjects who were older than those in the latter studies and who also were more skillful readers. In a lexical decision task with college-age deaf subjects (10th-grade reading level), Hanson and Fowler (1987) found that rhyming stimulus word pairs (*gave–cave*) facilitated a response and, for some of the subjects nonrhyming, look-alike pairs (*cave–have*) inhibited a response. Kelly (2003b) replicated this experiment with college-age skilled deaf readers (post-high school reading level) and found the rhyme facilitation effect, but not the inhibition effect. Hanson, Goodell, and Perfetti (1991) found involvement of phonology during sentence comprehension when they examined the performance of deaf college students (reading level 8 years, 7 months) while they made semantic acceptability judgments about tongue-twister sentences. When words are processed phonologically, it is more difficult to make semantic judgments about sentences such as "The sparrow snatched the spider swiftly off the ceiling" compared to control sentences.

Hauser (2000) examined college-age deaf students (11th-grade reading level) and found a similarity effect on a task requiring recall of phonemically similar words. LaSasso, Crain, and Leybaert (2003) studied two groups (one signing, one users of cued speech) of highly skilled college-age deaf readers and found a high level of accuracy generating rhyming words. These findings are consistent with a conclusion that the phonological knowledge of deaf readers develops relatively late.

Phonological Knowledge May Be Nonstandard

One issue that emerges from the research on deaf readers and English phonology pertains to the nature of the phonology that a deaf person learns and uses. Earlier in the chapter, it was observed that phonetic deviations noticeable in the speech of some deaf people may suggest possible concomitant differences in the representations of phonology that they form. Hanson and Fowler (1987) speculated that the phonological knowledge of deaf people may be useable during word reading even though it may be nonstandard. Hauser (2000) put this theory to the test when he investigated whether deaf readers' phonological representations may be different from those of hearing readers. During a

reading-for-recall task, the investigator found different levels of electrical activity for labial words (pronunciation of phonemes called for lip
movement) compared to nonlabial words for the hearing subjects but
not for the deaf subjects. The differences in the muscle activity
between the two groups of subjects suggested that the deaf readers'
version or versions of phonological representations were not necessarily the same phonetically as those of the hearing subjects.

If indeed deaf readers have internalized versions of phonology that
are nonstandard, it will influence how phonology serves word recognition, and it will affect the validity of tasks intended to detect effective
use of phonology during word reading. For example, failure to find
slower lexical decision times for words with an irregular grapheme–
phoneme correspondence simply may not reflect that deaf readers are
not encoding words phonologically. The measurement used in the
majority of the studies reviewed seemed to focus principally on the
sound-based aspect of phonology, although the previous discussion of
the input available to deaf children stressed the visual and somatosensory aspects of phonological acquisition, as well as the altered auditory input. Measurement intended to tap phonological knowledge
should be sensitive to representations based on these multiple sources.
Likewise, when tasks use words as stimuli to examine phonological
knowledge rather than the extent of lexical knowledge, there should be
confirmation that those words are already familiar to the subjects.

Future Research on Deaf Readers' Phonological Processing

One general observation emerging from the research reviewed is that
research with deaf readers has not yet capitalized on a number of paradigms that have produced insights related to the role of phonology
with hearing readers. One of these paradigms is the longitudinal
approach used by Stanovich, Nathan, and Zolman (1988) that clarified
the initial competence that leads to effective sight-word learning.
Existing research on deaf readers suggests that their development of
phonological knowledge is delayed. However, because of the cross-
sectional nature of these studies, it is uncertain whether the younger
readers were simply delayed in their acquisition of phonological knowledge at the time of testing, or whether, because of qualitative differences from those who achieved competence, their phonological competence would remain limited. Longitudinal research is needed to
document early competence profiles, subsequent learning experiences,
and the trajectory of growth in phonological knowledge.

Another approach that could prove fruitful is the one used in the
Share (1999) research, which studied the nature of the analytical pro-

cessing that results in words being learned as sight words. For hearing children, again, this appears to involve analytical phonological processing. Studies are needed to determine the nature of the representations that skilled deaf readers activate automatically during sight-word reading, leading in turn to activation of meaning. Specifically, phonological knowledge may develop in deaf readers as a partial consequence of their early reading experience, and subsequent reading development may be fostered by this late-developing phonological awareness. An alternative is that although phonological knowledge may develop over time as a by-product of another, more dominant mechanism (e.g., orthographic knowledge), it remains passive during reading, rarely recruited to support the speed and accuracy of word recognition. Again, at present, because of the absence of direct investigation, this remains an area of uncertainty.

With the exception of the Kelly (2003b) and the LaSasso et al. (2003) studies, the research related to phonological knowledge did not include highly skilled deaf readers. More studies of skilled deaf readers would have a greater likelihood of revealing whether phonological processing can be instrumental to sight-word learning and recognition. In order to test for the participation of phonological knowledge in fluent word recognition, it usually is necessary for subjects to possess a lexicon of sight words. Development of such a sight-word vocabulary is more likely with more mature readers. The same more gradual rate of acquisition is likely to be true of phonological competence itself, so waiting until readers are more mature may provide a greater likelihood of detecting phonological knowledge if indeed it is crucial to the performance of deaf readers. It may seem reasonable to study younger deaf readers, for example, 11-year-olds, who are reading on grade level compared to hearing children. However, at these lower levels of achievement, it is not possible to rule out that these children are leveling off before reaching levels of sight-word performance that would be considered competent. The uncertainty associated with this possible leveling off is avoided by studying readers performing at the post-high school level. Once the nature and role of phonological knowledge are determined with more mature readers, then longitudinal studies can turn to mapping the trajectory of development with younger readers.

Orthographic Knowledge

Orthographic competence allows a person to recognize words based on what their letters look like, that is, without resorting to sounding out the words intentionally and methodically. Referring to hearing readers, Cunningham et al. (2002) observed that "the ability to form, store, and access orthographic representations may be able to account for some of the residual variance in word recognition skills not explained by phonological factors" (p. 186). The importance of this largely visual faculty is intuitively compelling for deaf readers because many rely on specialized attention to visual detail and on the identification of visual patterns during face-to-face conversations in sign language and during speechreading.

Orthographic knowledge can occur at the lexical and the sublexical levels. Readers who are proficient in lexical orthographic competence are able to recognize a relatively large number of words as sight words. Again, according to research by Cunningham et al. (2002) and Share (1999), a word becomes represented as one that is recognized automatically not because of repeated visual scrutiny, but rather through visual scrutiny combined with phonological analysis. The research with hearing readers suggests that lexical-level orthographic reading of a word results in activation of its phonological representation, which leads in turn to activation of its meaning. Thus, orthographic reading is not necessarily an entirely visual process.

Another kind of orthographic knowledge is that which is sublexical, and this extends beyond familiarity with specific words. Readers can store knowledge of salient English letter patterns that, in theory, can be deployed in order to represent new words and activated in order to recognize words that are already in the lexicon. According to Rapp (1992), recurring patterns that may be noticed and applied to word recognition include morphemes, which are meaning-based. They can also include syllables, onset and rime, and word body; these are elements most closely associated with spoken language. Other sublexical patterns are those that manifest a salience that is more visual in nature, and these can include consonant clusters and vowel clusters.

The salience of visual orthographic patterns can be affected by "single-letter positional frequency" (how often a certain letter tends to appear in a certain serial position within words) and "bigram frequency" (how often two particular letters tend to be adjacent to each other in English words). Through experience, readers come to recognize some letter patterns as more word-like than others. Siegel, Share, and Geva (1995) measured knowledge of sublexical English letter patterns through a word-likeness task in which readers selected which of two letter strings (e.g., *filv* or *filk*) were more word-like. Combinations of two letters that rarely appear together in English syllables, "bigram troughs," have been theorized to be the bases for making syllable divisions within words. For example, in the word *anvil*, two bigrams are high frequency, *an* (289) and *vi* (324), while *nv* is a bigram trough with a frequency of only 5 according to counts in the Kucera and Francis

(1967) corpus of 1 million words, as reported in Rapp (1992). As another instance of a potentially salient orthographic pattern, the two exterior letters of a word may be especially helpful to its recognition (Jordan, Thomas, Patching, & Scott-Brown, 2003). Word recognition also can be affected by the visual distinctiveness (rarity) of a word's shape as it is formed by the configuration of the ascending, descending, or neutral orientations of its constituent letters (Lete & Pynte, 2003).

The ability to induce orthographic patterns such as these has been linked by Bowers and Wolf (1993) to performance on the rapid automatized naming task. Slow naming of familiar items on a list, such as letters or digits, may signal disruption of these processes and explain difficulty inducing orthographic patterns. These findings constitute further evidence that the visual aspects of words can be instrumental to word recognition and could be particularly so for readers highly attuned to the visual channel, such as those who are deaf.

Orthographic Knowledge and Deaf Readers

There has not been an abundance of research on the orthographic knowledge of deaf readers, even though the primarily visual component of this processing links it strongly to their visual orientation. A number of studies did find evidence of orthographic/visual processing as being predominant in younger deaf readers. Harris and Moreno (2004) administered the word-likeness task of Siegel et al. (1995) (*filk–filv*) to two groups of deaf students, one an average of 8 years of age and the other an average of 14 years, 2 months old. For both groups of deaf subjects, orthographic performance predicted reading age, indicating the relative importance of a visual strategy for processing words. Dyer et al. (2003) examined the performance of deaf children (average age 13 years) related to rapid automated naming (RAN), which Bowers and Wolf (1993) have linked to the ability to induce salient letter patterns. RAN results indicated that the deaf subjects were as fast as chronological-age controls and faster than reading-age controls, suggesting that they did not face obstacles to detection of orthographic patterns. Results from the Merrills et al. (1994) study of deaf children between the ages of 11 and 15 suggest that subjects relied on visual information, although it was relatively slow and inaccurate.

These combined results are in accord with the studies of the phonological knowledge of young deaf readers. The latter work found minimal phonological knowledge among subjects, so it stands to reason that young deaf readers would rely more on visual information, as the studies of orthography show. It must be noted, however, that the pro-

nounced reliance on orthographic information was clearly not sufficient for effective reading, because the reading comprehension of the
subjects in these studies was as uniformly deficient as it was in the studies of phonological knowledge.

Studies of more mature deaf readers examined both lexical and
sublexical orthographic knowledge. Hanson (1995) found some evidence of relatively developed lexical-level orthographic competence in
more mature college deaf readers, and this may have contributed to
their relatively high reading ability, which, on the average, was a grade
equivalent of 11 years, 7 months. Hanson (1986) also examined the
sublexical orthographic knowledge of deaf college students classified
with either good or poor speech, and found that those with good
speech skills were more sensitive to legal and illegal letter patterns.
In another study of sublexical orthographic knowledge, Olson and
Nickerson (2001) examined whether deaf readers were sensitive to
speech-based syllable boundaries in spite of their limited access to
speech, or whether they would tend to divide words based on their sensitivity to the orthographic pattern studied by Rapp (1992), the bigram
trough. The investigators hypothesized that deaf readers, because of
their relative isolation from English phonology, would tend to divide
words based on visual, orthographic considerations. The findings indicated that subjects were not sensitive to the bigram trough as a location
where words ought to be divided. Subjects were college age and their
mean reading grade equivalent was 6.5, so it is unknown whether
highly skilled deaf readers may be sensitive to the bigram trough.
These initial studies suggest the importance of orthographic knowledge to deaf readers, but they also indicate a clear need for a systematic
research effort in the future.

Future Research on Deaf Readers' Orthographic Processing

There are questions that remain unanswered related to deaf readers'
orthographic knowledge at both the lexical and sublexical levels. At the
lexical level, the research does not yet show whether deaf readers who
are highly skilled at comprehending text are also highly skilled readers
of sight words. In order to show whether lexical-level orthographic
knowledge is indeed a key element in the skill repertoire of accom-
plished deaf readers, there is a need for a research design that includes
a comparison group of hearing readers matched on comprehension
ability and then measures speed and accuracy of recognition of known
sight words. Caution needs to be taken in applying existing measures of
lexical orthographic knowledge, such as those presented by Olson et al.
(1994), because those techniques place a premium on phonological

competence, which could either artificially inflate or diminish performance depending on subject hearing status, thus complicating interpretation of results.

We do not know conclusively the importance of lexical orthographic knowledge to deaf readers, and, even more so, the research has not revealed the kind and amount of processing that is required to represent a given word so that it is recognized as a sight word. Research simply showing the number of exposures needed for sight-word learning to occur would be of some value. A related question is whether and how long apparent learning at the time of initial training tends to endure. More useful would be research showing the kind of processing that is needed in order to achieve the enduring representation of sight words in the lexicon. Does it result from the application of sublexical orthographic knowledge? For hearing readers, the analytical processing that results in sight-word representations appears to be phonological in nature (e.g., Cunningham et al., 2002; Ehri & Saltmarsh, 1994; Share, 1999). Whether phonological processing is the route to lexical orthographic learning for skilled deaf readers, however, we still do not know.

As part of this research effort, it needs to be determined whether the word-learning mechanisms used by deaf readers may differ qualitatively depending on their reading competence and development. Among hearing readers, Ehri (1994) has noted that children make a qualitative change in how they represent words once they acquire the alphabetic principle and stop trying to represent words based on some isolated distinguishing visual feature. This invites the question of whether deaf readers on the path to competence make a similar transition in their processing mechanisms, or do they simply use one single strategy throughout the course of their lexical development?

In this chapter we have repeatedly referred to the prospect that skilled deaf readers may deploy sublexical orthographic patterns to foster their learning of new words as well as to activate those words when encountered in the future. This implies that if hearing readers use sublexical phonological patterns to sound out new words and then activate them later, then deaf readers who are skilled orthographically apply their knowledge of salient letter patterns in order to "sight out" words when they are initially encountered, forming representations in the lexicon that are amenable to activation as sight words when seen in the future. It is reasonably clear how the process of sounding out words serves the learning efforts of hearing children: by gaining command of letter–sound correspondences they can translate the nonlinguistic data of print into the form of highly familiar speech. However, we have not specified the familiar form into which deaf readers convert print after they have gained reasonable command of many useful letter patterns. Thus, this is an area that requires both thought and research.

At this point, we do not know whether adroit use of recurring letter patterns is a mechanism that does result in sight-word learning among deaf readers, and thus we do not know the letter patterns that are truly salient and conducive to the kind of learning that enables fluent activation of meaning when reading a known word. It is likely that the research conducted with hearing readers related to the privileged status of exterior letters (Jordan et al., 2003), the salience of word shape (Lete & Pynte, 2003), and the distinctiveness of the bigram trough (Rapp, 1992) will provide useful guidance regarding which visual aspects of words are most helpful in word recognition by deaf readers. Just as we do not know the letter patterns that are salient, research also has not learned how salient patterns are noticed and added to a deaf reader's repertoire, in a way analogous to the differentiation of phonemes by hearing children. The rarity of skilled deaf readers suggests that no matter how this acquisition of knowledge does occur, for the average deaf reader it will not happen spontaneously. This indicates the need for research on instructional techniques that will make this information routinely accessible to the many deaf learners who struggle with reading.

POSSIBLE ALTERNATE SOURCES OF COMPREHENSION PROBLEMS

It is highly likely that many deaf readers also experience deficits related to other aspects of competence that are critical to successful comprehension, and that skilled deaf readers enjoy a significant advantage in these same areas. We believe, however, that addressing these areas instructionally will be futile while word recognition remains weak, and also that, in some ways, problems in these areas may actually stem from word recognition deficits. We believe, moreover, that insights related to the word recognition of skilled deaf readers have a higher potential to inform the larger field of reading comprehension research than do those related to these alternate sources of comprehension problems.

Syntactic Knowledge

The text comprehension problems of deaf readers stem partly from their difficulties analyzing the syntactic relations among the words in various kinds of English sentences. Quigley, Wilbur, Power, Montanelli, and Steinkamp (1976) found distortions of meaning that can occur because many deaf readers possess only limited knowledge related to certain syntactic structures, such as those of passive-voice sentences and sentences that contain relative clauses. For example, upon reading the passive-voice sentence "The boy was hit by the girl," many deaf readers would conclude that the boy was guilty of the violence. After reading the relative clause sentence "The boy who kissed the girl ran away," many deaf readers would wrongly identify the girl as the one who took flight. More recently, Kelly (2003b) found that deaf readers who were skilled comprehenders of extended text also demonstrated significantly better comprehension of relative clause sentences than did average deaf readers, even though the groups demonstrated virtually equal comprehension when reading control sentences written in less complex syntax and composed of exactly the same content words. The implication is that accurate processing of sentence-level syntax distinguishes deaf readers who demonstrate high levels of comprehension when reading larger texts.

Kelly (1996) found that, as a consequence of limited syntactic knowledge, deaf readers are unable to capitalize fully on their vocabulary knowledge to aid text comprehension. Specifically, for the adolescent deaf readers in the study, those in the highest quartile of syntactic performance demonstrated a relationship between word knowledge and text comprehension—a correlation of .70—that was double that demonstrated in the lower three quartiles. In other words, readers at the higher levels of syntactic knowledge were better able to make meaningful connections among known words than were those at the lower levels of syntactic competence. Beyond distortions of sentence meaning stemming from limited syntactic knowledge, Kelly (1998, 2003b) found that syntactic processing by deaf readers with low text comprehension can be very slow, intentional, and labor-intensive, and he concluded that this lack of automaticity likely diverts cognitive resources needed for text-level comprehension. It is also likely that an extended experience of successful reading comprehension may improve syntactic performance.

There are multiple explanations offered for the nonstandard syntactic knowledge that leads to text comprehension problems. Most obviously, deaf readers encounter very limited opportunity to use and practice English syntax in face-to-face communication because the conventions of American Sign Language, the version most common in the United States, differ significantly from those of English. Regarding these differences, Charrow (1981) observed:

> ASL lacks many of the features that make English what it is: articles, plural markers, tense markers, certain prepositions, passives, heavy use of subor-

dinate clauses. . . . ASL has many syntactic features that English lacks: simultaneous signs, tense and number inflections on time words, inflections for habitualness, the repetition of action, the ability to "spatialize" . . . and many others. (p. 112)

With differences like these in mind, Goldberg, Ford, and Silverman (1982) observed from their perspectives as highly experienced teachers of English composition to deaf students that ASL interferes with the acquisition of correct English because its forms are so remote from English.

The interplay between American Sign Language and English also has been advanced as a source of the syntactic difficulties of deaf readers and writers. Charrow (1981) and more recently Bragg and Channon (2005) have argued that there exists a "Deaf English," although the forms of this language have not yet been clearly defined. They argued that these forms result from the interaction of the conventions of ASL and English. In support of a nonstandard "competence" that is rather stable and thus resistant to instruction, Quigley, Power, and Steinkamp (1977) observed that there are "distinct syntactic structures, apparently rule ordered, that appear consistently and persistently in the language comprehension and production of deaf subjects" (p. 79).

Other factors that may contribute to syntactic limitations were alluded to in the earlier discussion of hearing loss and the consequent difficulty of developing an adequate lexicon of English words. For one thing, phrasal grouping of words and special sentence forms, such as questions, are accompanied and reinforced in speech by aspects of prosody, like intonation and rhythmic structure of the utterances, for which the acoustic information is not easily accessible to many deaf readers. The earlier discussion of word recognition problems also is relevant to syntax. If, as we have argued, many deaf readers face serious obstacles to representing a critical mass of words in their lexicons, then it will be enormously difficult for them to recognize and apply the conventional patterns for combining words in ways that are meaningful and grammatical. They simply will not have enough words to work with syntactically.

To conclude the discussion of the possible causes of deaf readers' syntactic problems, there has been comment in the research literature that comprehension problems that appear to be syntax-related may actually stem from more basic deficiencies. Lilo-Martin, Hanson, and Smith (1992), for example, found that low levels of sentence comprehension can occur even when deaf readers demonstrate appreciable knowledge of relative clause sentences *in sign language*. They speculate that low comprehension when reading printed relative clause sentences is a consequence of processing difficulties stemming from a phonological-processing deficit. These findings are in accord with earlier work (e.g., Smith, Macaruso, Shankweiler, & Crain,1989) linking poor hearing readers' phonological and syntactic processing deficits, discussed in this volume by Oakhill and Cain (Chapter 2).

Efforts to help deaf readers improve their syntactic knowledge have been both direct and indirect. Kelly, Saulnier, and Stamper (2000) reported significant gains in comprehension of relative clause and passive-voice sentences when conventional workbook practice was combined with the entertainment appeal and unambiguous meaning of Keystone Kop silent films. There was also evidence, however, that the improved comprehension came at the cost of slow, intentional analysis of target sentences, the kind of resource-dependent language processing that can jeopardize text-level comprehension while reading larger passages.

An indirect method of attempting to improve syntactic performance is Repeated Reading, a method developed by Dowhower (1987). According to this approach, students read texts multiple times to improve fluency. Ensor and Koller (1997) have been partially successful using this method with deaf readers. The method does seem to improve reading fluency, but this improvement in reading rate does not result from more automatic word recognition, according to Kuhn and Stahl (2000) in their review of the method's use with hearing readers. Kelly (2003a) reasoned that Repeated Reading may improve fluency because its conditions may be conducive to detection and practice of syntactic patterns. According to this line of thinking, repeated reading of the words in practice texts increases familiarity with them and frees processing resources ordinarily needed for word recognition, allowing investment of additional attention in the detection and practice of syntactic patterns. This reasoning is a reminder that for any method of teaching syntactic knowledge to be successful, the learner will require a reasonably well-developed lexicon.

Discourse Comprehension

Chamberlain and Mayberry (2000) identify another kind of competence that may be critical to the performance of skilled deaf readers, one that is an element of the "simple view" of reading proposed by Hoover and Gough (1990). Many thought processes critical to reading comprehension can be demonstrated in face-to-face communication by people who cannot read. These processes include noting salient details, drawing inferences, analyzing, synthesizing, and evaluating. In their two-component simple view, Hoover and Gough (1990) refer to competent face-to-face comprehension as "linguistic comprehension" when the listener takes lexical-level information and derives sentence- and discourse-level interpretation from it. The second of the two components is decoding, that is, when a reader converts letter strings into lexical information. According to Hoover and Gough (1990), decoding and linguistic competence are interactive (in their language, "multiplicative") in their contributions to reading comprehension; if either aspect of competence is deficient, the contribution of the other to reading performance will be correspondingly limited. In order for reading comprehension to be at a high level, both decoding and discourse comprehension must be well developed.

Within discourse comprehension we also include world knowledge, a person's fund of the kind of cultural information described by Hirsch (1987) as contributing significantly to reading comprehension. Listeners, signers, and readers can more effectively navigate convoluted syntax, arcane vocabulary, abstract conceptualizations, and even flawed discourse itself if they enjoy in-depth knowledge of the topic. For example, normally mediocre readers with a passion for bird watching may demonstrate exceptional comprehension of a challenging passage about the intricacies of "one good tern," while performing quite poorly on a valid standardized measure of reading ability. At the same time, readers who score high on standardized measures may read haltingly and with relatively limited comprehension when the topic is foreign to them.

Hoover and Gough (1990) found a correlation between face-to-face listening comprehension and reading comprehension to be .46 for first graders, increasing to .71, .80, and .87 for 2nd, 3rd, and 4th graders, respectively. They concluded that as decoding competence increased in each successive grade, the contribution of linguistic (discourse) comprehension to reading comprehension became progressively greater.

Chamberlain and Mayberry (2000) have applied the simple view of reading as a framework for considering the comprehension of deaf readers, and they have shown some evidence that the skilled performance of deaf readers stems partly from discourse competence in sign language. Studies reported in Chamberlain and Mayberry (2000) showed correlations between the sign language comprehension and reading comprehension of deaf readers that were similar to those reported by Hoover and Gough (1990) for hearing readers. For the deaf readers, the correlations between reading and signing comprehension ranged from .43 to .80 (excluding one correlation reported by Moores et al., 1987, which was not significant). Aware of findings such as these, Kuntz (2006) called for educators of deaf children to "see literacy with new eyes," and asserted that discourse skills used in signing are critical to reading comprehension.

Discourse comprehension during signing may well be influential in the comprehension of deaf readers, because there is evidence that the prevalence of deficient reading comprehension noted earlier is matched by the prevalence of conditions that are not conducive to acquisition of discourse skills in sign language. In their report of a survey involving over 20,000 deaf children, Mitchell and Karchmer (2005) indicate that in homes where both parents were hearing (79% of the sample), the percentage who reported regularly using signing in the home was only approximately 26%. Chamberlain and Mayberry (2000) may understate the prevalence, if not the nature of the problem, when they observe, "Indeed, some deaf children may have limited experience with discourse beyond a rudimentary level in any language as a consequence of impoverished opportunities for discourse exchanges with adults and peers; an inability to comprehend narration on a face-to-face basis may contribute significantly to their reading difficulties" (p. 246).

In considering the importance of discourse comprehension to reading comprehension, as suggested by the correlations seen earlier, it is also worth noting that it is not clear what the direction of influence is between discourse and reading comprehension. It is entirely plausible that early partial achievement in reading comprehension could foster refinements in thinking and the acquisition of substantive new knowledge that could result in higher level face-to-face comprehension. It is also important to return to the Hoover and Gough (1990) premise that the contribution of discourse skill to reading comprehension is enormously dependent on word-decoding competence, that is, automatic word recognition. As long as a deaf reader faces the obstacles to word recognition described earlier in this chapter, then even well-developed discourse skill will be of limited help to reading comprehension.

Comprehension Strategies

It could be that a potentially useful approach to helping average deaf readers achieve a high level of reading comprehension is to train them to read strategically. A strategic approach to reading takes into account the cognitive resources of the reader as well as the cognitive demands of the task, and deploys available resources in a manner that meets the challenges of the task in order to maximize comprehension. Comprehension strategies can include monitoring comprehension during reading, surveying a text in advance of reading to get its gist, or generating prior questions that the text will likely answer. The research focused on deaf readers' comprehension strategies appears to be principally of two types: either studies that examine deaf readers' spontaneous use of reading strategies, or those that examine attempts to stimulate strategy use.

Turning first to those that attempted to determine deaf readers' spontaneous use of strategies, it should be noted that those strategies used by typical deaf readers are not likely to achieve effective reading comprehension, given the prevalent low levels of comprehension reported earlier. Kelly, Albertini, and Shannon (2001) found that college-age deaf readers professed a better understanding of what they read than they were able to demonstrate. In other words, their strategic comprehension monitoring was deficient, a finding consistent with the theory of Kruger and Dunning (1999) that people who are relatively unskilled at certain tasks tend to overestimate their ability. Schirmer (1993) found that whether a story was well formed or not tended to affect the elaboration strategies that deaf children used when commenting on the story. Schirmer, Bailey, and Schirmer-Lockman (2004) tested the use of verbal protocols to identify deaf children's reading, and found evidence of comprehension monitoring. Walker, Munro, and Rickards (1998) found that deaf readers demonstrated the strategic flexibility to respond effectively to both literal and inferential questions in three different kinds of texts, although their performance was lower than hearing controls at each age level tested.

There is evidence from a study by Kelly (1995) that average deaf readers (i.e., third-grade reading level) without prompting do make use of their world knowledge when they are reading comprehensible texts. Average high school-age deaf students also read with significantly greater speed and comprehension when they read about familiar topics compared to those that were unfamiliar. The same was true of skilled deaf readers in the study, who were reading at a level comparable to same-age hearing readers. While it is not likely that the average readers in this study enjoyed world knowledge that in any way approached the reserves of the skilled readers, it can be said that they tended to make spontaneous use of the prior knowledge that was available to them. In addition, the less-skilled readers also seemed to spontaneously retrieve information learned in earlier parts of the text in order to facilitate processing. The evidence supporting this was that the reading speed of the average readers declined significantly when an experimental manipulation temporarily purged subjects' working memory of information from prior text. (Without warning they were required to solve an arithmetic problem before returning to the reading passage.) Again, the low comprehension of so many deaf readers suggests that the facilitation stemming from use of prior text information is not adequate for supporting effective comprehension.

The other category of studies related to reading strategies includes those that investigated intentional efforts to foster deaf readers' use of comprehension strategies. Most of this research, however, does not address whether any improvements in comprehension extended to passages that were not part of training exercises conducted by the teacher or experimenter. Schirmer and Woolsey (1997), for example, found that deaf children are able to analyze, synthesize, and evaluate text information even when the teacher does not first elicit information related to story details. Al-Hilawani (2003) found that three different teacher approaches to orchestrating class reading of a text (the key word approach, the modified reciprocal teaching approach, and the basic reading approach) produced differential effects regarding understanding of classroom passages. Similarly, Jackson, Paul, and Smith (1997) found that different types of probes for eliciting prior knowledge affected deaf readers' ability to answer comprehension questions about text-explicit and text-implicit information. Schirmer (1995) found that using mental imagery as a metacognitive strategy stimulated productive modes of thinking while reading the classroom materials.

What these studies have in common is a failure to investigate whether the strategic manipulations of the teachers produced changes in the reader strategies that carried over to the comprehension of future passages read without teacher assistance. A departure from this is a study by Kelly et al. (2001) who found that "strategy review instruction" improved comprehension of a posttraining passage for one portion of their sample, namely, those with relatively high reading ability.

The failure of strategy instruction to improve the comprehension of the less-able deaf readers in the Kelly et al. (2001) study is not surprising in light of interactive theories of reading processes. There is research indicating that less-skilled deaf readers do not have an abundance of disposable cognitive resources to be strategically managed in the service of reading comprehension. Research by Kelly (2003b), for example, found that less-skilled deaf readers demonstrated significantly lower automaticity during reading than did those with high levels of comprehension. By definition, low automaticity indicates completion of a task in a manner that is resource-dependent, and if resources are depleted by certain obligatory basic reading tasks, like word recognition and syntactic processing, then minimal resources will be available to invest in higher level comprehension operations. Although instruction in reading strategies may help deaf readers to a certain extent, if automaticity of word recognition is low, the contribution to improved comprehension will not be substantial.

EDUCATIONAL IMPLICATIONS

The previous sections indicate that typical deaf readers do face multiple obstacles to reading comprehension, impediments that may represent resources for the minority of deaf readers who comprehend at a high level. These discussions also suggest, however, that deficient word recognition may be responsible for difficulties developing syntactic knowledge and applying discourse or strategic knowledge. These constitute additional reasons to consider fluent word recognition to be the most pressing instructional need of deaf children.

Gough (1996) suggests that for hearing children, the usual sequence is to acquire phonemic awareness, to learn letter–phoneme correspondences and some of the rules governing them, and then to embark as an independent reader in order to induce over time the regularities of phonology, rules that "must number in the hundreds or even thousands" (p. 13). Because the alphabet represents the phonemes of speech, which these children have been using successfully for years prior to starting to read, they are capitalizing on a strength. It is important to reemphasize that the alphabet is related to speech in a manner that is systematic, and, equally important, speech ordinarily is a highly developed, automatized skill. For deaf children at the age when reading normally begins, processing of phonology is far from a strength; indeed, it is a pronounced weakness. Their representations of the English phonemes are impoverished, and, as a consequence, their lexicons of phonologically represented words are small. What are their alternatives for developing rapid word recognition?

Rather than struggle with limited phonological knowledge early in their reading development, it may be that young deaf readers must turn to a paired-associate/logographic approach to learning words. Their development of a repertoire of some hundreds or even thousands of words learned this way may provide the lexicon necessary to begin acquiring phonological knowledge. It is not likely that the acquisition of phonological forms will arise spontaneously from a rudimentary vocabulary. In order to overcome the obstacles described earlier, it will require intervention at least as concentrated as what Shaywitz (2003) described to be necessary for dyslexic hearing readers. However, because of the field's lack of a successful track record, it is not clear what form these interventions ought to take. As the earlier discussion of the effects of hearing loss on phonological knowledge suggests, multiple avenues of information are potentially involved, and, depending on a person's hearing loss profile, each of these may be the focus of productive instruction. However, given that phonological knowledge might not be a particular asset to learning words at the outset of learning to read, it may be that early instructional planning might defer introduction of phonological awareness as an instructional objective until some useable lexicon has been developed, even if it is based on a logographic, paired-associate learning strategy.

While the need to develop a rudimentary vocabulary prior to development of phonological knowledge might require young deaf readers to learn words initially as intact, unanalyzed letter combinations, it is not likely that such paired-associate learning will be the long-term route to skilled sight-word reading. The comprehension of many deaf readers levels off at approximately the third- or fourth-grade level, and this may be a consequence of never deviating from a strategy for learning words that uses an exclusively paired-associate method. As each new word is added to the lexicon, memory of those learned previously becomes more difficult, and the addition of new words with spellings similar to those of existing vocabulary increases the chances of confusions. These burdens on memory place limits on the size of the vocabulary available for use during reading.

Another possible strategy for developing the beginnings of a lexicon is to associate a word as an intact unit with either the manual sign for the word or the finger-spelled version of the word. Sign language and finger spelling are both indispensable for communication, language development, and instruction, and they may participate in some way in the learning and representation of printed words by skilled deaf readers. But any strategy that relies exclusively on making connections between unanalyzed words and either the manual sign for the word or its finger-spelled version is not likely to lead to skillful sight-word reading, even though both signing and finger spelling appear to qualify as systems that are as familiar to deaf readers as speech is to hearing readers.

For many deaf readers, manual sign language is a well-learned system that is part of their linguistic profiles, and this may invite speculation that sight words might be learned by associating them with the commonly accepted sign for the word. However, associating the letters of a word with its corresponding sign imposes the same memory burden as associating a word's pronunciation with its unanalyzed letters. The combinations of letters that make up printed words simply are not related systematically to the signs for those words. Thus, it is not possible to convert the printed letters of a word into a sign for the word or into the phonemes of the sign for the word. For example, the signs for the words *tops, spot,* and *pots* are quite different from each other even though the three words share exactly the same letters and phonemes. It is possible to learn the printed word that corresponds to the generally accepted sign for that word, but there is no systematic relationship between the two; it is simply another instance of paired-associate learning that is vulnerable to the limitation of memory, posing an ever greater obstacle to word recognition performance as the list of known words increases.

It is possible to finger-spell any word that appears in print because there is a separate hand shape for each letter of the alphabet. Instances of finger spelling do occur with some regularity in face-to-face communication, so this is a system that is well known by deaf readers, inviting consideration that finger spelling could be a resource that would allow learning of sight words. However, the predominant way that the manual alphabet relates systematically to printed words is the same way that the printed alphabet does, and that is as a representation of the phonemes of spoken English. The letters of the finger-spelled alphabet may be well known, just as the letters of the printed alphabet may be well known, but the manual alphabet is just an alternate version of the printed alphabet, which is only a surrogate for the phonemes of spoken English. Unless the finger-spelled word can be translated into the phonemes of the word, then it must be remembered through its sign or perhaps a picture that depicts what it means, presenting the same burden on memory as paired-associate learning.

One of the studies conducted with older deaf readers suggests that phonological knowledge can develop as a result of an intervention with appropriate methods, intensity, and duration. It is possible that this learning can occur relatively early in life given the right conditions. The deaf subjects from the LaSasso et al. (2003) study who demonstrated the best rhyming skill and reading ability were those who had been long-time users of cued speech (CS), which may qualify as an intervention that is appropriate for helping deaf people acquire representations of English phonological forms. CS is described by LaSasso et al. (2003) as "a mode of communication for visually conveying traditionally spoken languages at the phonemic level" (p. 251). During conversations, CS "cuers" make use of eight different hand shapes positioned at one of four facial locations and combined with the mouth shapes made when a word is spoken in order to unambiguously convey all of the phonemes of English. Prior to the study, cuers in the LaSasso et al. research had been using CS as a method of face-to-face communication for at least 10 years and some for their entire lives. Thus, this experience likely fostered acquisition of English phonological forms, which may have contributed to their high level of reading comprehension. Just how early these readers developed phonological knowledge that aided their word recognition is not known. It must be pointed out that the noncuers in this study also were comprehending text at a post-high school level, and they demonstrated over 80% accuracy on the rhyming task that tapped phonological competence. CS is apparently not the only route to competence related to phonology and comprehension.

FINAL COMMENTS

To conclude this chapter, we return to the fact that printed English is alphabetic, and readers are at a distinct disadvantage if they cannot capitalize on the patterns of English phonology in order to learn words initially and activate the meanings of familiar words. Phonological patterns are, however, not the only ones present among the letters of printed English. But theory about the induction and application of patterns that are orthographic in nature has been tested with only a fraction of the empirical research devoted to the examination of phonological knowledge. The availability of deaf people who are skillful readers thus represents a distinct opportunity to refine our understanding of how both orthography and phonology participate in word recognition, and this may be an instance of reciprocal illumination between research with deaf readers and the larger field of reading research.

It is entirely possible that the reading of skilled deaf readers does depend on application of well-developed phonological knowledge. Phonological knowledge was evident in the performance of relatively mature deaf readers who are skilled, suggesting that this type of knowledge may contribute to the word recognition of skilled deaf readers. However, phonological knowledge as well as reading performance was limited in the younger deaf readers in the studies reviewed, and this suggests that phonology does not come into play at the outset of reading development. This is not surprising, given the obstacles to acquisition of phonology described earlier in this chapter. In order to determine conclusively whether phonological knowledge is enabling a skillful level of performance by deaf readers, the field needs research embodying the same thoroughness and ingenuity that characterizes investigations into the role of phonology with hearing readers. The need for a concerted research effort is not confined to this quarter.

If research on the use of phonology by deaf readers is a need, then work on their ability to induce orthographic patterns is a need that is urgent. Even the literature related to hearing readers' use of orthographic knowledge is still rather limited, and discussions are rather abstract when describing precisely how orthographic patterns are detected, incorporated into the reader's repertoire, and then deployed to sight-out new words and activate the meanings of known words. Again, obstacles to the acquisition of phonological forms and a heavy reliance on the visual channel for communication suggest that if an instrumental, if not predominant, role for orthography is to be found anywhere, it will be among skilled deaf readers. Thus, research in this direction could make a distinct contribution to the knowledge base in the larger field of reading research. More importantly, it will bring us closer to finding ways to help the vast majority of deaf readers who struggle to comprehend written text.

ACKNOWLEDGMENTS

We are grateful to Robert C. Johnson and Elizabeth S. Parks for their valuable comments on earlier versions of this chapter.

REFERENCES

Al-Hilawani, Y. (2003). Clinical examination of three methods of teaching reading comprehension to deaf and hard-of-hearing students: From research to classroom applications. *Journal of Deaf Studies and Deaf Education*, *8*(2), 145–156.

Allen, T. (1986). *Understanding the scores: Hearing-impaired students and the Stanford Achievement Test* (7th ed.). Washington, DC: Gallaudet University, Gallaudet Research Institute, Center for Assessment and Demographic Studies.

Allington, R. (1980). Poor readers don't get to read much in reading groups. *Language Arts*, *57*(8), 872–876.

Auer, E., & Bernstein, L. (1997). Speechreading and the structure of the lexicon: Computationally modeling the effects of reduced phonetic distinctiveness on lexical uniqueness. *Journal of the American Acoustical Society*, *102*(6), 3704–3710.

Berent, I., & Perfetti, C. (1995). A rose is a REEZ: The two-cycles model of phonology assembly in reading English. *Psychological Review*, *102*(1), 146–184.

Bernstein L., Demorest, M., & Tucker, P. (2000). Speech perception without hearing. *Perception and Psychophysics*, *62*(2), 233–252.

Boothroyd, A. (1984). Auditory perception of speech contrasts by subjects with sensorineural hearing loss. *Journal of Speech and Hearing Research*, *27*(1), 134–144.

Bowers, P., & Wolf, M. (1993). Theoretical links among naming speed, precise timing mechanisms and orthographic skill in dyslexia. *Reading and Writing*, *5*(1), 69–85.

Bragg, L., & Channon, R. (2005, March). *Describing Deaf English*. Paper presented at the Conference on College Composition and Communication, San Francisco.

Carpenter, P., & Just, M. (1981). Cognitive processes in reading: Models based on readers' eye fixations. In A. Lesgold & C. Perfetti (Eds.), *Interactive processes in reading* (pp. 177–213). Hillsdale, NJ: Erlbaum.

Chamberlain, C., & Mayberry, R. (2000). Theorizing about the relation between American sign language and reading. In C. Chamberlain, J. Morford, & R. Mayberry (Eds.), *Language acquisition by eye* (pp. 221–259). Mahwah, NJ: Erlbaum.

Charrow, V. (1981). The written English of deaf adolescents. In M. F. Whiteman (Ed.), *Writing: The nature, development, and teaching of written communication: Vol. 1. Variation in writing* (pp. 179–188). Hillsdale, NJ: Erlbaum.

Cox, R., Matesich, J., & Moore, J. (1988). Distribution of short-term rms levels in conversational speech. *Journal of the Acoustical Society of America, 84*(3), 1100–1104.

Cunningham, A., Perry, K., Stanovich, K., & Share, D. (2002). Orthographic learning during reading: Examining the role of self-teaching. *Journal of Experimental Child Psychology, 82*(3), 185–199.

Dowhower, S. (1987). Effects of repeated reading on second-grade transitional readers' fluency and comprehension. *Reading Research Quarterly, 22*(4), 389–406.

Dyer, A., MacSweeny, M., Szczerbinski, M., Green, L., & Campbell, R. (2003). Predictors of reading delay in deaf adolescents: The relative contributions of rapid automatized naming speed and phonological awareness and decoding. *Journal of Deaf Studies and Deaf Education, 8*(3), 215–229.

Ehri, L. (1994). Development of the ability to read words: An update. In R. Ruddell, M. Rapp, & H. Singer (Eds.), *Theoretical models and processes of reading* (4th ed., pp. 323–358). Newark, DE: International Reading Association.

Ehri, L. (1997). Sight word learning in normal readers and dyslexics. In B. Blachman (Ed.), *Foundations of reading acquisition and dyslexia: Implications for early intervention* (pp. 163–189). Mahwah, NJ: Erlbaum.

Ehri, L., & Saltmarsh, J. (1995). Beginning readers outperform older disabled readers in learning to read words by sight. *Reading and Writing, 7*(3), 295–326.

Ehri, L., & Wilce, L. (1985). Movement into reading: Is the first stage of printed word learning visual or phonetic? *Reading Research Quarterly, 20*(2), 163–179.

Ensor, A., & Koller, J. (1997). The effect of the method of repeated readings on the reading rate and word recognition accuracy of deaf adolescents. *Journal of Deaf Studies and Deaf Education, 2*(2), 61–70.

Erber, N. (1979). Speech perception by profoundly hearing-impaired children. *Journal of Speech and Hearing Disorders, 44*, 255–270.

Fisher C. (1968). Confusions among visually perceived consonants. *Journal of Speech and Hearing Research, 11*, 796–804.

Gallaudet Research Institute. (1991). *Stanford Achievement Test, 8th edition: Hearing impaired norms booklet.* Washington, DC: Author.

Gallaudet Research Institute. (1996). *Stanford Achievement Test, 9th edition: Norms booklet for deaf and hard of hearing students.* Washington, DC: Author.

Gallaudet Research Institute. (2004). *Stanford Achievement Test: Norms booklet for deaf and hard of hearing students.* Washington, DC: Author.

Gallaudet Research Institute. (2005). *Regional and national summary report of data from the 2003–2004 Annual Survey of Deaf and Hard of Hearing Children and Youth.* Washington, DC: Author.

Goldberg, J. P., Ford, C., & Silverman, A. (1982, May). *Deaf students in ESL composition classes: Challenges and strategies.* Paper presented at the 16th Annual TESOL Convention, Honolulu.

Gough, P. (1996). How children learn to read and why they fail. *Annals of Dyslexia, 46*, 3–20.

Grant, K., Walden, B., & Seitz, P. F. (1998). Auditory–visual speech recognition by hearing-impaired subjects: Consonant recognition, sentence recognition, and auditory–visual integration. *Journal of the Acoustical Society of America, 103*(5), 2677–2690.

Hanson, V. (1986). Access to spoken language and the acquisition of orthographic structure: Evidence from deaf readers. *Quarterly Journal of Experimental Psychology A: Human Experimental Psychology, 38A*(2), 193–212.

Hanson, V. (1995). Linguistic influences on the spelling of ASL/English bilinguals. In L. Feldman (Ed.), *Morphological aspects of language processing* (pp. 211–224). Hillsdale, NJ: Erlbaum.

Hanson, V., & Fowler, C. (1987). Phonological coding in word reading: Evidence from hearing and deaf readers. *Memory and Cognition, 15*(3), 199–207.

Hanson, V., Goodell, E., & Perfetti, C. (1991). Tongue-twister effects in the silent reading of hearing and deaf college students. *Journal of Memory and Language, 30*(3), 319–330.

Hanson, V., Liberman, I., & Shankweiler, D. (1984). Linguistic coding by deaf children in relation to beginning reading success. *Journal of Experimental Child Psychology, 37*(2), 378–393.

Harcourt Assessment. (2003). *Stanford Achievement Test: Tenth edition.* San Antonio, TX: Harcourt Assessment.

Harris, M., & Moreno, C. (2004). Deaf children's use of phonological coding: Evidence from reading, spelling, and working memory. *Journal of Deaf Studies and Deaf Education, 9*(3), 254–268.

Hauser, P. (2000). *Deaf readers' phonological encoding: An electromyogram study of covert reading behavior.* Unpublished PhD dissertation, Gallaudet University, Washington, DC.

Hirsch, E. D. (1987). *Cultural literacy: What every American needs to know.* Boston: Houghton Mifflin.

Hoover, W. A., & Gough, P. B. (1990). The simple view of reading. *Reading and Writing, 2*(2), 127–160.

Izzo, A. (2002). Phonemic awareness and reading ability: An investigation with young readers who are deaf. *American Annals of the Deaf, 147*(4), 18–28.

Jackson, D., Paul, P., & Smith, J. (1997). Prior knowledge and reading comprehension ability of deaf adolescents. *Journal of Deaf Studies and Deaf Education, 2*(3), 172–184.

Jeffers J., & Barley M. (1971). *Speechreading (Lipreading)*. Springfield, IL: Thomas.

Jordan, T., Thomas, S., Patching, G., & Scott-Brown, K. (2003). Assessing the importance of letter pairs in initial, exterior, and interior positions in reading. *Journal of Experimental Psychology: Learning, Memory, and Cognition, 29*(5), 883–893.

Just, M., Carpenter, P., & Masson, M. (1982). *What eye fixations tell us about speed reading and skimming* (Technical Report). Pittsburgh, PA: Carnegie Mellon University.

Kelly, L. (1993). Recall of English function words and inflections by skilled and average deaf readers. *American Annals of the Deaf, 138*(3), 288–296.

Kelly, L. (1995). Processing of bottom-up and top-down information by skilled and average deaf readers and implications for whole language instruction. *Exceptional Children, 61*(4), 318–334.

Kelly, L. (1996). The interaction of syntactic competence and vocabulary during reading by deaf students. *Journal of Deaf Studies and Deaf Education, 1*(1), 75–90.

Kelly, L. (1998). Using silent motion pictures to teach complex syntax to adult deaf readers. *Journal of Deaf Studies and Deaf Education, 3*(3), 217–230.

Kelly, L. (2003a). Considerations for designing practice for deaf readers. *Journal of Deaf Studies and Deaf Education, 8*(2), 171–186.

Kelly, L. (2003b). The importance of processing automaticity and temporary storage capacity to the differences in comprehension between skilled and less skilled college-age deaf readers. *Journal of Deaf Studies and Deaf Education, 8*(3), 230–249.

Kelly, L., Saulnier, K., & Stamper, L. (2000). Lessons through laughter: Drilling without killing. *Odyssey: New Directions in Deaf Education, 2*(1), 26–27.

Kelly, R., Albertini, J., & Shannon, N. (2001). Deaf college students' reading comprehension and strategy use. *American Annals of the Deaf, 146*(5), 385–400.

Kruger, J., & Dunning, D. (1999). Unskilled and unaware of it: How difficulties in recognizing one's own incompetence lead to inflated self-assessments. *Journal of Personality and Social Psychology, 77*(6), 1121–1134.

Kucera, H., & Francis, W. (1967). *A computational analysis of present-day American English*. Providence, RI: Brown University Press.

Kuhn, M., & Stahl, S. (2000). *Fluency: A review of developmental and remedial practices* (State-of-the-Art Papers, Research Summaries, Reviews of the Literature on a Topic) (ERIC Document Reproduction Service No. ED438530).

Kuntz, M. (1998). Literacy and deaf children: The language question. *Topics in Language Disorders, 18*(4), 1–15.

Kuntz, M. (2006, March). *Seeing literacy with new eyes*. Paper presented at Revolutions in Sign Language Studies: Linguistics, Literature and Literacy, Washington, DC.

LaSasso, C., Crain, K., & Leybaert, J. (2003). Rhyme generation in deaf students: The effect of exposure to cued speech. *Journal of Deaf Studies and Deaf Education, 8*(3), 250–270.

Lete, B., & Pynte, J. (2003). Word-shape and word-lexical-frequency effects in lexical-decision and naming tasks. *Visual Cognition, 10*(8), 913–948.

Lillo-Martin, D., Hanson, V., & Smith, S. (1992). Deaf readers' comprehension of relative clause structures. *Applied Psycholinguistics, 13*(1), 13–30.

Massaro, D. (1998). *Perceiving talking faces: From speech perception to a behavioral principle*. Cambridge, MA: MIT Press/Bradford Books.

Matys, S., Bernstein, L., & Auer, E. (2002). Stimulus-based lexical distinctiveness as a general word-recognition mechanism. *Perception and Psychophysics, 64*(4), 667–679.

Merrills, J., Underwood, G., & Wood, D. (1994). The word recognition skills of profoundly, prelingually deaf children. *British Journal of Developmental Psychology, 12*(3), 365–384.

Mitchell, R., & Karchmer, M. (2005). Parental hearing status and signing among deaf and hard of hearing students. *Sign Language Studies, 5*(2), 231–244.

Monsen R. (1983). The oral speech intelligibility of hearing-impaired talkers. *Journal of Speech and Hearing Disorders, 48*(3), 286–296.

Moore, B. (1996). Perceptual consequences of cochlear hearing loss and their implications for the design of hearing aids. *Ear and Hearing, 17*(2), 133–161.

Moores, D., Kluwin, T., Johnson, R., Cox, P., Blennerhassett, L., Kelly, L., et al. (1987). *Factors predictive of literacy in deaf adolescents with deaf parents. Factors predictive of literacy in deaf adolescents in total communication programs* (Project No. NIH-NINCDS-83–19. Final Report to National Institute of Neurological and Communicative Disorders and Stroke). Washington, DC: Gallaudet Research Institute.

Olson, A., & Nickerson, J. (2001). Syllabic organization and deafness: Orthographic structure or letter frequency in reading? *Quarterly Journal of Experimental Psychology A: Human Experimental Psychology, 54A*(2), 421–438.

Olson, R., Forsberg, H., Wise, B., & Rack, J. (1994). Measurement of word recognition, orthographic, and phonological skills. In G. R. Lyon (Ed.), *Frames of reference for the assessment of learning disabilities: New views on measurement issues* (pp. 243–277). Baltimore: Brookes.

Quigley, S., Power, D., & Steinkamp, M. (1977). The language structure of deaf children. *Volta Review, 79*(2), 73–83.

Quigley, S., Wilbur, R., Power, D., Montanelli, D., & Steinkamp, M. (1976). *Syntactic structure in the language of deaf children*. Urbana: University of Illinois, Institute for Child Behavior and Development.

Rapp, B. (1992). The nature of sublexical orthographic organization: The bigram trough hypothesis examined. *Journal of Memory and Language, 31*(1), 33–53.

Reitsma, P. (1989). Orthographic memory and learning to read. In P. Aaron & R. Joshi (Eds.), *Reading and writing disorders in different orthographic systems* (pp. 51–73). New York: Kluwer Academic/Plenum Press.

Ronnberg, J., Samuelsson, S., & Lyxell, B. (1998). Conceptual constraints in sentence-based lipreading in the hearing-impaired. In R. Campbell, B. Dodd, & D. Burnham (Eds.), *Hearing by eye: Vol. 2: The psychology of speechreading and auditory–visual speech* (pp. 143–153). Hove, UK: Psychology Press.

Rumelhart, D. (1977). Toward an interactive model of reading. In S. Dornic (Ed.), *Attention and performance* (Vol. 6, pp. 573–603). Hillsdale, NJ: Erlbaum.

Schirmer, B. (1993). Constructing meaning from narrative text: Cognitive processes of deaf children. *American Annals of the Deaf*, *138*(5), 397–403.

Schirmer, B. (1995). Mental imagery and the reading comprehension of deaf children. *Reading, Research and Instruction*, *34*(3), 177–188.

Schirmer, B., Bailey, J., & Schirmer-Lockman, A. (2004). What verbal protocols reveal about the reading strategies of deaf students: A replication study. *American Annals of the Deaf*, *149*(1), 5–14.

Schirmer, B., & Woolsey, M. (1997). Effect of teacher questions on the reading comprehension of deaf children. *Journal of Deaf Studies and Deaf Education*, *2*(1), 47–56.

Share, D. (1995). Phonological recoding and self-teaching: The *sine qua non* of reading acquisition. *Cognition*, *55*(2), 151–218.

Share, D. (1999) Phonological recoding and orthographic learning: A direct test of the self-teaching hypothesis. *Journal of Experimental Child Psychology*, *72*(2), 95–129.

Shaywitz, S. (2003). *Overcoming dyslexia*. New York: Knopf.

Siegel, L., Share, D., & Geva, E. (1995). Evidence for superior orthographic skills in dyslexics. *Psychological Science*, *6*(4), 250–254.

Smith, S. T., Macaruso, P., Shankweiler, D., & Crain, S. (1989). Syntactic comprehension in young readers. *Applied Psycholinguistics*, *10*, 429–454.

Stanovich, K. (1980). Toward an interactive-compensatory model of individual differences in the development of reading fluency. *Reading Research Quarterly*, *16*, 32–71.

Stanovich, K., Nathan, R., & Zolman, J. (1988). The developmental lag hypothesis in reading: Longitudinal and matched reading-level comparisons. *Child Development*, *59*, 71–86.

Stanovich, K., & Siegel, L. (1994). Phenotype performance profile of children with reading disabilities: A regression-based test of the phonological-core variable difference model. *Journal of Educational Psychology*, *86*(1), 24–53.

Sterne, A., & Goswami, U. (2000). Phonological awareness of syllables, rhymes, and phonemes in deaf children. *Journal of Child Psychology and Psychiatry*, *41*(5), 609–626.

Sutcliffe, A., Dowker, A., & Campbell, R. (1999). Deaf children's spelling: Does it show sensitivity to phonology? *Journal of Deaf Studies and Deaf Education*, *4*(2), 111–123.

Van Orden, G. (1987). A ROWS is a ROSE: Spelling, sound, and reading. *Memory and Cognition*, *15*(3), 181–198.

Van Orden, G., Johnston, J., & Hale, B. (1988). Word identification in reading proceeds from spelling to sound to meaning. *Journal of Experimental Psychology: Learning, Memory, and Cognition*, *14*(3), 371–386.

Van Tasell, D. J. (1993). Hearing loss, speech, and hearing aids. *Journal of Speech and Hearing Research*, *36*(2), 228–244.

Walker, L., Munro, J., & Rickards, F. (1998). Literal and inferential reading comprehension of students who are deaf or hard of hearing. *Volta Review, 100*(2), 87–103.

Waters, G., & Doehring, D. (1990). The nature and role of phonological information in reading acquisition: Insights from congenitally deaf children who communicate orally. In T. Carr & B. Levy (Eds.), *Reading and its development: Component skills approaches* (pp. 323–373). San Diego: Academic Press.

Wauters, L. N., Van Bon, W., & Tellings, A. (2006). Reading comprehension of Dutch deaf children. *Reading and Writing, 19*(1), 49–76.

PART IV

Conclusions

CHAPTER 10

Cognitive Bases of Children's Language Comprehension Difficulties

Where Do We Go from Here?

KATE CAIN

JANE OAKHILL

In this volume we have brought together a collection that details the current state of knowledge about the written and spoken language problems experienced by different populations of children. This final chapter has several intentions. First, we want to offer a simple summary: We think it is important to draw together the main findings and common themes that emerge from the various chapters. Second, we intend to assess the theoretical implications of this body of work: How do the findings from different populations, using a diverse set of methodologies, inform models of written and spoken language comprehension and development? Third, we need to consider practical matters: What are the implications for educational practice and remediation? Essentially, how might this body of knowledge inform good (or better) practice? Fourth, our final intention is bound up in the other three: to stimulate future research that leads to a better understanding of the causes of comprehension failure and how best to remediate it.

MAIN FINDINGS AND COMMON THEMES

This collection demonstrates that language comprehension can pose significant problems for children diagnosed with what appear to be very distinct types of difficulty and disorder. Language comprehension problems are found in children with predominantly social cognition and communication difficulties such as children with autism spectrum disorders (ASD) and those with specific and pragmatic language impairment (SLI/PLI); in children characterized by behavioral impairments such as those with attention-deficit/hyperactivity disorder (ADHD); in children with sensory impairment or neurological injury; and even in children with no apparent diagnosed difficulty, such as children with specific comprehension problems. So our first question might be: Is there a common profile of language ability that emerges?

One answer to this question is "No": Some of the populations have impairments rooted at one level of language processing whereas others do not. Consider the example of word-reading skills, a topic considered by many authors and which we know might limit reading comprehension (Hoover & Gough, 1990; Oakhill & Cain, Chapter 1). The children with hearing impairment described by Kelly and Barac-Cikoja (Chapter 9) have pronounced word-reading difficulties, which may be the primary cause of their written language comprehension problems, whereas elevated word-reading ability forms part of the definition of the hyperlexia experienced by some of the children with ASD considered by Leekam (Chapter 4). The populations that were the focus of other chapters were selected to rule out word reading as an obvious cause of their poor reading comprehension. For example, the children with specific comprehension difficulties who were the subject of Cain and Oakhill's discussion (Chapter 2) were matched to peers for word-reading accuracy, as were the children with spina bifida myelomeningocele (SBM) in the studies described by Barnes, Johnston, and Dennis (Chapter 7). In a similar vein, Swanson, Howard, and Sáez (Chapter 6) compared two groups of poor comprehenders with learning disabilities (LD) in reading: those with and those without word-reading impairments. However, in other work it was noted that many children have poor comprehension *and* poor word reading, for example, children with SLI and children with PLI (Botting, Chapter 3). Thus, some poor comprehenders have word-reading difficulties and some do not.

It is not our purpose here to provide an exhaustive list of all the skills that were assessed in each chapter and to summarize performance on each one. We think it is more informative to consider whether or not there is a deficit common to these different populations. If we reword the question posed earlier to, "Is there a deficit found in each of these different populations?" we can answer "Yes." That common deficit is language comprehension failure and, with the exception of individuals with hearing impairment, these very different populations experience both written *and* spoken language comprehension deficits. Indeed, the work on children with ADHD conducted by Lorch, Berthiaume, Milich, and van den Broek (Chapter 5) has focused on the comprehension impairment itself and developed the televised viewing methodology to measure comprehension, rather than rely on the traditional assessments of reading and listening comprehension. Cook, Chapman, and Gamino's (Chapter 8) research on children with traumatic brain injury (TBI) has used discourse production as an index of language comprehension (see also the work on children with specific comprehension difficulties by Cain & Oakhill, Chapter 2).

Thus a main theme and a common finding is that language comprehension problems are not modality-specific: Children who experience difficulties understanding written text will usually experience similar problems understanding spoken discourse.

THEORETICAL IMPLICATIONS

We next consider the theoretical implications that arise from the similarities and differences in this collected research.

Implications for Models of Language Comprehension

First, we find substantial support for a model of reading ability, such as the simple view of reading (Hoover & Gough, 1990), which proposes that reading ability is the product of word-reading ability and listening comprehension. For children with hearing impairment, poor word-reading skills will overtax limited processing resources and lead to reading comprehension failure. For many of the other populations considered, children who have difficulties understanding extended tracts of written text will likely experience difficulties understanding spoken discourse as well. So when reading comprehension fails, the cause might not necessarily lie at the word-reading level: Comprehension of spoken language is often impaired as well.

Our own work on children with specific comprehension difficulties arose from the identification of reading comprehension difficulties in otherwise typically developing children. When researchers consider theoretical models of comprehension, they often talk about theories of *text* comprehension. One reason for this is that adequate comprehension of written text for educational purposes is a focus of a literate society. However, theories of comprehension do not distinguish between comprehension of written text or spoken discourse: The product is the same. The outcome of skilled comprehension is more than simply memory for the words and propositions in the text or discourse: it is a representation of a text's meaning that is coherent, integrated, and complete—a mental model (Johnson-Laird, 1983) or a situation model (Kintsch, 1998).

Children with comprehension problems do not produce accurate, coherent, or complete representations of meaning. For example, they do not always take context into account. As a result, they may interpret figurative expressions such as idioms, for example, "It's raining cats and dogs," in their literal sense, which has been seen in children with ASD, children with specific comprehension difficulties, and children with SBM. Children with poor comprehension often fail to generate inferences to go beyond the meanings of individual sentences, to link up ideas within a text, and to incorporate their own background knowledge to make full sense of the text. We see evidence of these specific difficulties in the work on children with ADHD by Lorch and colleagues (Chapter 5), among others (see also the chapters on children with SLI [Botting, Chapter 3], children with specific comprehension difficulties [Cain & Oakhill, Chapter 2], and children with SBM [Barnes et al., Chapter 7]). In essence, children with comprehension problems generally fail to represent the gist of the overall meaning of the text, as described in the work on TBI by Cook and colleagues (Chapter 8).

In addition, the processes necessary to construct this representation of meaning are the same for both written text and spoken discourse. This idea has been explored most fully in the literature on adults' comprehension. Gernsbacher has shown that adults with comprehension difficulties fail to build adequate representations of meaning for narratives presented in a range of modalities: written, spoken, and pictorial (see Gernsbacher, 1990, for a review of this work). Similarly, work reviewed in this volume has demonstrated that children with reading comprehension difficulties experience difficulties with the comprehension of spoken language in both conversational and narrative formats; see the chapters on ASD (Leekam, Chapter 4) and specific comprehension difficulties (Cain & Oakhill, Chapter 2), respectively. Many children also experience comprehension difficulties in other presentation formats, such as picture sequences (children with SLI) and televised narratives (children with ADHD). We would argue that it is the process of comprehension generally, rather than the process of understanding information presented in a specific modality, that fails. One implication is that we need to embrace this generality in our models of language comprehension.

Implications for Our Understanding of the Product and the Process of Comprehension

The construction of this meaning-based representation and the processes that support its construction is the focus of many chapters. Lorch and colleagues (Chapter 5) consider the central elements in the representation of a story's meaning: the types of causal relations among events and the overall structure of causal relations. Even children as young as 4 years of age are sensitive to the causal relations between story events: they are more likely to recall events that are causally connected to several events than events that have few antecedents or consequences. Children with ADHD do not show the same sensitivity to causality between story events as their peers. Similarly, Cook et al. (Chapter 8) find that children with TBI are less likely to include key information in their narratives and show impairments in the overall organization of episodic information. For these children, the ability to structure meaning appears to be qualitatively impaired.

Research on children with specific comprehension deficits reviewed by Cain and Oakhill (Chapter 2) has investigated particular skill deficits that might affect the construction of a meaning-based representation: inference and integration, monitoring, and knowledge of story structure. Inferences are necessary to construct a coherent representation of meaning, comprehension monitoring can alert the individual to the need to generate an inference, and explicit awareness about text structure can help the individual to invoke relevant background information and schemas to facilitate their construction of a meaning-based representation. These skills are impaired in children with specific comprehension problems (Cain & Oakhill, Chapter 2). Work with other populations supports the importance of these component skills: the inference, monitoring and discourse structure skills of children with SBM and children with ADHD are impaired, and children with SLI fail to generate the inferences necessary to fully understand a narrative. Thus, many of these populations have difficulties with the specific skills that aid the construction of an integrated and coherent representation of the meaning of a text or discourse.

Three chapters deal explicitly with the cognitive resources that might underpin these difficulties. Swanson's work has focused on the memory processes that might impair comprehension. As we have discussed, the construction of meaning-based representations involves more than simply storing word and sentence meanings: ideas have to be integrated, both within the text and from background knowledge. Swanson et al. (Chapter 6) have established that comprehension failures in children with learning disabilities are associated with information-processing deficits that affect the ability to store and process information simultaneously, for example, executive processing or working memory. Their deficit contrasts with that of children who experience both word-reading and reading comprehension difficulties. The latter group experience specific problems with storing information in short-term memory as a phonological code. Swanson et al. explain how the ability to coordinate processing resources can limit the ability to perform tasks such as inference, integration, and monitoring of comprehension, which are essential to building a representation of meaning. Their work is supported by the research on children with specific comprehension deficits (see Cain & Oakhill, Chapter 2).

Two other chapters discuss how limited information-processing capacity might impair specific comprehension processes related to building a representation of meaning. Barnes et al. (Chapter 7) have studied how comprehension in children with SBM might fail because of poor memory resources. Similar to Swanson's work with children with LD, Barnes et al. find that these children's short-term memory is intact, but they are impaired on memory tasks that tax working memory. Further, they find that comprehension difficulties of children with SBM are more pronounced on inference and comprehension-monitoring tasks when the information that has to be integrated is separated by several sentences in a text. Barnes et al. relate these findings to the process of constructing meaning-based representations of written and spoken text. The ability to use processing resources to manipulate and organize information during text comprehension is also discussed by Cook et al. (Chapter 8) as a factor in the comprehension difficulties of children who have experienced TBI. They emphasize the importance of memory systems that enable the integration of incoming information with that retrieved from long-term memory, to update the unfolding representation of meaning.

Another difficulty that might lead to written and spoken language comprehension difficulties is a failure to appreciate how language is used to convey meaning, which results in difficulties with the use and comprehension of language in *context*, rather than with structural or semantic aspects of language. Children with ASD have poor social cognition and pragmatic language difficulties. They often fail to take turns in conversation and to grasp the intended meaning in a conversation or text. Their problems with the pragmatics of language may go some way to explaining why the high-functioning individuals with ASD who can read often fail to fully understand the meaning of the text (see

Leekam, Chapter 4). Children with SLI are often noted for their structural language impairments. However, they, in common with children with ASD and also with children with PLI, often fail to understand the meaning intended by the writer or speaker (see Botting, Chapter 3). For example, they make inappropriate inferences and often interpret figurative expressions as literal, despite the inconsistency with the context. Both groups fail to use context to help with the interpretation of meaning. Other populations not noted for pragmatic language deficits have difficulties that can be related to use of context. For example, Barnes et al. (Chapter 7) describe how children with SBM are slower to suppress meanings of ambiguous words that are not relevant to the sentential context.

Implications for Theories of Comprehension Development

Unfortunately, we have much less to say about theories of comprehension development and how children acquire the ability to construct meaning-based representations. As we discussed in Chapter 1, evidence-based models of comprehension development are relatively incomplete, particularly when compared to our knowledge about the skills that promote the development of word-reading ability. Comprehension depends on many different cognitive skills, processes, and knowledge (Oakhill & Cain, Chapter 1). Research in the past two decades has come a long way in identifying the skills that facilitate skilled comprehension. The task now it to disentangle the relative contributions of each. To date, there are simply too few longitudinal studies with comparable measures to develop a full and accurate picture of which skills promote comprehension development and which skills simply develop alongside it. We also find that in some studies, the potentially important and interesting variables—notably, language measures—are relegated to the status of "control variables" (see Oakhill & Cain, Chapter 1, for further discussion of this point).

Nevertheless, we have a good body of knowledge on which to build and have established some key facts that should guide future research. First, there is an independence in the development of language skills: The skills that underpin word reading and reading comprehension are dissociated in many populations with reading comprehension difficulties (e.g., children with ASD, LD, PC, and SBM) and in the course of development (see Oakhill & Cain, Chapter 1). This finding provides strong evidence that the language comprehension skills common to understanding both written and spoken language are impaired in these populations. Second, and related to this point, is the fact that comprehension skills develop early: Basic spoken language skills support later reading comprehension skills. Evidence for this comes, for example, from the strong relation found between preschool assessments of narrative comprehension and later reading comprehension (see Oakhill & Cain, Chapter 1). We identify how we might use this knowledge in the next section.

PRACTICAL IMPLICATIONS

Educators and practitioners want to know what are the practical implications of these academic endeavors: How can we best remediate poor comprehenders? How do we prevent comprehension failure? In this section we consider possible causes of poor comprehension and we review suggestions for remediation and teaching that arise from the work in this volume.

Possible Causes of Language Comprehension Failure

One conclusion about the causes of poor comprehension that arises from this volume is not particularly satisfactory: Comprehension may fail for a variety of reasons. We must point out that most of the research discussed in this volume has been correlational in design and cannot establish the causes of poor comprehension (see Cain & Oakhill, Chapter 2, for a discussion of the methodologies used to identify causal relations). However, identification of skill strengths and weaknesses in the different populations is the foundation for research designed to identify causality.

There are similarities and differences in the language and cognitive profiles of these populations, and the similarities might provide some clues to causality. For example, some children appear to have a memory impairment, but the nature of this impairment is not the same for all populations. Children with SLI and PLI often have impaired storage capacity, whereas the other populations experience difficulties on memory tasks that tap both storage and processing. Children with SLI, PLI, and ASD have difficulties with the social use of language: it is not clear the extent to which these difficulties arise in other populations. Many children have specific problems with inference making (those with PC, SBM, and TBI); some also have difficulties with the recall of explicit information from text (those with ASD and SLI). As discussed earlier, some children may experience reading comprehension failure because of poor word-reading abilities, but others do not. In each chapter, it becomes clear that not just one skill is impaired in each population. As Oakhill and Cain (Chapter 1) demonstrated in their analysis of the research on comprehension development, comprehension of language is dependent on many aspects of knowledge, cognitive skills, and processes. Perhaps it is not surprising that many populations show several comprehension-related skill deficits.

Remediation of Comprehension Failure

The only population for whom a truly effective remedy might be found is the population of children with specific comprehension difficulties described by Cain and Oakhill (Chapter 2); by definition, if intervention works, they will no longer be defined by their comprehension failure. For other populations, successful comprehension intervention will not remedy the nature of the developmental disorder or fix the neurological injury. However, intervention can be used to teach strategies to support language comprehension, which may help children to circumvent their problems, if not to alleviate the underlying reason for comprehension failure. Thus, intervention can help to minimize educational and social consequences of language comprehension failures.

Although the underlying causes of many children's comprehension failure have not been established, we can still make clear suggestions about what types of intervention might work for children with language comprehension difficulties. There are interventions that support and improve children's ability to understand text, such as metacognitive training (see Barnes et al., Chapter 7). These interventions do not necessarily tackle the original source of the comprehension problem—for example, reverse a memory deficit or integration weakness—but they may be effective in providing supports and scaffolds that negate its effect.

Cook et al. (Chapter 8) suggest a multilevel approach to remediation of the language comprehension difficulties of children with TBI, based on the evaluation of the strengths and weakness of oral summaries produced by a child, Emma, whose progress was followed for several years. Early on, Emma was good at remembering specific pieces of information from a story but the information recalled reads like a set of isolated statements rather than a set of causally related events. Misinterpretations of a character's actions were also evident in her recall summaries. At the 3-year evaluation, improvement in performance was apparent: Emma demonstrated use of inferencing to extract the gist of the story, even though she continued to experience difficulties organizing a coherent sequence of information. Cook et al. suggest the use of titles and main ideas prior to presentation of a text to help activate background knowledge of the topic. They suggest that recalls should be produced immediately after reading or listening to text, followed by a summarization task that requires the combination of ideas included in the recall. Thus, the individual is guided in the process of extracting the gist of the text from the specific surface details. A similar approach to helping children to identify what is more important and less important in stories and training in inference-making skills is proposed by Lorch et al. (Chapter 5).

Preventing Comprehension Failure

How can this research inform teaching practice in general? The primary focus on comprehension in educational settings is on reading comprehension. It is clear that we must be careful not to focus solely on word-reading skills in beginning reading instruction. Reading comprehension will not develop automatically and effortlessly once children have been taught to read words, and we need to consider how comprehension skills can be nurtured from an early age. Furthermore, if the same skills support the comprehension of written and spoken language, we do not need to wait for word-reading fluency before introducing comprehension-based work in the curriculum. This volume has demonstrated that children use the same skills to understand the causal structure of events in written, televised, and cartoon-based narratives. Work to engage children in the identification of causality, main events, and the extraction of the gist can be conducted with different media at different ages. Many of the suggestions for skills-based teaching to remediate comprehension problems can be incorporated into the daily classroom for all children.

IMPLICATIONS FOR FUTURE RESEARCH

In this final section, we identify some ideas for future research that arise from the work in this volume. To avoid repetition, we introduce some new ideas here that may also be considered to be theoretical implications. First, we consider the consequences of poor language comprehension and how future research might shed light on these. Second, we focus on how to further our understanding of the causes of poor comprehension.

Consequences of Poor Language Comprehension

Language comprehension problems are important and deserve the attention of academics, educators, therapists, and policymakers. In the absence of good language comprehension skills, an individual's academic and employment opportunities are limited. However, first we need to establish what happens to poor comprehenders: Do their language comprehension difficulties diminish over time, or do they become more pronounced, as do the difficulties of poor readers (Stanovich, 1986). The answer to this question has important implications for the focus of our intervention-based research.

Chapter 9 on deaf readers by Kelly and Barac-Cikoja reports data on the reading comprehension levels of deaf readers derived from large-scale norming studies of approximately 4,000 readers. The figures are dismal: The reading comprehension of 10-year-old deaf readers was approximately 4 years below grade level and that of 17-year-olds was 8 years behind. These studies are not longitudinal in nature, but strongly suggest that for these children comprehension problems increase over time. These findings indicate that effective and early interventions are a priority for this population.

Few longitudinal studies have followed atypically developing children with language comprehension problems over time. The findings of the studies of children with specific comprehension difficulties reviewed by Cain and Oakhill (Chapter 2) were contradictory: some research indicates that poor comprehenders might recover, while other work suggests that without intervention their problem will persist. Methodological differences in how poor comprehenders were identified for these studies make the difficulties hard to compare. For that reason, it hard to comment on the importance of developing effective interventions and what their focus should be.

In addition, few longitudinal studies examine how comprehension difficulties might affect other areas of attainment. An exception is the research on the consequences of SLI presented in Botting's Chapter 3. This work indicates that areas of attainment that appear to preserved at the time of a diagnosis of SLI, such as nonverbal IQ, may actually decline over time. Thus, the profile of cognitive strength and weakness may vary at different points in development. Skills that were once in the "normal" range, and therefore not causally related to the language comprehension problems, may be identified as a weakness at a later point in development. Such findings have implications for the diagnosis of developmental disorders.

Future research needs to consider longitudinal research designs to identify the consequences of early comprehension problems and the associated deficits that might arise.

Causes of Poor Comprehension

We have come a long way in identifying possible causes of poor comprehension. Swanson and colleagues (Chapter 6) have established the specific aspects of memory that are impaired in LD poor comprehenders. Barnes and colleagues (Chapter 7) have identified weaknesses in mathematical calculations that might stem from the same underlying causes of language comprehension failure in children with SBM. Kelly and Barac-Cikoja's (Chapter 9) review of deaf readers' difficulties clearly points to difficulties at the word-processing stage of reading; however, the different contributions made by phonological and orthographic processes is clearly a central topic for future research.

As stated previously, much of the research to date has been correlational: it provides snapshots of skills that are associated with poor comprehension in different groups, but does not identify the causal direction of influence between these skills. Future research needs to disentangle cause and effect in relation to comprehension problems: Are comprehension difficulties simply comorbid with a population's primary deficit or do the comprehension difficulties arise from that primary deficit? For example, do the attentional difficulties of children with ADHD cause their language comprehension problems or they do simply co-occur? Longitudinal research is needed to address these issues.

In future longitudinal studies, we must also consider the dynamics of development. This point is made by both Botting (Chapter 3) and Leekam (Chapter 4). The latter notes that "causes of impairment are . . . multidimensional and interact with each other in complex, non-linear ways." What may be a general difficulty at one point may develop into a more specific impairment later in time. Leekam discusses Bates's (2004) analysis of how language impairments might emerge from deficits in abilities that are not part of the language system, such as early attentional or perceptual skills. Thus, the similar outcome of poor language comprehension might arise from different skill deficits in different populations.

Our analysis appears to be steering us in the direction of longitudinal research studies, which are costly, in terms both of time and money. However, if we want to understand the development of a skill, we need to study the process of change over time. We need to design research that enables us to clarify the roles of specific early language skills and their role in subsequent development, rather than simply treating these skills as influences on performance that need to be controlled, as is sometimes the case.

FINAL THOUGHTS

We have reached an exciting point in research on language comprehension development. Independent groups of researchers working with different groups of children are reaching a consensus on the key skills and processes that enable comprehension to take place and the nature of the meaning-based representation produced by these children and the ways in which it might be deficient. They have developed innovative tasks to assess comprehension and produced a body of knowledge that provides a solid foundation for future work. The aim of that work must be to develop a better understanding of the cognitive bases for comprehension failure: Why does comprehension fail and what can we do to prevent it?

REFERENCES

Bates, E. (2004). Explaining and interpreting deficits in language development across clinical groups: Where do we go from here? *Brain and Language, 88,* 248–253.

Gernsbacher, M. A. (1990). *Language comprehension as structure building.* Hillsdale, NJ: Erlbaum.

Hoover, W. A., & Gough, P. B. (1990). The simple view of reading. *Reading and Writing, 2,* 127–160.

Johnson-Laird, P. N. (1983). *Mental models.* Cambridge, UK: Cambridge University Press.

Kintsch, W. (1998). *Comprehension: A paradigm for cognition.* New York: Cambridge University Press.

Stanovich, K. E. (1986). Matthew effects in reading: Some consequences of individual differences in the acquisition of literacy. *Reading Research Quarterly, 21,* 360–406.

Index